INDIVIDUALIZED SUPPORTS FOR STUDENTS WITH PROBLEM BEHAVIORS

The Guilford School Practitioner Series

EDITORS

STEPHEN N. ELLIOTT, PhD
Vanderbilt University

JOSEPH C. WITT, PhD
Louisiana State University, Baton Rouge

Recent Volumes

Individualized Supports for Students with Problem Behaviors:
Designing Positive Behavior Plans
LINDA M. BAMBARA and LEE KERN

Think First: Addressing Aggressive Behavior in Secondary Schools
JIM LARSON

Academic Skills Problems Workbook, Revised Edition
EDWARD S. SHAPIRO

Academic Skills Problems: Direct Assessment and Intervention,
Third Edition
EDWARD S. SHAPIRO

ADHD in the Schools, Second Edition:
Assessment and Intervention Strategies
GEORGE J. DUPAUL and GARY STONER

Helping Schoolchildren Cope with Anger:
A Cognitive-Behavioral Intervention
JIM LARSON and JOHN E. LOCHMAN

Child Abuse and Neglect: The School's Response
CONNIE BURROWS HORTON and TRACY K. CRUISE

Traumatic Brain Injury in Children and Adolescents:
Assessment and Intervention
MARGARET SEMRUD-CLIKEMAN

Schools and Families: Creating Essential Connections for Learning
SANDRA L. CHRISTENSON and SUSAN M. SHERIDAN

Homework Success for Children with ADHD:
A Family–School Intervention Program
THOMAS J. POWER, JAMES L. KARUSTIS, and DINA F. HABBOUSHE

Individualized Supports for Students with Problem Behaviors

DESIGNING POSITIVE BEHAVIOR PLANS

◆ ◆ ◆

Linda M. Bambara
Lee Kern

◆

gp

THE GUILFORD PRESS
New York   London

© 2005 The Guilford Press
A Division of Guilford Publications, Inc.
72 Spring Street, New York, NY 10012
www.guilford.com

Printed in the United States of America

This book is printed on acid-free paper.

Last digit is print number: 9   8   7   6   5   4

Library of Congress Cataloging-in-Publication Data is available from the publisher.

ISBN 1-59385-118-9

About the Authors

♦

Linda M. Bambara, EdD, received her doctorate in special education from Vanderbilt University with an emphasis in severe disabilities. She is currently Professor of Special Education at Lehigh University and Executive Director of Lehigh Support for Community Living, a university-affiliated program that supports adults with disabilities to live in their communities. For more than 15 years, Dr. Bambara has actively promoted positive behavior supports for school-age children and adults with developmental disabilities through research, advocacy, and consulting. Her other interests include enhancing self-management, self-determination, and community participation for people with severe disabilities. Dr. Bambara has published numerous articles and book chapters in these areas, including two books on positive behavior support. She serves on five editorial boards of professional journals in developmental disabilities, including the *Journal of Positive Behavior Interventions*, and is the past editor-in-chief of *Research and Practice for Persons with Severe Disabilities*, formerly the *Journal of the Association for Persons with Severe Handicaps (JASH)*.

Lee Kern, PhD, received her doctorate in special education from the University of South Florida and is currently Professor of Special Education at Lehigh University. Dr. Kern has worked in special education for more than 20 years as a classroom teacher, behavior specialist, and consultant. Her research interests focus on severe challenging behavior, functional assess-

v

ment, and curricular interventions, primarily with individuals with social, emotional, and behavioral needs. She has published numerous articles and book chapters in these areas and has received several grants from the Department of Education and the National Institute of Mental Health to research strategies to address children's behavioral challenges. Dr. Kern is currently Associate Editor of *Education and Treatment of Children, Journal of Behavioral Education,* and *Journal of Positive Behavior Interventions* and serves on the editorial boards of five educational journals.

Contributing Authors

♦

Mendy Boettcher, PhD, Yale Child Study Center, Yale University School of Medicine, New Haven, Connecticut

Lauren Brookman-Frazee, PhD, Child and Adolescent Services Research Center, Department of Psychiatry, University of California, San Diego, California

Shelley Clarke, MA, Department of Child and Family Studies, University of South Florida, Tampa, Florida

Glen Dunlap, PhD, Department of Child and Family Studies, University of South Florida, Tampa, Florida

Lise Fox, PhD, Department of Child and Family Studies, University of South Florida, Tampa, Florida

James Halle, PhD, Department of Special Education, University of Illinois, Urbana–Champaign, Illinois

Joshua Harrower, PhD, Department of Child and Family Studies, University of South Florida, Tampa, Florida

Robert H. Horner, PhD, Educational and Community Supports, University of Oregon, Eugene, Oregon

Don Kincaid, EdD, Department of Child and Family Studies, University of South Florida, Tampa, Florida

Tim Knoster, EdD, Department of Exceptionality Programs, Bloomsburg University, Bloomsburg, Pennsylvania

Lynn Kern Koegel, PhD, Department of Counseling, Clinical, and School

Psychology, College of Education, University of California, Santa Barbara, California

Robert L. Koegel, PhD, Department of Counseling, Clinical, and School Psychology, College of Education, University of California, Santa Barbara, California

Freya Koger, PhD, Special Education Program, College of Education, Lehigh University, Bethlehem, Pennsylvania

Teri Lewis-Palmer, PhD, Educational and Community Supports, University of Oregon, Eugene, Oregon

Raymond G. Miltenberger, PhD, Department of Psychology, North Dakota State University, Fargo, North Dakota

Stacy Nonnemacher, MEd, Special Education Program, College of Education, Lehigh University, Bethlehem, Pennsylvania

Robert E. O'Neill, PhD, Department of Special Education, University of Utah, Salt Lake City, Utah

Joe Reichle, PhD, Department of Communication Disorders, University of Minnesota, Minneapolis, Minnesota

Kristin Starosta, MEd, Special Education Program, College of Education, Lehigh University, Bethlehem, Pennsylvania

George Sugai, PhD, Educational and Community Supports, University of Oregon, Eugene, Oregon

Anne W. Todd, MS, Educational and Community Supports, University of Oregon, Eugene, Oregon

Preface

♦

WHAT IS THIS BOOK ABOUT?

Individualized Supports for Students with Problem Behaviors: Designing Positive Behavior Plans describes a process for developing individualized positive behavior supports (PBS) for students with disabilities who engage in problem behaviors. Many students with disabilities do not respond well to general school or classroom behavior management systems, which puts them at risk for exclusion from typical school experiences and settings. For these students, this book describes effective solutions through PBS. PBS is first and foremost about understanding the student and identifying environmental "reasons" or determinants for problem behavior through a process called functional assessment. Once the student and his or her challenging behaviors are understood, PBS involves developing individualized interventions that change problem contexts and teach the student alternative skills for dealing with problem situations. PBS is effective because it directly alters those conditions that contribute to a student's problem behavior. In addition, it creates comprehensive lifestyle supports to effect long-term change and student and family satisfaction over time. Currently, PBS has a substantial research base demonstrating its effectiveness among students with diverse disabilities and problem behaviors across a variety of school, home, and community settings.

WHAT IS THE PURPOSE OF THIS BOOK?

This book provides school-based practitioners with detailed information on how to design individualized behavior support plans for students consistent with the requirements of the Individuals with Disabilities Education Act (IDEA'97). Although other excellent resources on PBS now exist, few books actually detail the process from beginning to end and provide practitioners with a compendium of assessment and intervention strategies in one volume. This book emphasizes a team-based approach involving teachers, parents, support specialists, administrators, the student with disabilities, and others who are responsible for student outcomes and success. Our goal is to walk readers through the PBS process by providing an array of assessment tools and intervention strategies, guiding questions, and detailed case examples that team members may consider when developing support plans for individual students. The process is sufficiently adaptable to address the diverse needs of students across disabilities, abilities, ages and grade level, and problem behaviors. Specifically, key features of the book include:

- A step-by-step collaborative teaming process for developing individualized PBS plans, including procedures for conducting a functional assessment.
- Examples of research-based, practical interventions and supports for each component of a comprehensive behavior support plan, including antecedent and setting event interventions, alternative skill training, responses to problem behaviors, and long-term supports.
- Numerous case examples illustrating the process of PBS with a wide array of students across different disabilities and problem behaviors.
- Critical self-check questions designed to help teams think carefully through the process.
- Practitioner-friendly planning forms that are applicable to school settings.

FOR WHOM IS THE BOOK WRITTEN?

This book was written with two audiences in mind. First, it is intended for school-based professionals serving on individual student teams. We hope the book provides sufficient detail for professionals such as teachers, school administrators, behavior support specialists, and school psychologists who are called upon to lead or contribute to the design of behavior support plans. Although this book was developed with school professionals in mind, it is also a valuable resource to any member of a student's team, especially parents who are interested in the details of the process. Given that the book is intended to speak to readers with diverse experiences and backgrounds, we tried to avoid extensive special education or technical terminology to facilitate understanding among all who may be involved in the behavior support process.

Second, this book is designed to serve as a college text for preservice professionals, especially special education teachers, school psychologists, and behavior specialists at the undergraduate or graduate level. (Advanced graduate students may benefit from having supplemental materials, especially research examples, added to their course readings.) We organized the book to fit a typical course sequence in PBS, giving special consideration to time-honored topics for class sessions. The book may also be appropriate as a supplemental text for courses in classroom management, behavior management, home–school interventions, and applied behavior analysis.

HOW IS THE BOOK ORGANIZED?

The chapters are organized sequentially, with each chapter building upon previous ones to lay out the conceptual underpinnings, processes, and extensions of PBS beyond individualized supports in school settings. Because books, like behavior support plans, are enhanced by the contributions of others, we invited leading PBS experts and researchers to author or coauthor selected chapters to showcase their particular areas of expertise and interest. Contributors worked collaboratively so that each chapter contributes to describing a cohesive process presented throughout the book.

The first five chapters provide the philosophical foundation for PBS, present an overview of the behavior support process, and outline many of the basic concepts that are central to developing individualized supports for students with disabilities. Chapter 1, by Linda M. Bambara, describes the history and essential characteristics of PBS. In Chapter 2, Glen Dunlap, Joshua Harrower, and Lise Fox set forth a conceptual framework for understanding how problem behaviors may be governed by events in the environment. This framework provides an essential practical structure for guiding the assessment and intervention process described in this book.

In Chapters 3 and 4, Linda M. Bambara, along with Stacy Nonnemacher and Freya Koger in Chapter 4, overviews the five-step process for designing a PBS plan. These steps, which are discussed in detail later in the book, include prioritizing and defining problem behavior; conducting a functional assessment; developing hypothesis statements; developing a behavior support plan; and implementing, evaluating, and modifying the support plan. Chapter 4 situates this five-step process within the context of problem-solving teams. It describes why collaboration is essential to the design of support plans and how the five-step process can be part of a teaming process that builds commitment and capacity among its members. Chapter 5, written by Raymond G. Miltenberger, is the last of the introductory chapters. In it, he describes strategies for measuring behavior change. Although at first glance it would appear that a chapter on behavior change would be better suited for the end rather than the beginning of the book, we elected to place it with the other overview chapters because measuring student progress and behavior change is ongoing and is needed before supports are implemented, during the functional assessment process, and after supports are in place to determine whether modifications in the support plan are needed. This chapter provides readers with the basics on how to measure target behaviors, including both problem behaviors and desired alternatives. Later in the book, we build upon these basics by discussing how progress monitoring may be used to make changes in the support plan.

In addition to describing the behavior support process in the first set of chapters, we introduce two features that are carried out across the book. First, beginning in Chapter 3, we introduce two students, Malik and Bethany, who represent composite case examples based on our personal experiences. The stories of Malik and Bethany and the development of their support plans are presented at the end of selected chapters. These case illustrations are intended to demonstrate the application of the content within that chapter as well as how the complete PBS process is applied to individual students. Malik's and Bethany's fully developed support plans appear at the end of Chapter 11. Readers are encouraged to flip back and forth between chapters to get a sense of how the five-step process and components of a behavior support plan work together for these students. Because we are interested in illustrating the process in its application for students with the most comprehensive needs, these support plans may be more extensive than necessary for most students.

The second feature, Commonly Asked Questions, is introduced in Chapter 4 and appears at the end of selected chapters. In this feature, we anticipate some of the issues commonly faced by school practitioners and offer answers based on the research literature and our applied experience.

Chapters 6 through 11 describe the core steps for developing individualized behavior supports. Using case examples, these chapters detail the process and describe numerous strategies for assessment and intervention. Lee Kern, Robert E. O'Neill, and Kristin Starosta begin by describing the process for gathering functional assessment information in Chapter 6. The assessment process continues in Chapter 7, in which Lee Kern discusses how to make sense of the gathered assessment information. Specifically, she outlines a process for summarizing assessment information into hypothesis statements, which will then be used to inform the development of a behavior support plan. Next, Chapters 8 through 11 describe the four major components of a behavior support plan; each chapter provides detailed considerations for selecting the best supports for individual students. In Chapter 8, Lee Kern and Shelley Clarke discuss antecedent and setting event interventions. Alternative skill interventions, including teaching replacement, coping and tolerance, and general adaptive skills as alternatives to problem behavior, are presented by James Halle, Linda M. Bambara, and Joe Reichle in Chapter 9. In Chapter 10, Lee Kern follows with guidelines on how to respond to problem behavior while still remaining positive, instructive, and respectful of students. In Chapter 11, Tim Knoster and Don Kincaid address the last component of a behavior support plan, long-term supports, which are typically overlooked in school settings. Long-term supports consist of making broad lifestyle changes for the student and strategies for ensuring the maintenance of a support plan across time and settings. Building upon the basics of progress monitoring introduced in Chapter 5, this chapter also discusses considerations for modifying behavior support plans based on assessments of meaningful outcomes.

The book closes with two chapters that describe extensions of the PBS support process emphasized throughout the book. Because families of children with disabilities also face behavioral challenges, Lynn Kern Koegel, Robert L. Koegel, Mendy Boettcher, and Lauren Brookman-Frazee illustrate the process of developing behavior supports for home and community settings. These authors stress the importance of establishing parent–professional partnerships, a critical principle for working with families regardless of whether behavior supports are developed for home or school. Finally, Robert E. Horner, George Sugai, Anne W. Todd, and Teri Lewis-Palmer present a model of *schoolwide* PBS, in which the basic principles of PBS are applied to entire schools to prevent discipline problems. Although there will always be students with disabilities who require individualized supports, the schoolwide model may reduce the overall number of children requiring intensive supports in any one school. Perhaps just as importantly, a schoolwide model, in which all school personnel are exposed to the basic values and principles of PBS, can create a positive school culture in which individualized student supports can flourish and teams feel supported.

We believe the PBS process described in this book is imperative for meeting the needs of individuals with challenging behavior. Although the process may seem overwhelming at first glance, as educators begin to approach problem behaviors in preventative, proactive, and instructive ways, the strategies become much more feasible and even a part of routine practice. Further, an inordinate amount of time is spent reacting to problem behaviors. The process described in this book is designed to replace the extensive time and effort that is spent with reactive strategies, generally with little payoff. We are convinced, with a growing literature base to support this assertion, that in the end, this approach will significantly improve the lives of students with disabilities and/or challenging behaviors over the long term and will allow educators to experience greater satisfaction as a result of improved child outcomes and increased time to devote to the important job of instructing our nation's students.

We are indebted to a great number of individuals for the ideas and materials in this book. The strategies and suggestions contained here are based upon the empirical and conceptual literature on PBS, and shaped by our continuous dialogue with countless professional colleagues, students, and parents of children with disabilities who are committed to implementing respectful and positive supports. In fact, the case examples are based upon our personal clinical and research experiences. We are especially grateful for the opportunity to learn directly from the many individuals with disabilities whom we have known over the years. Finally, we would like to thank the authors and coauthors of the chapters in this book, who worked patiently with us to describe a cohesive process for support plan development.

Contents

◆

CHAPTER 1

◆ ◆ ◆

Evolution of Positive Behavior Support

◆

LINDA M. BAMBARA

Of all the social and learning problems displayed by students with disabilities, *problem or challenging behaviors* remain the most formidable. Such behaviors can take many forms. Some students engage in angry outbursts, tantrums, or attempts to hurt others or themselves. Other students disrupt classroom activities, have difficulty following instructions, do not cooperate with others, or break school rules. Conversely, students may display problem behaviors through extreme passivity or social withdrawal, or may engage in forms of self-stimulation (such as repetitive rocking or hand flapping), which seem to isolate them from others. Problem behaviors can take many forms; however, what defines a problem behavior is not the form that it takes, but its impact on a student and the social systems in which the student lives and learns.

By definition, problem or challenging behaviors are *problems* because they interfere with students' educational and social well-being, and present formidable *challenges* to school personnel and families responsible for students' education and care. For instance, when students engage in such behaviors in school, educational activities for all students are frequently disrupted. For an individual student, problem behaviors can interfere with learning and negatively affect the student's social, emotional, and cognitive development. Moreover, problem behaviors can prevent students from forming friendships and interfere with their social acceptance and inclusion in school life (e.g., Farrington, 1991; Hanson & Carta, 1996; Kauffman, Lloyd, Baker, & Riedel, 1995). In fact, problem behaviors are often the number one reason why students are removed from their neighborhood schools and placed in alternative settings, such as special schools or residential facilities (Kaufman et al., 1995). At home, a child's problem behaviors can have a pervasive impact on all aspects of family functioning, making it difficult (and in some cases impossible) for the family to carry out and enjoy typical family activities, such as shopping, attending church, and sharing family meals (Fox, Vaughn, Wyatte, & Dunlap, 2002). Problem behaviors can create sibling conflicts, affect how family members relate to one another, and interfere with the family's ability to form friendships outside the home (Turnbull & Ruef, 1996, 1997). Without proper intervention or support, problem behaviors often continue well into adulthood, resulting in significant economic, social, and overall quality-of-life implications for the individual (Kazdin, Mazurick, & Bass, 1993; Walker, Colvin, & Ramsey, 1995).

Fortunately, recent developments in special education and psychology have sparked a new, effective approach for addressing the serious problem behaviors of students with disabilities. *Positive behavior support* (PBS) is a comprehensive intervention approach that stresses prevention of problem behavior through systematic and careful educational programming. PBS first emerged in the mid-1980s as an alternative to the highly punitive and restrictive behavior management interventions used to stop very difficult behaviors (e.g., self-injury, self-stimulation, and aggression) displayed by individuals with severe disabilities (Evans & Meyer, 1985; Meyer & Evans, 1989; Horner et al., 1990). Since its inception, PBS has been used successfully to support students across various disabilities and behavior problems in a variety of school, home, and community settings (e.g., Carr et al., 1999). In addition, the principles of PBS have been expanded from an intervention approach designed primarily for individual students to an approach that can be applied to an entire school, as described in Chapter 13 (see also Sugai et al., 2000). As PBS evolves, it continues to gain widespread national support. The 1997 legislation amending the Individuals with Disabilities Education Act (IDEA '97; Public Law 105-17), for example, directs teachers to consider positive strategies when designing behavior intervention plans for individual students.

In this book, we describe a process for designing PBS plans for individual students who present persistent and difficult challenging behaviors. We also recommend this process for emerging behavior problems. Before we introduce this process, however, it is important to understand the underlying assumptions and philosophy of PBS. This chapter provides an important foundation for the rest of the book. After defining PBS, we describe the historical influences on it—where we have been and how our views of problem behaviors and behavioral interventions have changed over the years. Next, we describe the characteristics of and problems with conventional approaches to behavior management. Finally, we define and describe the key features, assumptions, and goals of PBS. We end with a brief discussion of how PBS is included in IDEA '97 and how its concepts are applied to entire schools.

WHAT IS PBS?

PBS is a problem-solving approach to understanding reasons for problem behavior and designing comprehensive interventions that are matched to hypotheses about why problem behavior is occurring and to the individual's unique social, environmental, and cultural milieu. A critical goal of PBS is not just to reduce problem behaviors in the short term, but also to create long-lasting change that will have an impact on the individual's overall quality of life. PBS is characterized by educative, proactive, and respectful interventions that involve teaching the student alternative skills to problem behaviors and changing environments that contribute to problem behaviors. PBS blends best practices in behavioral technology, educational methods, and ecological systems change with person-centered values, in order to achieve outcomes that are meaningful and relevant to the student with disabilities, his or her family, and others who are involved in the student's education.

According to an old adage, in order to fully understand where we are going, it is best to understand where we have been. To amplify our definition of PBS, we now trace some of the major influences on PBS, which have fostered new ways of thinking about problem behaviors and behavior management.

MAJOR INFLUENCES ON PBS

At least four major influences emanating from advances in behavioral psychology, special education, and the community service system for people with disabilities facilitated the development of PBS (Carr et al., 2002; Jackson & Panyan, 2002; Meyer & Park, 1999). These influences are applied behavior analysis, person-centered planning, self-determination, and inclusion.

Applied Behavior Analysis

PBS is rooted in *applied behavior analysis*, defined as the systematic or scientific application of behavioral or operant psychology to solve problems of social importance or significance (Baer, Wolf, & Risley, 1968). Applied behavior analysis is characterized by precise measurement and a systematic, scientific approach to learning and behavior change. As the foundation of PBS, applied behavior analysis provided the theoretical framework and many of the strategies used in PBS to understand and change problem behaviors. It can be credited for making at least three major contributions to PBS (Carr et al., 2002).

First, applied behavior analysis provided a conceptual framework for understanding human behavior and learning. The four-term contingency model (described in Chapter 2) explains how human behavior, including problem behavior, is learned and influenced by environmental events and consequences. This model provides a useful and important structure for identifying environmental determinants of problem behavior and designing effective interventions aimed at changing environments and teaching new skills.

Second, applied behavior analysis can be credited for numerous effective teaching and behavior management interventions used in special education and PBS. Most effective teaching interventions, including direct instruction (e.g., Carnine, Silbert, & Kame'enui, 1997) and systematic instruction (e.g., Snell & Brown, 2000), used to teach students with disabilities academic, communication, social, and community life skills are based on behavioral principles and practices. In addition, most behavior management interventions used to change behaviors of students with disabilities, such as curriculum modifications (e.g., Dunlap, Kern & Worchester, 2001), contingency contracting (e.g., Cooper, Heron, & Heward, 1987), social problem solving (e.g., Hune & Nelson, 2002), and self-management strategies (e.g., King-Sears & Carpenter, 1997), are rooted in applied behavior analysis.

Third, applied behavior analysis was responsible for introducing the principles and methods of *functional analysis*, and the concept of *behavior function*, into the framework of PBS. What is currently known in PBS as *functional assessment* or *functional behavioral assessment* (as coined by IDEA '97) originated from functional analysis, an experimental method used to identify the purpose or function of behavior by examining how behavior is reinforced by the consequences that follow it (Iwata, Dorsey, Slifer, Bauman, & Richman, 1982). A pivotal point in applied behavior analysis was the discovery that problem behavior can be *socially motivated* (Carr, 1977). That is, problem behaviors are shaped by other people's social responses to them, and thus they serve a *communicative function* in their intent to change or influence the action of others (e.g., Carr & Durand, 1985). Beginning in the mid-1980s, this understanding led to an expansion of functional assessment procedures designed to identify the communicative function of behavior and to indicate effective interventions—ones aimed not at punishment, but at teaching new communicative alternatives. Furthermore, functional assessment expanded to include an analysis of antecedent events, not just consequences of behavior. This ultimately led to broader, more comprehensive interventions focused on changing the problem environments that provoke problem behaviors in individuals. Functional assessment, teaching alternative skills, and changing problem environments are now the cornerstones of PBS.

The contributions of applied behavior analysis to PBS are substantial. The interventions derived from applied behavior analysis tell us how to change behaviors, but our values and vision for people with disabilities are better suited for telling us what is important to change and exactly how that should happen (Carr et al., 2002). Developments in person-centered planning, self-determination, and inclusion have helped to shape the values and vision of PBS, and have encouraged new ways of thinking about educational practice, behavior management, and people with disabilities in general.

Person-Centered Planning and Values

Person-centered planning (PCP) originated within the community service system for children and adults with developmental disabilities during the late 1980s (e.g., O'Brien, 1987). PCP provides both a process and a value base for developing supports for people with disabilities. As a process, it involves the focal student with disabilities and a broad array of significant people in the student's life (e.g., family members, teachers, friends) in a collaborative teaming effort. Through collaborative discussions, team members create a vision for a desirable future or better school, community, or home life for the focal student, based on the student's strengths, interests, and preferences. Over time, team members plan and work together to figure out what services, interventions, supports, and resources are needed to make the vision become a reality. Since its inception, a number of PCP processes have been designed specifically for school and community settings. These include Lifetyle Planning (O'Brien, 1987), Personal Futures Planning (Mount, 2000), Planning Alternative Tomorrows with Hope (PATH; O'Brien & Pearpoint, 2003), and Making Action Plans (MAPS; Forrest & Pearpoint, 1992). Additional information on PCP is provided in Chapter 11.

The underlying values of PCP greatly influenced PBS by changing our thinking about how interventions and supports should be designed for people with disabilities. At least four important value-based contributions were made. First, PCP shifted our thinking away from *program-centered supports* (i.e., developing a program that students must fit into) to *person-centered supports* (i.e., doing what is in the best interest of the individual). To be person-centered requires understanding the person's unique needs and preferences and then designing interventions from this base, rather than prescribing interventions developed for others or for the convenience of the educational program. Instead of forcibly fitting a student into a pre-existing program that is not appropriate, person-centered values require educators to do what it takes to rearrange existing services, or to create new ones if necessary, to meet the unique needs of the student.

Second, person-centered values underscored the importance of targeting *quality of life* as both the guiding vision for planning and the intervention outcome. Person-centered values helped educators to realize that the purpose of any educational or behavior intervention is not just to change behavior per se, but rather to enhance quality of life by making positive lifestyle changes for the student. Quality of life for individuals with disabilities is the same as that for all people. It includes participating in meaningful and enjoyable activities in school and community settings; the feeling of belonging or being an accepted member of a group; having good relationships with peers, family members, and friends; having the opportunity to make choices and direct one's life; and having the skills and abilities to pursue dreams and engage in activities that are personally meaningful or important (O'Brien, 1987). With quality of life as a guiding value, educators have increasingly argued that behavioral interventions must change from a narrow focus on behavior change to a more complex focus, including interventions that promote improved lifestyles for students (e.g., Berkman & Meyer, 1988; Risley, 1996).

Third, person-centered values influenced the way we, as a field, came to view people with disabilities. By emphasizing "the person," person-centered values helped us increasingly to see that people with disabilities are people first, with more similarities to all people than differences. With regard to educational and behavior management interventions, this view forced us to recognize that the standards for intervention acceptability are best judged by what we (people without disabilities) would want for ourselves in similar circumstances. Person-centered values tell us that when people with disabilities are viewed as people first, there can be no room for a double standard of intervention acceptability—one that is acceptable for "us," and another for "them." In addition to diminishing the differences among people, person-centered values encouraged us as educators to place greater emphasis on the gifts or capacities of people with disabilities than on their deficits. Thus, instead of taking a deficit-fixing approach to intervention (i.e., attempting to change or remediate all the qualities that make a person different), person-centered values guide us to see what a person can do and what his or her interests are, so that intervention efforts may be focused on enhancing the student's quality of life.

Finally, person-centered values underscored the importance of teaming and collaboration not just among professionals, but among family members and friends of the person with disabilities. Meaningful lifestyle change cannot occur when a few professionals dictate behavior intervention plans that target one or two problem behaviors. Making a meaningful difference across environments, particularly for students with pervasive behavioral difficulties, requires the synergy and commitment of many significant people in a student's life.

Self-Determination

Just as significant in changing our thinking about educational and behavioral interventions for people with disabilities was the educational movement in *self-determination*. Similar to PCP, the self-determination movement grew out of the community services system for adults with disabilities, but is now emphasized in schools for all students with disabilities. For instance, IDEA '97 requires that students with disabilities be involved in their transition planning for postschool life. Numerous self-determination curricula are now available for school use that teach students with disabilities how to express their preferences, set educational goals, plan for their future, and participate in their individualized education program (IEP) and transition planning meetings (Malian & Nevin, 2002).

Fostering self-determination among students with disabilities means that educators are responsible for teaching the skills and creating opportunities that will empower students to become the "primary causal agents" in directing and controlling their lives, especially as they achieve adulthood (Wehmeyer, Agran, & Hughes, 1998). Self-determination is inherently linked to quality of life (e.g., Wehmeyer & Palmer, 2003). If a goal of education is to enhance quality of life, then who better than the person with disabilities to determine what a good life should be? Although there is no known formula, single approach, or curriculum for enhancing the development of self-determination, professionals recommend that the following elements be infused in educational programming:

- Listening to students' preferences, interests, and dreams for the future, and wherever possible, incorporating them into educational planning and instruction (Browder & Bambara, 2000). When students are given opportunities to pursue their interests, self-determination is encouraged.
- Teaching specific skills for self-determination that will enable stu-

dents to exert greater control over the direction of their lives. These include skills for choice and decision making, problem solving, self-regulation or self-management, assertiveness, and self-advocacy (Wehmeyer et al., 1998).

• Creating opportunities for student involvement in educational planning and decision making. This may range from infusing opportunities for daily choice making into daily school or home routines to involving students in conducting their assessments, planning for their future, and leading their own IEP meetings (e.g., Bambara, Cole, & Koger, 1998; Malian & Nevin, 2002).

The emphasis on self-determination influenced PBS and educational programs for students with disabilities in general in several important ways (Meyer & Park, 1999). First, as in PCP, educators were no longer viewed as the sole experts in developing interventions or educational plans for students with disabilities. By involving students with disabilities in the planning process and incorporating their preferences into programming, professionals were encouraged to form partnerships with a new group of consumers—the students themselves. Furthermore, when students with disabilities could not speak for themselves, educators were obligated to ask family members or other advocates to speak on the students' behalf. In either case, the focus on student involvement reinforced the person-centered values that student preferences and choice are critical components in educational planning, and that students with disabilities should be respected as active participants in the educational process (Meyer & Park, 1999).

Second, the self-determination movement held educators responsible not just for teaching skills, but for *empowering students* by removing environmental barriers to self-determination and teaching specific self-determination skills that would lead to the pursuit of personal preferences and control. Increasingly, problem behaviors were viewed as acts of self-determination created by individuals' lack of alternative skills for achieving desired outcomes, as well as by restrictive environments that failed to respond appropriately to individuals or provide opportunities for self-expression and control (e.g., Brown, Gothelf, Guess, & Lehr, 1998). For example, numerous studies beginning in the 1980s (see Kern et al., 1998) conducted with individuals with disabilities have shown a direct link between the absence of choice and problem behaviors displayed by these individuals. The emphasis in self-determination encouraged educators to reconsider their views of problem behaviors. From the perspective of self-determination, problem behaviors were to be not just eliminated, but understood in terms of what individuals are trying to achieve or control. Furthermore, eliminating problem behaviors without teaching students alternative ways of acting upon their environment, or without changing environments that provided little opportunity for choice and control, was viewed as inhibiting the students' rights to self-determination.

Inclusion

Inclusion also influenced the values and practices of PBS by setting new standards for service delivery and behavioral interventions. *Inclusion* is the movement toward the full participation of individuals with disabilities in typical school and community settings. In the educational system, inclusion means placing students with disabilities in general education programs in their neighborhood schools, rather than in segregated schools or classrooms, and changing systems so that specialized supports can be fully integrated and coordinated within general educational settings (Carr et al., 2002; Sailor, 1996). In the community arena, inclusion means doing away with segregated group homes and sheltered workshops, and replacing them with individualized supports that will allow individuals with disabilities to live in homes and work in jobs of their own choice, and to participate in and become accepted members of their local community.

Inclusion differs substantially from the earlier *mainstreaming* or *integration* practices, in which individuals with disabilities were placed in segregated environments for educational or behavioral "remediation," and then reintegrated into mainstream settings once certain educational and behavioral standards were met. In contrast, in an inclusion model intervention or support is provided to an individual with disabilities as a *member* of the general education classroom or inclusive community setting. Rather than removing the individual for remediation, educators bring specialized services, including instruction and accommodations, to the individual *within* the inclusive setting.

The emphasis on inclusion fostered the values that all students with disabilities, even those with challenging behaviors, belong in general education settings, and that students' welfare is the responsibility of the general education community and not just special education. Second, the inclusion movement challenged educators to provide behavior support without compromising students' right to inclusive lifestyles (Meyer & Park, 1999). In other words, to be truly helpful to a student with disabilities, behavioral interventions must be made portable and acceptable to everyday settings. If dangerous behaviors prohibit the student from participating in inclusive settings for any length of time, then the goal is to consider how to bring behavior supports into these settings so that the student can return to them. These values stand in sharp contrast to educational practices that place students with difficult behavioral challenges in segregated classrooms or schools for the treatment or remediation of problem behavior. From an inclusion perspective, segregated schools not only deny students their right to typical school experiences, but also prevent them from acquiring the critical experiences needed for them to be successful in future general educational environments (e.g., to form friendships with nondisabled peers, to participate in general education classrooms, to play active roles in school clubs and activities).

The inclusive school movement also fostered the value that ongoing environmental accommodations are critical features of behavior management supported by law. In other words, making appropriate accommodations and adaptations in school curricula, practices, and routines as required by IDEA '97 to keep students in general education classrooms applies not just to academics, but to behavior support as well. This value obligates educators to change classroom conditions that contribute to problem behaviors, so that students can participate in and benefit from the experiences of general education settings. In essence, this value encourages educators to meet students with disabilities halfway (Jackson & Panyan, 2002). The burden of successful inclusion falls not just on the individuals with disabilities to demonstrate certain target skills, but also on the social and educational environments to make changes for the students to support their learning and participation in inclusive settings.

To summarize, the developments in applied behavior analysis, PCP, self-determination, and inclusion have had a substantial impact on the way we have come to view people with disabilities, problem behaviors, and acceptable interventions—and thus have influenced the development of PBS. Increasingly, our field has come to do the following:

- View people with disabilities with dignity and respect, especially in terms of their interests, preferences, and capacity to be full and self-directing citizens of inclusive communities.
- View problem behaviors not just as deficits that reside within an individual, but as problems that are promoted and maintained by poor environments.
- Hold new standards for intervention outcomes (e.g., quality of life, inclusion) and acceptability (e.g., interventions must fit inclusive settings).
- View intervention in terms of environmental adaptations and support, rather than just remediation of skill deficits.
- View individuals who are not special education professionals (e.g., family members, general education teachers, peers, community members, and the person with disabilities) as co-collaborators and partners in intervention design.

PROBLEMS WITH CONVENTIONAL APPROACHES
TO BEHAVIOR MANAGEMENT

As our values, standards, and vision for educational practice have evolved, conventional approaches to behavior management commonly used to address problem behaviors of students with disabilities in both school and nonschool settings have increasingly fallen from favor. Most conventional behavior management strategies are based on behavioral interventions developed in the 1960s and 1970s, and to this day form the basis of typical school discipline practices used for students both with and without disabilities. However, as professionals, parents, and advocates for people with disabilities have recognized the critical problems and shortcomings with conventional interventions, acceptance of PBS has increased. These problems are discussed below.

Limited Long-Term Effectiveness and Outcomes

Conventional approaches to behavior management are limited with respect to their long-term effectiveness and ability to promote meaningful lifestyle outcomes for individuals with disabilities. Characteristically, conventional behavior management approaches are *reactive, consequence-based*, and *short-term-focused*. The primary goal of conventional behavior management is to stop future occurrences of a problem behavior quickly, or to get it quickly under control so that intervention may be faded as soon as possible. To reduce a problem behavior, most conventional approaches rely on implementing punishing consequences while or soon after the student engages in the behavior. Punishment may involve taking something positive away (e.g., no recess) or introducing an unpleasant or negative event (e.g., sending the student to the principal, after-school detention).

Most school discipline practices are consequence-based, and no doubt can be highly effective for many students with and without disabilities. One day of after-school detention, for example, can deter lateness for a good number of students. However, when schools rely wholly on predominantly punitive approaches, students do not fare well. Furthermore, for students with disabilities who present persistent behavioral challenges, the effects are often merely suppressive or temporary at best. Many years of accumulated research studies (e.g., Scotti, Evans, Meyer, & Walker, 1991; Scotti, Ujcich, Weigle, Holland, & Kirk, 1996) have shown us that conventional interventions often fail to maintain their effectiveness once punishing consequences are terminated or eliminated. In other words, when an intervention is taken away, problem behavior frequently returns. Unfortunately for many students with disabilities who present persistent behavioral challenges, this often results in a steady diet of constant punishment in an attempt to control repeated episodes of problem behavior—an outcome that does little to contribute to the students' quality of life. Furthermore, research tells us that reductions of a problem behavior obtained in one situation are not likely to occur in new settings and situations unless the intervention is added to the new settings. In other words, when conventional approaches are effective, the effects are often only limited to the circumstances in which the intervention is being currently implemented. Thus we cannot expect gains achieved by conventional approaches in one setting to generalize to other settings in which a student participates.

In addition to poor long-term outcomes, conventional behavior management approaches are limited in their ability to create lifestyle improvements for students. As our standards for acceptable practice and meaningful outcomes evolved, this limitation came to light. Clearly, interventions that promote lifestyle outcomes such as positive relationships with others and successful participation in inclusive settings require more than a focus on eliminating problem behaviors. Logically, there is little reason to expect lifestyle improvements when interventions narrowly focus on stopping problem behaviors. Stopping problem behaviors, particularly for students with a history of being denied access to inclusive settings, is not enough. Valued lifestyle outcomes require a much more comprehensive approach to intervention.

Nonfunctional Interventions

A second related problem with conventional interventions is their largely nonfunctional approach to behavior change (Carr, Robinson, & Palumbo, 1990). Most conventional behavior management practices were developed before we fully realized that problem behavior is functional and environmentally determined. Thus, when using a conventional approach, educators often select interventions on the basis of behavior topography or the form of the behavior, with little or no consideration given to potential reasons for or environmental influences of problem behavior. In Mrs. Jones's classroom, for example, any student who fails to turn in his or her completed homework assignments on time does not go to recess. Typical school practice dictates that the same consequences should be applied to any student that engages in the same misbehavior. At one time, researchers and other behavior experts encouraged teachers to select interventions on the basis of behavior topography, because research had shown particular interventions to be effective with certain types of behavior problems. For example, Louise Kent's (1974) language program for children with autism encourages teachers to use overcorrection techniques (i.e., physically guiding students to overpractice "correct" behaviors) to eliminate "interfering self-stimulatory behavior," because research has shown overcorrection to work with other students who engage in self-stimulation.

The limitations of this nonfunctional approach explain why conventional behavior management interventions frequently result in failure for many students with disabilities. The problem is that when we select an intervention on the basis of a student's behavior only, and ignore the environmental reasons for the problem behavior, we can, at best, temporarily stop the behavior; we cannot stop it for good, *because the reasons for it continue to exist.* As long as the environmental conditions remain unchanged, the student will be motivated to respond in some way to get his or her needs met. Some students, after being punished, will choose to respond by engaging in socially appropriate or desired behaviors if they have the skills. However, for the vast majority of students with severe social, cognitive, academic, and/or communication deficits, few or no options may be available to them except continuing to engage in some type of problem behavior to respond to difficult events. All too often, once students with disabilities are punished for one type of problem behavior, a new problem behavior will crop up because they lack socially appropriate alternatives or because they are unable to exert change (i.e., the students are being punished for a problem that lies in the environment).

Consider Mark, a fourth grader in Mrs. Jones's classroom, who repeatedly fails to turn in his homework assignments. Despite many days of sitting in the principal's office while his classmates go outside for recess, Mark continues not to hand in his assignments. A closer look at Mark and his home situation provides some clues as to why this is happening. Mark, a student with learning disabilities, often struggles with his assignments and concentrates best in a quiet setting. He lives with his mother and 2-year-old sister. Because his mother works full-time, he attends an after-school program until his grandmother can pick him up at 6:15 each night. Mark is given about 45 minutes to do homework at the after-school program, but he finds the commotion of other children fooling around too distracting to concentrate. At his grandmother's house, Mark eats dinner, helps with the dinner dishes, and waits for his mother to take him home at 7:30. Once at home, Mark's mom usually asks him to watch his baby sister for about an hour each night as she quickly gets her home in order after a long, busy day (e.g., gets the mail, listens to phone messages, takes out the garbage, washes breakfast dishes). By about 9:00 each night, as soon as his baby sister is put to bed, Mark and his mom sit down at the kitchen table to do his homework. Unfortunately, even though it is now quiet and Mark's mom is available for assistance, both Mark and his mom are typically exhausted from their long day. Now cranky, Mark easily becomes frustrated. He cries, whines, screams for help, and then rejects help when his mother tries to offer assistance ("Go away! I don't need you!"). Sometimes Mark's mother is able to persist and helps him complete at least some of his homework. But on most nights—too tired to struggle with Mark, and knowing that Mark is too tired to concentrate—she sends him off to bed, hoping that tomorrow will bring a better day.

If Mrs. Jones continues to punish Mark for not handing in his homework assignments, we can predict that two things will happen. First, Mark will still not complete his homework. Punishment will not teach Mark how to do his homework, nor will it address the circumstances that make it impossible for him to complete his assignments. Second, we can predict that both Mark and Mrs. Jones will change their behaviors in response to this difficult situation. After being repeatedly punished for a situation that he cannot change, Mark is likely to become extremely angry, frustrated, or anxious. He may try to avoid school by feigning illness, or he may increasingly withdraw from all classroom activities. He may cause a disruption before homework assignments are due, hoping to divert his teacher's attention. Or, when told that he must stay in during recess, Mark may scream and shout at his teacher ("This is stupid! I hate you!"). As Mrs. Jones realizes that her intervention is ineffective and Mark is getting increasingly incorrigible, she is likely to try a more punishing or intrusive strategy to control all of Mark's escalating problem behaviors, such as an intrusive token or point system where Mark can earn regular classroom privileges for being good, and is denied others for problem behaviors. Conventional behavior management supports the use of more intrusive or punishing interventions when less intrusive methods fail, but even the most punishing intervention is not likely to change Mark's habits if the reasons for his problem behaviors remain unchanged. Mrs. Jones's interventions can only go so far in her fourth-grade classroom. As Mark's problem behaviors escalate to the point of causing severe classroom disruptions, Mrs. Jones will ask that he be permanently removed from her classroom. Depending on how Mark's problem behaviors are viewed by the team that has developed his IEP, Mark may be placed in a special classroom or special school where teachers are trained specifically to deal with students who have serious problem behaviors.

Mark's story illustrates what can happen when a nonfunctional approach to behavior management is used. For many students both with and without disabilities, conventional behavior management approaches result in failure when the environmental reasons for problem behavior are left unaddressed. Although we have focused on punishment in this example, the same outcome can be expected for any intervention, even positive ones, that fail to address the reasons for problem behavior. For instance, reinforcing Mark with extra stickers and class privileges when he does complete his homework may be a powerful motivator, but it is doomed for failure when Mark, under the circumstances, still cannot get his homework done. Admittedly, Mark's story is overly simplistic, but it does unfortunately typify what happens with many students when conventional interventions fail.

Moral and Ethical Issues

Still another problem with conventional behavior management interventions has to do with the moral and ethical concerns raised by exposing students with disabilities to highly intrusive and punishing interventions. An unfortunate and most disturbing by-product of using nonfunctional methods is that interventionists often resort to more and more intrusive interventions in an effort to find one powerful enough to stop a problem behavior once and for all. Historically, students with disabilities who present the most difficult behavior challenges (e.g., aggression, property disruption, self-injury, self-stimulation) and/or who have the most severe disabilities (e.g., cognitive and social/emotional) have been exposed to the most intrusive interventions (commonly referred to as *aversive interventions*), largely in treatment settings other than public schools. For example, in 1987, Guess, Hemstetter, Turnbull, and Knowlton reviewed the research to that date on behavioral interventions for individuals with severe cognitive disabilities, and identified an array of aversive interventions used with this population. Some examples included visual screening (e.g., covering a child's eyes with a cloth or a helmet shield), taste or smell aversives (e.g., spraying lemon juice or hot pepper sauce in a child's mouth, breaking an ammonia capsule under a child's nose), white noise (e.g., forcing a child to wear a helmet that produced repetitive noise at uncomfortable decibels), overcorrection (forcing a child to practice exaggerated forms of appropriate behavior), and contingent electric shock—all of which were applied after an individual engaged in some form of problem behavior. Students with behavior disorders were also exposed frequently to aversive interventions. Some of the most common interventions used with these children were physical restraint, time out in seclusion, and highly restrictive token economies where almost all of the child's activities were controlled by the interventionist.

The primary concern about such aversive interventions is that they fall outside the boundaries of acceptable ways of treating people, especially children. Simply put, regardless of their potential to control problem behavior in the short term, aversive interventions violate standards of moral decency and are therefore unacceptable. As emphasized by Singer, Gert, and Koegel (1999), moral people should not intentionally inflict any of the five kinds of moral harm—death, pain, loss of ability, loss of freedom, or loss of pleasure—as a form of "treatment." Perhaps with the exception of death (although some children have died as a result of inappropriate uses of physical restraint), aversive interventions are regularly associated with four of the five harms.

What came to be known as the *nonaversive movement* started in the early 1980s, when many advocates and professionals began to argue that aversive interventions—those that cause pain, extreme stress, and/or severe stigmatization, and are deemed inappropriate for students without disabilities—should be eliminated from use. As a result, numerous professional organizations, such as TASH (formerly The Association for Persons with Severe Handicaps), the Council for Exceptional Children (CEC), the American Association on Mental Retardation (AAMR), and the National Association of School Psychologists (NASP), have supported the cessation of highly intrusive forms of interventions. In addition to raising moral arguments, professional organizations noted other severe limitations with aversive interventions: (1) their limited effectiveness (e.g., suppressive effects and limited long-term outcomes); (2) their potential for misuse and misapplication (e.g., indiscriminately using aversive interventions for *any* problem behavior, physically restraining students for inappropriately long periods of time); and (3) their power to destroy the trust and positive relationships needed between teachers and students to enhance the students' growth and learning.

Coupled with the shifts of thinking about behavioral and educational practices, the nonaversive movement spurred the birth of PBS. Professionals sought new ways of addressing problem behaviors with new standards and a new vision for success. This is not to say that aversive interventions have completely been eliminated today. In fact, research continues to investigate the effects of the Self-Injurious Behavior Inhibiting System (SIBIS), an electric shock system, on students with severe disabilities who engage in certain forms of problem behaviors (e.g., Linsheid & Reichenbach, 2002). On the whole, however, special education has come to accept alternative approaches to conventional interventions, paving the way for PBS.

KEY FEATURES OF PBS

PBS embodies contemporary values and best practices in behavior intervention. When teachers, parents, and other interventionists use PBS for individuals with disabilities, they use a much broader approach than simply implementing consequences aimed at decreasing or eliminating problem behaviors (Janney & Snell, 2000), although the reduction of problem behaviors is certainly one important goal. The ultimate goal PBS is to effect meaningful, long-lasting changes that will result in improvements in individuals' lifestyles. In many ways, PBS attempts to address the critical limitations of conventional behavior management. In contrast to conventional approaches, PBS includes the key features listed in Table 1.1 and discussed below.

Ecologically Oriented

PBS is governed by two interrelated assumptions about problem behaviors. First, the way a person behaves in a given situation is a function of the interaction between the person and conditions of the environment (Janney & Snell, 2000). Problem behaviors are not caused by disabilities—they are not the results of attention deficit disorder, autism, emotional/behavior disorders, or mental retardation, for example. Rather, from an ecological and behavioral perspective, problem behaviors occur because certain environmental events or conditions provoke and support them. The second assumption is that a problem behavior serves a useful purpose or function for a person. The behavior is undesirable and at times harmful to the person or others, but it is not "maladaptive." Rather, it is an adaptive response to current environmental conditions. From the individual's perspective, a problem behavior "works" to achieve desired outcomes, given the current situation. For example, it can help the person to avoid a difficult situation, get assistance from the teacher, or initiate an interaction if he or she is feeling bored. Regular use of a problem behavior often signals that the person has no other effective means for getting his or her needs met. The implication of both these assumptions is that the first step toward behavior change requires looking toward the environment for explanations for the problem behavior.

Assessment-Based

If interventions are to be effective, then they must address or be linked to environmental reasons for problem behaviors. PBS interventions are guided by functional assessments. A functional assessment focuses on understanding the relationship among environmental events, the person's response, and the purpose or function that problem behavior serves for the individual. In addition to functional assessments, PBS incorporates person-centered approaches to assessment. Emphasis is placed on learning about the student's preferences, strengths, and current lifestyle at home and in school, as well as the student's and family's vision for the future. This information focuses PBS on achieving important lifestyle outcomes for the student.

TABLE 1.1. Key Features of Positive Behavior Support (PBS)

PBS is ...	
• Ecologically oriented	• Comprehensive
• Assessment-based	• Team-based
• Preventive and educational	• Respectful
• Lifestyle- and inclusion-focused	• Long-term-focused

Customized

When interventions are designed around the reasons for problem behavior and a student's preferences and interests, they are customized or uniquely tailored to the individual. Unlike conventional approaches, PBS involves no expectation that the same intervention will work or be appropriate for another student, unless of course another student has similar needs and preferences. PBS interventions are customized in another important way: In addition to being tailored to an individual's needs and preferences, they are tailored to fit the person's unique school, home, or community setting. In order for such interventions to be carried out by teachers or parents, they must be made practical and realistic by fitting into typical settings. Supports must be designed so that they do not interfere with daily routines, must take into consideration the day-to-day demands placed on teachers and parents, and must match cultural expectations and family values.

Preventive and Educational

Once problem behaviors are understood in terms of their purposes and the environmental conditions that support them, the primary aims of PBS are not to punish, but to prevent and teach. Prevention is achieved by changing the environmental conditions that contribute to challenging behaviors, which from students' perspective are often stressful and problematic. The purpose for teaching is to give students alternative ways of achieving desired outcomes during problem situations and the skills needed to change problem situations in the future. When preventing and teaching are the aims of intervention, reductions in problem behavior occur as by-products of changed environments and new learned skills. Furthermore, students learn skills that can be applied across many situations and that contribute to long-term success.

Lifestyle- and Inclusion-Focused

PBS focuses on achieving broad-based outcomes that will result in overall lifestyle change. It seeks to reverse the negative conditions influenced by problem behaviors or created by restrictive interventions and segregated educational settings. Emphasis is placed on improving friendships with peers, increasing involvement in typical school activities, increasing participation in family and community activities, improving interactions with siblings and parents, increasing opportunities for self-determination, and enhancing personal satisfaction or happiness. When broad outcomes are the focus, PBS includes interventions geared toward facilitating inclusion and enhancing quality of life.

Comprehensive

With emphasis on prevention, teaching alternative skills, and improving lifestyle, PBS plans are characteristically comprehensive. Conventional behavior management plans typically include a single intervention, usually consequence based, aimed at reducing problem behavior. In a PBS plan, multiple intervention strategies are included in order to (1) prevent problem behaviors, (2) teach alternative skills, (3) respond to problem behaviors when they occur, and (4) facilitate lifestyle improvements for the student.

Team-Based

PBS interventions require a team effort involving parents, teachers, school administrators, behavior support specialists or school psychologists, the student with disabilities, and other interested parties. Team members collaborate or work together to conduct assessments, design the PBS plans, and carry out and evaluate the interventions. A team-based approach is essential to share critical information and expertise across team members, and to ensure that interventions are practical and realistic. Most importantly, a team approach is needed to assure that intervention goals are indeed meaningful to all team participants, especially family members and the student with disabilities.

Respectful

PBS interventions do not stigmatize, humiliate, or inflict pain. Rather, they are always age-appropriate and normalized, and are designed with the goal of promoting a positive image of the person in inclusive settings. Moreover, PBS is respectful in its emphasis on understanding the person; understanding problem behavior from the individual's perspective; and being responsive to the student's needs, preferences, and interests.

Long-Term-Focused

PBS recognizes that many people with disabilities will require lifelong supports to help them to succeed in new situations. Unlike conventional behavior management interventions, where the focus is on short-term treatment (i.e., stopping problem behaviors quickly), PBS takes on a long-term focus. PBS interventions are modified over time and build upon previous years' successes. A long-term focus is necessary to ensure that lifestyle changes are realized and, furthermore, to ensure that new problem behaviors do not develop in the future as a function of poor environments or lack of skills in new situations. With continual environmental adaptations and teaching for new situations, long-term prevention and success can be achieved.

SCHOOLWIDE POSITIVE BEHAVIOR SUPPORT

Many school staff members will wonder whether individualized PBS as described in this book is necessary for all students with disabilities who present challenging behaviors. Given its comprehensiveness, the answer, to the relief of many, is no; however, many of the underlying philosophies, values, and general practices of PBS are relevant for *all* children—with and without disabilities. Historically, schools have relied on punitive approaches for controlling problem behaviors, but they could be so much more effective if they focused instead on understanding reasons for problem behaviors, rewarding positive/prosocial behaviors, and arranging school contexts where students are encouraged to behave in prosocial ways.

One of the more recent developments of PBS is its application to an entire school. In what is known as *schoolwide positive behavior support* (see Chapter 13; Horner & Sugai, 2000; and Sugai et al., 2000), many of the fundamental features of individualized PBS are adapted so that they can be applied at a school level to address the behavior of all students, whether or not they have disabilities. Schoolwide PBS emphasizes stating clear expectations for positive student behaviors; creating incentive or rewards for positive behaviors; and changing trouble-prone environments (e.g., school cafeteria, hallways) so that they promote, rather than discourage, positive student interactions. One goal of schoolwide PBS is to prevent serious problem behaviors and decrease the overall number of students who may require individualized supports. Although most students will be responsive to general school practices, there will always be a small percentage of students who will require the more intensive, individualized supports described in this book. In these cases, the second purpose of schoolwide PBS is to create a supportive school culture that will encourage and sustain individualized efforts. Individualized PBS is most likely to be effective when all teachers, parents, and the school administrator understand and accept the importance of PBS practices and values.

PBS AND IDEA '97

Individualized PBS is encouraged by IDEA '97 in several important ways. First, when developing a student's IEP, the team is required to consider "positive behavior interventions" in cases where the student's challenging behavior interferes with his or her learning or that of others. The IEP team may consider other interventions (e.g., medications), but positive behavior interventions are *required by law* to be considered (Turnbull, Wilcox, Stowe, & Turnbull, 2001). Second, in cases where a student's educational placement is threatened by repeated school suspensions or expulsion, the school must conduct a functional behavioral assessment if it has not already been done. In addition, the IEP team must convene to review the student's behavioral intervention plan and determine whether it is appropriate. In other words, in cases where severe disciplinary action is being considered, IDEA '97 requires the IEP team to reconsider the appropriateness of a student's support plan (i.e., is it working?) and reasons for problem behavior via functional assessment as the primary course of action. The PBS interventions described in this book may go beyond what is needed for most students or required by law; however, the regulations and language of IDEA '97 require them in some form (Turnbull, Stowe, Wilcox, Raper, & Hedges, 2000; Turnbull et al., 2001).

SUMMARY

In this chapter, we have explored the evolution of PBS. After providing a definition of PBS, we have shown how advances in applied behavior analysis, PCP, self-determination, and inclusion have influenced the development of PBS in terms of its practices and values. Moreover, we have discussed how advances in these areas have radically changed our views of students with disabilities, problem behaviors, and behavior interventions. Next, we have discussed the critical limitations of conventional behavior management practices for students with disabilities. Finally, we have described the essential assumptions and characteristics of PBS, and discussed its continued development and acceptance in schools.

PBS is more than just a collection of positive, nonpunitive behavior management strategies. It provides a philosophical and value-based approach for understanding reasons for problem behaviors and designing interventions that are ultimately respectful and meaningful to students with disabilities and their families. This value base, coupled with continued advances in behavioral technology, is likely to shape the continued evolution and applications of PBS in years to come.

REFERENCES

Baer, D. M., Wolf, M. M., & Risley, T. R. (1968). Some current dimensions of applied behavior analysis. *Journal of Applied Behavior Analysis, 1,* 91–97.
Bambara, L. M., Cole, C., & Koger, F. (1998). Translating self-determination for adults with developmental disabilities. *Journal of The Association for Persons with Severe Handicaps, 23,* 18–37.

Berkman, K. A., & Meyer, L. H. (1988). Alternative strategies and multiple outcomes in the remediation of severe self-injury: Going "all out" nonaversively. *Journal of The Association for Persons with Severe Handicaps, 13,* 76–86.

Browder, D. M., & Bambara, L. M. (2000). Home and community. In M. E. Snell & F. Brown (Eds.), *Instruction of students with severe disabilities* (5th ed., pp. 543–589). Upper Saddle River, NJ: Merrill.

Brown, F., Gothelf, C. R., Guess, D., & Lehr, D. (1998). Self-determination for individuals with the most severe disabilities: Moving beyond chimera. *Journal of The Association for Persons with Severe Handicaps, 23,* 17–26.

Carnine, D. W., Silbert, J., & Kame'enui, E. J. (1997). *Direct instruction reading* (3rd ed.) Upper Saddle River, NJ: Merrill.

Carr, E. G. (1977). The motivation of self-injurious behavior: A review of some hypotheses. *Psychological Bulletin, 84,* 800–816.

Carr, E. G., Dunlap, G., Horner, R. H., Koegel, R. L., Turnbull, A. P., Sailor, W., et al. (2002). Positive behavior support: Evolution of an applied science. *Journal of Positive Interventions, 4,* 4–16.

Carr, E. G., & Durand, M. V. (1985). Reducing problem behaviors through functional communication training. *Journal of Applied Behavior Analysis, 18,* 111–126.

Carr, E. G., Horner, R. H., Turnbull, A. P., Marquis, J. G., McLaughlin, D. M., McAtee, M. L. (1999). *Positive behavior support for people with developmental disabilities: A research synthesis.* Washington, DC: American Association on Mental Retardation.

Carr, E. G., Robinson, S., & Palumbo, L. W. (1990). The wrong issue: Aversive versus nonaversive treatment. The right issue: Functional versus nonfunctional treatment. In A. C. Repp & N. Singh (Eds.), *Perspectives on the use of nonaversive and aversive interventions for persons with developmental disabilities* (pp. 361–379). Sycamore, IL: Sycamore.

Cooper, J. O., Heron, T. E., & Heward, W. L. (1987). *Applied behavior analysis.* Columbus, OH: Merrill.

Dunlap, G., Kern, L., & Worchester, J. (2001). Applied behavior analysis and academic instruction. *Focus on Autism and Other Developmental Disabilities, 16,* 129–136.

Evans, I. M., & Meyer, L. H. (1985). *An educative approach to behavior problems: A practical decision model for interventions with severely handicapped learners.* Baltimore: Paul H. Brookes.

Farrington, D. P. (1991). Childhood aggression and adult violence: Early precursors and later-life outcomes. In D. J. Pepler & K. H. Rubin (Eds.), *The development and treatment of childhood aggression* (pp. 5–29). Hillsdale, NJ: Erlbaum.

Forest, M., & Pearpoint, J. C. (1992). Putting all kids on the MAP. *Educational Leadership, 50,* 26–31.

Fox, L. Vaughn, B. J., Wyatte, M. L., & Dunlap, G. (2002). "We can't expect other people to understand": Family perspectives on problem behavior. *Exceptional Children, 68,* 437–450.

Guess, D., Helmstetter, E., Turnbull, R. H., & Knowlton, S. (1987). *Use of aversive procedures with persons who are disabled: An historical review and critical analysis.* Seattle, WA: The Association for Persons with Severe Handicaps.

Hanson, M. J., & Carta, J. J. (1996). Addressing the challenges of families with multiple risks. *Exceptional Children, 62,* 200–212.

Horner, R. H., Dunlap, G., Koegel, R. L., Carr, E. G., Sailor, W., Anderson, J., et al. (1990). Toward a technology of "nonaversive" behavioral support. *Journal of The Association for Persons with Severe Handicaps, 15,* 125–132.

Horner, R. H., & Sugai, G. (2000). School-wide behavior support: An emerging initiative. *Journal of Positive Behavior Interventions, 2,* 231–232.

Hune, J. B., & Nelson, C. M. (2002). Effects of teaching a problem solving strategy on preschool children with problem behavior. *Behavior Disorders, 27,* 185–207.

Iwata, B. A., Dorsey, M. F., Slifer, K. J., Bauman, K. E., & Richman, G. S. (1982). Toward a functional analysis of self-injury. *Analysis and Intervention in Developmental Disabilities, 2,* 1–20.

Jackson, L., & Panyan, M. V. (2002). *Positive behavioral support in the classroom: Principles and practices.* Baltimore: Paul H. Brookes.

Janney, R., & Snell, M. E. (2000). *Teachers' guides to inclusive practices: Behavioral support.* Baltimore: Paul H. Brookes.

Kauffman, J. M., Lloyd, J. W., Baker, J., & Riedel, T. M. (1995). Inclusion of all students with emotional and behavioral disorders?: Let's think again. *Phi Delta Kappan, 76,* 542–546.

Kazdin, A. E., Mazurick, J. L., & Bass, D. (1993). Risk of attrition in treatment of antisocial children and families. *Journal of Clinical Child Psychology, 22,* 2–16.

Kent, L. (1974). *Language acquisition program for the severely retarded.* Champaign, IL: Research Press.

Kern, L., Vorndram, C. N., Hilt, A., Ringdahl, J. E., Adelman, B. E., & Dunlap, G. (1998). Choice as an intervention to improve behavior: A review of the literature. *Journal of Behavioral Education, 8,* 151–169.

King-Sears, M. E., & Carpenter, S. L. (1997). *Teaching self-management to elementary students with developmental disabilities.* Washington, DC: American Association on Mental Retardation.

Linsheid, T. R., & Reichenbach, H. (2002). Multiple factors in the long-term effectiveness of contingent electric shock treatment for self-injurious behavior: A case example. *Research in Developmental Disabilities, 23,* 161–177.

Malian, I., & Nevin, A. (2002). A review of the self-determination literature. *Remedial and Special Education, 23,* 68–74.

Meyer, L. H., & Evans, L. M. (1989). *Nonaversive intervention for behavior problems: A manual for home and community.* Baltimore: Paul H. Brookes.

Meyer, L. H., & Park, H. (1999). Contemporary, most promising practices for people with disabilities. In J. R. Scotti & L. H. Meyer (Eds.), *Behavioral intervention: Principles, models, and practices* (pp. 25–45). Baltimore: Paul H. Brookes.

Mount, B. (2000). *Person-centered planning.* New York: Graphic Futures.

O'Brien, J. (1987). A guide to life-style planning: Using The Activities Catalog to integrate services and natural support systems. In B. Wilcox & G. T. Bellamy (Eds.), *A comprehensive guide to The Activities Catalog: An alternative curriculum for youth and adults with severe disabilities* (pp. 175–189). Baltimore: Paul H. Brookes.

O'Brien, J., & Pearpoint, J. (2003). *Person-centered planning with MAPS and PATH: A workbook for facilitators.* Toronto: Inclusion Press.

Risley, T. (1996). Get a life! In L. K. Koegel, R. L. Koegel, & G. Dunlap (Eds.), *Positive behavioral support: Including people with difficult behaviors in the community* (pp. 425–437). Baltimore: Paul H. Brookes.

Sailor, W. (1996). New structures and systems change for comprehensive positive behavioral support. In L. K. Koegel, R. L. Koegel, & G. Dunlap (Eds.), *Positive behavioral support: Including people with difficult behaviors in the community* (pp. 163–206). Baltimore: Paul H. Brookes.

Scotti, J. R., Evans, I. M., Meyer, L. H., & Walker, P. (1991). A meta-analysis of intervention research with problem behavior: Treatment validity and standards of practice. *American Journal on Mental Retardation, 96,* 233–256.

Scotti, J. R., Ujcich, K. J., Weigle, K. L., Holland, C., & Kirk, K. S. (1996). Interventions with challenging behavior of persons with developmental disabilities: A review of current research practices. *Journal of The Association for Persons with Severe Handicaps, 21,* 123–134.

Singer, G. H., Gert, B., & Koegel, R. (1999). A moral framework for analyzing the controversy over aversive behavioral interventions for people with severe mental retardation. *Journal of Positive Behavior Interventions, 1,* 88–100.

Snell, M. E., & Brown, F. (Eds.). (2000). *Instruction of students with severe disabilities* (5th ed.). Upper Saddle River, NJ: Merrill.

Sugai, G., Horner, R. H., Dunlap, G., Hieneman, M., Lewis, T. J., Nelson, C. M., et al. (2000). Applying positive behavior support and functional behavioral assessment in schools. *Journal of Positive Behavior Interventions, 2,* 131–143.

Turnbull, A. P., & Ruef, M. (1996). Family perspectives on problem behavior. *Mental Retardation, 34,* 280–293.

Turnbull, A. P., & Ruef, M. (1997). Family perspectives on inclusion lifestyle issues for people with problem behavior. *Exceptional Children, 63,* 211–227.

Turnbull, R. H., Stowe, M., Wilcox, B. L., Raper, C., & Hedges, L. P. (2000). The public policy foundations for positive behavioral interventions, strategies, and supports. *Journal of Positive Behavior Interventions, 2,* 218–230.

Turnbull, R. H., Wilcox, B. L., Stowe, M., & Turnbull, A. (2001). IDEA requirements for use of PBS. *Journal of Positive Behavior Interventions, 3,* 11–18.

Walker, H. M., Colvin, G., & Ramsey, E. (1995). *Antisocial behavior in school: Strategies and best practices.* Pacific Grove, CA: Brooks/Cole.

Wehmeyer, M. L., Agran, M., & Hughes, C. (1998). *Teaching self-determination to students with disabilities.* Baltimore: Paul H. Brookes.

Wehmeyer, M. L., & Palmer, S. B. (2003). Adult outcomes for students with cognitive disabilities three years after high school: The impact of self-determination. *Education and Training in Developmental Disabilities, 38,* 131–144.

CHAPTER 2

◆◆◆

Understanding the Environmental Determinants of Problem Behaviors

◆

GLEN DUNLAP
JOSHUA HARROWER
LISE FOX

Perhaps the most critical principle of intervention in positive behavior support (PBS) is that a plan of support should be based on a functional understanding of the problem behavior that caused the plan to be developed in the first place. The behavior support plan is not arbitrary; it is not photocopied from generic behavior management manuals; and its components are not dictated by previous experience or interventions with other individuals. Rather, the plan is based on the existing science of human behavior and, most importantly, on information that is derived from a functional assessment of the individual's identified problem behavior. The synthesis of the functional assessment information constitutes the *functional understanding* that is the foundation of the support plan. The purpose of this chapter is to describe the concepts and assumptions that serve as the basis for the functional assessment process and PBS.

Our aim in this chapter is to present a simple conceptual framework for understanding how problem behaviors may be governed by events in

25

the environment. In meeting that purpose, we discuss an empirically supported framework for understanding factors related to problem behavior, and we also describe the need for developing models or processes to broaden this understanding to include complex contexts and lifestyle issues. The framework is based on extensive research and the fundamental concepts of operant psychology and applied behavior analysis, and it has been demonstrated to be a very useful mechanism for guiding practical processes of assessment and intervention. Indeed, thousands of scientific studies have documented very conclusively that the framework's principles are valid, and that they can be used to develop effective strategies of intervention. An increasing proportion of this documentation is in the area of PBS (Carr et al., 1999).

Before we begin our description of the framework, it is important to acknowledge that it does not offer an absolutely comprehensive explanation for all problem behavior. We recognize the existence of interactive neurophysiological and psychological variables that are not yet understood. For instance, it is clear that neurophysiological factors extending beyond currently known environmental variations are involved in the governance of some self-injury, as well as of obsessive, repetitive, and compulsive behaviors (Romanczyk & Matthews, 1998; Schroeder, Oster-Granite, & Thompson, 2002). However, at the present time, this knowledge has not been developed to the point that such variables can be identified, measured, or made useful in the processes of practical assessment and intervention. Although the practical science of addressing challenging behaviors is substantial, it will remain deficient until we acquire a much better understanding of the interactive and neurophysiological factors that contribute greatly to the development and occurrence of all behavior.

One additional caveat is in order before we introduce the conceptual framework. This involves the fact that our understanding at this point in the field's development is focused largely on the immediate environmental influences on behavior. The lens we use for assessment provides a sharp but narrow view—a view that can be considered microscopic. The value of this lens lies primarily in its power to generate prediction and control of behavior on a moment-to-moment basis. This value should not be underestimated, because this is the traditional level of intervention, and it is indisputably vital for concerns related to instruction and contingency management. However, it is not the only perspective needed to construct the understanding that is the basis for effective PBS and truly meaningful lifestyle outcomes. In order to address these broader and more substantial goals, our micro-level understanding needs to be situated in the context of a more macro-level view of a person's life. This view looks well beyond the influences of specifically defined behaviors to the fulfillment, preference, satisfaction, and value a person derives from his or her life arrangements. Such arrangements include social relationships, living circumstances, opportunities for setting and achieving goals, satisfaction and stimulation in work or school, and other circumstances that, in the aggregate, define a person's quality of life. Having an understanding of a person's quality of life, and of the vision and plans that have been considered for its enhancement, is the necessary context in which to carry out the processes of functional understanding and support plan development. This macro level of understanding is especially urgent when it comes to goal setting and intervention planning. Indeed, some authors have indicated that these life arrangement variables probably account in one way or another for the vast majority of behavior problems, and that if life arrangements could be made perfectly satisfactory, very few behavioral problems would remain for focused intervention (Risley, 1996; Turnbull & Turnbull, 1990).

In PBS, there is a growing appreciation of the critical need to understand the particular impact that macro-level (lifestyle) variables can have on specific challenges of behavior (Carr, Carlson, Langdon, Magito-McLaughlin, & Yarbrough, 1998; Carr et al., 2002; Risley, 1996). It is clear that the effect is important, but the processes of macro-level assessment, understanding, and support have not been analyzed or conceptualized in the precise manner that characterizes assessment and intervention at the micro or molecular level. Very useful guidelines have been developed for examining life arrangements (see Chapter 11; Kincaid & Fox, 2002; and Turnbull & Turnbull, 1996), and these guidelines show promise for providing a context for the development and implementation of an effective, assessment-based PBS plan. Still, for predictable change to be accomplished in the occurrence of specific, identified problem behaviors, the more focused lens that produces a functional understanding of more contextually immediate influences is mandatory.

The environmental determinants that are the topic of this chapter have been described many times by authorities in applied behavior analysis and PBS. The framework we present is not new. A distinction, however, may be that we seek to present the framework in such a way as to facilitate an understanding of behavior–environment relations as a means for developing an effective, assessment-based PBS plan. In the next section of the chapter, we present the basic assumptions or principles that serve as the scientific foundation for the framework. The bulk of the chapter is then devoted to a process for systematically considering aspects of the environment as these aspects influence the occurrence of behavior. This process is operationalized in the procedures of functional assessment, which are described in Chapters 6 and 7 of this book.

BASIC PRINCIPLES AND ASSUMPTIONS

An examination of the environmental determinants of problem behavior must begin with a delineation of the basic principles and assumptions that define behavior–environment relations. These principles constitute the core understanding of an operant science of behavior (Skinner, 1953), and they similarly represent the most fundamental concepts of PBS (see Table 2.1). The first principle is that behavior, whether it is desirable or undesirable, conforms to a set of natural laws and is therefore accessible to our understanding. This principle is a critical assertion because, without it, we would be obliged to concede that there is an arbitrariness to the occurrence and nonoccurrence of behavior, and that our efforts to comprehend and influence behavior change would ultimately be futile. If, however, we subscribe to the principle of lawfulness, we stipulate that human behavior is understandable and ultimately predictable. We can take this further. If behavior is lawful, we should theoretically be able to gain an understanding of all the pertinent laws, and thereby to possess knowledge of the variables that affect behavior. If we possess this knowledge and are able to observe the variables, then we should be able to predict when behavior will occur. And if we are able to issue such a prediction, and if we can exert control over those variables, then we should be able to reliably manage the occurrence of behavior. Of course, these are a lot of "ifs," and we are not anywhere close to such a position of understanding, but the point is that an assumption of lawfulness is pivotal to any empirically grounded quest to improve our capacity to support positive behavior. This assumption of lawfulness is the basis for all systematic considerations of human behavior, and it has been strongly validated by an immense amount of basic and applied research concerned with the behavioral sciences.

The second principle is that behavior is functional. This means that behavior occurs for a reason that serves the interests of the individual engaged in the behavior. In other words, behavior not only makes sense in the light of natural laws; it also makes sense from the perspective of the individual. A very simple (admittedly overly simple) way to look at it is that an individual engages in a behavior either to obtain something or to escape

---

TABLE 2.1. Three Basic Principles of Behavior

Behavior is . . .
- Lawful
- Functional (and communicative)
- Context-related

or avoid something (O'Neill et al., 1997); however, many authors have described different and more elaborate classifications (e.g., Donnellan, Mirenda, Maseros, & Fassbender, 1984; Maag & Kemp, 2003). Sometimes the purpose or function is readily apparent (e.g., an infant cries to escape an uncomfortably wet diaper), but at other times it is not immediately obvious. Often the purpose is beyond the individual's awareness or ability to explain, and the purpose is frequently complex and multifaceted (e.g., we perform work to earn a paycheck, but also because the work is linked to social relationships, feelings of accomplishment, etc.). In addition, the purpose may be inconspicuous because it is no longer relevant to the person's circumstances, but is rather an artifact of the individual's learning history. It is possible that this principle of functionality does not apply to all behaviors, though behaviors that are not developed and maintained by functional relations are not easy to identify.

A corollary of this second principle is that many behaviors are communicative. That is, the function of the behavior is to act on the social environment—to engage another person's assistance in obtaining or avoiding something—and is therefore an act of communication. This may be especially true for so-called "acting-out" behaviors (tantrums, aggression) that are conspicuously intended to spur the activity of others, but it has been demonstrated to be true also for many benign and even "internalizing" behaviors (e.g., Koegel, Dyer, & Bell, 1987). For instance, the behavior of looking away in the presence of a social initiation may be the communicative equivalent of saying, "Please go away, because I want to be alone." Table 2.2 provides examples of the possible functions behavior may serve.

The applied literature in PBS is rich in examples where the communicative functions of problem behaviors are clearly depicted (e.g., Carr, 1977; Donnellan et al., 1984; Carr & Durand, 1985; Horner & Budd, 1985). This literature demonstrates the unmistakable significance of communication as a functional intervention for problem behaviors (Carr et al., 1994). That is, if we teach alternative forms of communication that serve the same function as the problem behaviors, then the problem behaviors can be reduced or eliminated, because the individual has another effective way to satisfy the function (objective) of these behaviors.

Still, the principle that describes behavior as having a function transcends the communicative equation described above, and the applied importance has many more implications than communicative competence. For instance, in early applied research, Rincover, Cook, Peoples, and Packard (1979) showed that some forms of solitary toy play could replace stereotypic behaviors, if the forms of sensory stimulation produced by the stereotypy (e.g., repetitive noise making, gazing at visual stimuli) and by the toy play (e.g., playing an autoharp, blowing bubbles) were approximately equivalent.

TABLE 2.2. Categories of the Communicative Functions of Behavior

Function	Communicative message
Obtain attention/social interaction	"Pay attention to me." "I need help." "Can I play with you?"
Obtain materials/activities	"I want to use the computer." "I want the book." "I want to listen to music."
Obtain sensory stimulation	"This movement feels good." "This movement makes me feel calm."
Escape/avoid sensory stimulation	"This noise is too loud." "This classroom is too hot."
Escape/avoid attention/social interaction	"I don't want to talk to you." "I don't want you to look at me."
Escape/avoid materials/activities	"I don't want to do this work." "I don't want to be in the classroom." "I don't like this; I need a break."

The third principle that undergirds our understanding is that behavior is governed by the context in which it occurs. This principle asserts that behavior does not occur randomly; instead, it occurs in accordance with conditions in the environment. The environment presents circumstances that incite certain behaviors to occur and discourage others from occurring. The reason why the environment differentially inspires some behaviors and not others is probably that the functions of one type of behavior have been satisfied under those (or similar) conditions previously in the person's experience, whereas other functions have not been so satisfied. For example, a boy may respond to the presentation of difficult academic work by putting his head on his desk and pretending to sleep. This behavior results in the teacher's approaching him and offering assistance. Although the teacher may prefer that the student raise his hand and request assistance, the student has experienced a history of using the less desirable behavior effectively to bring about his desired outcome (i.e., assistance from the teacher).

Here it is appropriate to emphasize two points of definition. First, by environmental *context*, we refer to internal or external events or circumstances that are perceived by an individual (consciously or not) and may influence the individual's behavior. This definition emphasizes that the environment consists of physiological sensations and conditions (e.g., pain, arousal, exhaustion, hunger, fear), as well as sights, sounds, and other experiences produced by stimuli in the external surroundings. Second, the context consists of very many events and circumstances, and behavior is governed by the complex interaction of these events and circumstances. Some events in the immediate context may serve to trigger a particular behavior, whereas other circumstances may serve to increase the likelihood of a particular behavior. For instance, hunger may be a contextual circumstance increasing the chances that a behavior with the function of procuring food may occur. The sight or sound of a desired food item may be the trigger that actually occasions the behavior. Their interaction is the context that determines whether the behavior occurs.

Generally speaking, the immediate stimuli in the environment that set off a particular behavior are referred to as *antecedent stimuli* or *discriminative stimuli*—or, more colloquially, *triggering stimuli* or *triggers* (they are referred to as *antecedents* in the remainder of this book). These are typically very proximal events that are readily identified in the external environment (though it is quickly acknowledged that they may also be internal, and therefore more difficult to detect). Conditions or events that make a particular behavior more or less probable are referred to as *setting events* or *establishing operations* (Kantor, 1959; Michael, 1993). These include physiological and ecological conditions of relative deprivation, and other circumstances that alter the value of reinforcers, thus heightening the likelihood of behaviors that have the function of obtaining those reinforcers (see further explanation later in this chapter). A good deal of conceptual and empirical research has focused on these different aspects of the environmental context (e.g., Gardner, Cole, Davidson, & Karan, 1986; Michael, 1993), but the critical point we wish to emphasize is that behavior is determined to a great extent on the basis of these contextual situations and events.

DEVELOPING AN UNDERSTANDING OF PROBLEM BEHAVIOR

Understanding problem behavior means understanding the variables in the environment that govern the behavior's occurrence, nonoccurrence, and future probability. If we acquire such an understanding, we should be able to predict when, where, with whom, and under what circumstances the behavior will and will not occur (or will be more or less likely to occur). Furthermore, understanding problem behavior means understanding the purposeful nature of such behavior. Many researchers have hypothesized a link between nonverbal behavior and communication (e.g., Carr et al., 1994; Durand, 1990). In the area of typical child development, crying has long been understood as an early and primitive form of communication. Studies have shown that infants cry for a variety of reasons, such as seeking the attention of their mothers, obtaining certain tangible items, and escaping from unpleasant situations (Bayley, 1932; Wolff, 1969). In addition to crying, aggression has been suggested as a primitive form of communication. Brownlee and Bakeman (1981) observed that certain aggressive acts displayed by toddlers, such as hitting with an open hand, influenced other children in reliable ways, such as immediately terminating interaction. The authors suggested that the hitting was equivalent to saying, "Leave me alone." Also, lightly hitting toys tended to result in a positive social interaction, which the authors interpreted as expressing, "Hey, wanna play?" Furthermore, these observations held true for 2-year-olds, but not for 3-year-olds, who appeared to rely more on speech than on aggression to influence their peers.

Thus it appears that the typically occurring disruptive behaviors displayed by young children without disabilities may in fact occur for the same reasons and serve the same purposes as more severe and chronic problem behaviors. The difference then, perhaps, is that while most children tend to develop new communicative competencies and thus "outgrow" problem behaviors such as crying and aggression, some children who experience disabilities may not develop these same competencies over time. This notion appears to be supported by studies documenting the correlation between problem behaviors and lack of communication skills. For example, children with delays or impairments in communication are more likely to be described as aggressive, noncompliant, or hostile (Aram, Ekelman, & Nation, 1984; Baker & Cantwell, 1982; Cantwell, Baker, & Mattison, 1980; Caulfield, Fischel, DeBaryshe, & Whitehurst, 1989; Kaiser, Cai, & Hancock, 2002). In addition, among individuals diagnosed with mental retardation, those who were found to have relatively poor communication skills were rated as displaying higher levels of aggressive behavior than those who had better communication skills (Talkington, Hall, & Altman, 1971).

Similar findings have also been reported on the link between poor communication skills and self-injurious behaviors among children with autism (Shodell & Reiter, 1968). These findings have led to conclusions that such problem behaviors serve as primitive forms of communication by individuals lacking more sophisticated, effective, or socially acceptable ways to communicate. The implication is that if individuals with problem behaviors could learn more sophisticated, effective, and socially appropriate ways to communicate, then they would no longer need to engage in the problem behaviors. This is not to say that only people with communicative delays will engage in problem behaviors. In fact, under certain circumstances, people with competent communication skills will engage in problem behaviors. This may occur because the expression of those messages are difficult for an individual (e.g., it may be difficult to express frustration, anxiety, or anger directed at an authority figure) or because the appropriate communicative expressions are not likely to result in the desired outcome (e.g., a child may know from experience that a request for a break from a difficult math lesson is likely to be denied). Yet it very well may be that in certain situations the individual has simply not yet learned that verbal communication skills can be used to rectify a particular situation to his or her satisfaction.

It is also important to note that the fact that problem behavior may be *purposeful* does not imply that individuals *intentionally* use such behavior to influence others. There is no evidence to suggest that a person with problem behavior is strategizing along the lines of "This person is asking me to engage in an activity I find aversive; I think I will hit him, so I can go to the principal's office and avoid the activity altogether." Rather, viewing problem behavior as purposeful implies that problem behavior functions as if it were a form of communication, and thus is useful in the design and implementation of behavior support plans.

Clearly, developing a functional understanding of problem behavior has tremendous implications for the assessment of problem behavior and the design and implementation of behavior support plans. When problem behavior is viewed as serving a communicative function, the primary goal of assessment becomes identifying exactly what that function is, and under what circumstances the problem behavior is most (and least) likely to occur. Regarding the design and implementation of support plans, strategies that simply seek to suppress the behavior through the use of consequences are clearly inadequate and ill advised. Rather, through modifications to the environment and the teaching of new communication skills, the existence of problem behavior can be obviated.

Given a functional understanding of problem behavior, the resulting goal of assessment is to identify the purpose, or communicative function, that the problem behavior serves. To accomplish this goal, it is important to gain a clear understanding of the context in which problem behavior does (and does not) occur, the function that the behavior serves, and the functional alternatives that could potentially replace the problem behavior. A framework for developing such an understanding is based upon the *four-term contingency*, and upon an examination of each of these terms within the context in which the behavior occurs.

THE FOUR-TERM CONTINGENCY

Since problem behavior serves a communicative purpose, as manifested by bringing about some change in the environment, we can assume that problem behavior does not occur unless there is something "wrong" with the environment, which we refer to as the *context* in which behavior occurs. The context is defined as all events and stimuli in the internal and external environment that are perceived and have some influence on behavior.

Our understanding of environmental determinants is referenced to a behavioral equation that delineates the process of behavioral governance in terms of a four-term contingency. This equation is presented in Figure 2.1. In this figure, the context includes the *setting events* and the *antecedents*; the *maintaining consequences* indicate the stimuli from the environment that follow the *behavior*, and presumably produce the functional reinforcers that are responsible for the behavior's continued presence. The four-term contingency is the framework that organizes our understanding and prediction of behavior from the molecular viewpoint, and as we have indicated, this viewpoint is critical for producing effective behavior support plans. We reiterate, however, that this level of understanding must be couched in a larger, more holistic perspective that includes the broader considerations of health, safety, relationships, and the totality of lifestyle factors. These factors are discussed briefly near the end of this chapter, and in much more detail in Chapter 11 of this book.

Antecedent Events

Antecedent events are those stimuli that lead directly to the occurrence of problem behavior. These are usually immediate, simple, and discrete events that are said to evoke or trigger problem behaviors (Durand, 1990). These stimuli tend to be present during, or immediately prior to, the occurrence of problem behavior, and lead to its immediate occurrence. These direct events predict problem behavior by serving as a signal that reinforcement is available, given the occurrence of such behavior.

Examples of antecedent events can be summarized into (at least) four general areas (1) physiological, (2) cognitive/emotional, (3) physical envi-

Setting events + Antecedent events → Behavior →			Maintaining consequences
Student has fight on the bus before coming to school.	Teacher passes out pop quiz.	Student tears up paper and refuses to complete quiz.	Student is sent to office and does not return to classroom until second activity period.

FIGURE 2.1. Four-term contingency model and examples illustrating environmental influences on behavior.

ronment, and (4) social/activity events. Examples of antecedent events in the physiological area could include the immediate onset of pain, a full bladder, or illness that serves as a direct trigger for behavior (e.g., crying because the individual has an earache) (see Table 2.3). The unifying feature of antecedent events in this area is that something in the physiological makeup of the individual changes, thus evoking an immediate response that has previously been reinforced under similar conditions. An example from the cognitive/emotional category might be an onset of symptoms of a mental health disorder, or possibly a change in the emotional condition of the individual. In this case, the cognitive or emotional characteristics are what change, triggering problem behavior that has successfully recruited reinforcement in similar previous circumstances. For example, a student with an emotional disorder may periodically "hear voices," which serve as an antecedent for running out of the classroom. In the physical environment category, some examples of antecedent events may include furniture rearrangement, change in seating arrangement at school, distracting noises, or changes in classroom temperature. Again there is a change in the context, this time in the physical environment, which results in problem behavior. Various examples in the area of social/activity events may include presentation of academic demands, a request to complete a nonpreferred task, method of instruction delivery (e.g., written vs. oral instruction, large-group vs. individual instruction, etc.), delivery of corrective feedback, change in routine, teasing, social overtures, and so forth. This category simply shifts the focus of antecedent events to the area of social interactions or specific academic, work, leisure, or other activities.

The common theme among all of these examples is that a specific event occurs or is present in the context, resulting in an immediate display of problem behavior. This more immediate relationship between contextual events and problem behavior is the primary feature that distinguishes antecedent events from setting events. It is important to point out that whereas many examples of antecedent events involve changes in environmental stimuli (e.g., the onset or cessation of some contextual event), often an

TABLE 2.3. Examples of Possible Setting Events
and Antecedents to Problem/Behavior

Setting event	Antecedent
Fatigue	Instructional demand
Illness	Lack of social attention
Difficult social interaction	Removal of desired object
Medication side effects	Request

antecedent event will not consist of any clearly observable change. One fairly common example of this is when students have been alone (e.g., working or playing independently) and then engage in problem behavior that causes an adult to attend to them in some manner. Although it may be tempting to write this type of scenario off as having occurred "out of the blue," a closer examination of the immediate context will provide useful information. For example, the act of working independently for a certain period of time may be an antecedent event that triggers problem behavior, meaning that the antecedent event involves both the activity and the amount of time spent in that activity. In other words, there is always an antecedent event associated with a problem behavior. Whether or not that event is easily or readily observable, however, is another matter.

Setting Events

Setting events are events, circumstances, or stimuli that increase the probability of problem behaviors' occurring because they affect the value of the response to direct antecedent events. Specifically, setting events serve to alter the value of maintaining (reinforcing) consequences for particular responses in particular situations. For instance, if a setting event serves to make a child more tired and irritable, then escape from demanding schoolwork will be more valuable than if the child was not exposed to the setting event. Thus the child will be more likely to engage in problem behaviors (e.g., tantrums) that are maintained by escape when he or she is presented with academic instruction.

As opposed to antecedent events, setting events are typically characterized as more complex events, circumstances, or stimuli that set the stage for problem behavior, or increase the likelihood that problem behavior will occur, rather than immediately evoking its occurrence. They are conditions that may occur just before or simultaneously with problem behavior, or conditions that occur well prior to the onset of problem behavior. A distinguishing feature of setting events is that they do not, in and of themselves, evoke problem behavior. They rely on antecedent events to occasion the problem behavior. In fact, the presence of setting events increases the likelihood that problem behavior will occur following antecedent events that may not otherwise evoke problem behavior. Figure 2.2 depicts how the occurrence of a setting event can influence an individual's behavior. In this example, the first sequence depicts a brief interaction in a classroom, where Kara is obliged to wait for a computer to become available. The second sequence is characterized by a setting event in which an illness accompanied by a severe headache has deprived Kara of sleep. As a result, the value of completing her work without delay is heightened (as are her irritability and lack of patience), and this means that the delay in accessing a computer

Setting event	Antecedent	Behavior	Maintaining consequences
Absent	Kara moves to computer area and sees that all stations are full.	Kara signs name on board to indicate that she is waiting for her turn.	Student working on computer leaves, and Kara begins working.
Present Kara is up most of the night with a severe headache. She comes to class with dark circles under her eyes from lack of sleep.	Kara moves to computer area and sees that all stations are full.	Kara grabs student's shirt and pulls student from chair.	Student working on computer leaves, and Kara begins working.

FIGURE 2.2. Example of a behavioral sequence without and with the presence of a setting event.

station triggers Kara's assaultive behavior, rather than the more typical and socially sanctioned response of Sequence 1.

Examples of setting events can be summarized into the same four general areas as antecedents: (1) physiological, (2) cognitive/emotional, (3) physical environment, and (4) social/activity events. Examples of setting events in the physiological area include allergies, illness, and menses (see Table 2.3). The presence of allergy symptoms (setting event), for example, may increase the likelihood that when asked by the classroom teacher to read a book (antecedent event), a student may throw the book across the classroom to avoid that activity. The key in identifying the setting event as contributing to the onset of problem behavior is whether the request to read a book is one that is typically complied with when the student is not experiencing allergy symptoms. If not, we would view the teacher's request for the student to read a certain book—the antecedent event—as the salient context for problem behavior.

In the cognitive/emotional category, an example of a setting event may include a fight on the school bus earlier in the day that has resulted in an angry emotional state or bad mood. In this category, these internal events would have an indirect impact on problem behavior. So take, for example, the instance of one student's hitting a classmate at school. We learn that the student is in a bad mood, and we also happen to know that this student is typically receptive to this particular classmate's greetings. Thus we can conclude that the emotional state (i.e., the bad mood) is probably the influencing, albeit indirect, event leading to the student's hitting the classmate upon being greeted (antecedent event).

Examples in the physical category may include lighting (or lack thereof), noise level, fatigue, hunger, and so forth. An ongoing high level of background noise in a classroom may play a role in influencing the onset of problem behavior. If under these conditions, for example, a child is asked to engage in an activity, and due to the noise has trouble either hearing the instructions or concentrating on the task, the child may engage in problem behavior instead. Again, in this example it is not necessarily the instructions or the assigned tasks (antecedents) that trigger the problem behaviors; rather, it is their combination with the high noise level (setting event) that leads to the occurrence of problem behavior.

Lastly, in the social/activity category, one example would appear to be the extent of rapport between individuals. Take the scenario of a boy who is having difficulties and engaging in problem behavior when the classroom teacher works with him on daily living skills. In contrast, when the instructional assistant is engaging the student in the same daily living skills, he engages in minimal to no problem behavior. Perhaps the instructional assistant has been working with the student for 3 years, while the teacher has just begun working with the student, and when given the option the student consistently chooses to work with the assistant. This would be an example of rapport's influencing problem behavior as a setting event, since the activity and the instruction associated with it (antecedent events) do not elicit the problem behavior when the assistant is involved (or at least not to the same extent as when the setting event is present).

It is worth noting that a single event, circumstance, or stimulus can serve as either an antecedent event or a setting event, depending on the nature of the circumstance. Take the issue of being overheated and exhausted from physical exercise, for instance. On one hand, a student who becomes overheated and exhausted from physical exercise may immediately drop to the floor and refuse to stand. In this example, the state of exhaustion and being overheated serve as an antecedent event. On the other hand, another student may be overheated and exhausted, but does not display problem behavior unless that setting event is paired with the antecedent of being asked to engage in a challenging academic task. In this second example, the state of being exhausted and overheated serves as a setting event.

As a result of looking closely at the combination of antecedent and setting events for problem behavior, we gain a better understanding of the contexts in which such behavior occurs and those in which it does not occur. By understanding these circumstances in the environment, we begin to gain an understanding of the purposeful nature of problem behavior. Since the occurrence of behavior in a particular context indicates that it is likely that the behavior has been previously satisfied under similar conditions, these conditions can become a focus of intervention. For example, when it is observed that a student's problem behavior is triggered by the antecedent of instructional demands, the presentation of task demands becomes the context for intervention. Through the identification of contextual features (i.e., antecedents and setting events) that are associated with problem behavior, modifications and enhancements can then be made to obviate the need for the problem behavior's occurrence (as discussed in Chapter 8).

Maintaining Consequences

Although an understanding of the events that occur prior to problem behavior is essential to the functional understanding of problem behavior, it is not sufficient. In order to gain a full understanding, we must also consider the purpose or function that the problem behavior is serving, and the conditions following the behavior that reinforce and maintain it. As we have described before, problem behavior is functional in that it serves the interests of the individual engaged in the behavior. We can gain an understanding of how the individual's interests are being served by examining the consequences that follow the behavior's occurrence. The consequences that ordinarily follow the behavior are likely to be the maintaining consequences, and thus the function of the behavior. A baby crying because of a wet diaper results in recruiting an adult to change the diaper (escaping the unpleasantly wet diaper is the consequence). A girl who averts her eye gaze when approached by others avoids unwanted social interaction (avoidance of social contact is the maintaining consequence). A student who talks out during a difficult assignment accesses assistance from the teacher (in this instance, the provision of help is the likely maintaining consequence).

Although problem behavior is functional, and thus can be seen as being quite sensible, what makes it problematic is that it is deemed socially inappropriate. Despite its social inappropriateness, problem behavior is often the best (most effective, most efficient) way that a person has learned to achieve this function-specific satisfaction. The behavior results in access to, or avoidance of, events by the individual. These events are referred to as *maintaining consequences.*

Understanding problem behavior from a functional perspective means identifying why the behavior is occurring (its function), as well as what socially approved alternatives to the behavior might exist and why they do not occur instead. There are at least two possible reasons why socially approved alternatives either may not exist or do not occur: (1) Socially appropriate alternative skills are not currently in the individual's repertoire; or (2) socially appropriate skills are in the individual's repertoire, but are not effective or efficient in accessing the function-specific outcome of the problem behavior(s) in question (i.e., the environment is less responsive to socially appropriate skills than it is to problem behavior).

An important point to consider when we are developing an understanding of problem behavior is the very likely possibility that an individual simply does not possess the socially appropriate skills for a given situation, or is unable to use them when needed. If an individual does not possess these skills—regardless of whether the individual experiences a disability, a deprived environment, or some other experience—we can assume that the socially appropriate requisite skills simply have not been effectively taught. Given the lack of a particular socially appropriate skill, it is not surprising that problem behavior is displayed, since it may simply be the continued development of behavior that was highly successful during infancy and early childhood in satisfying the function-specific outcome. It is the most effective and efficient behavior that is available to obtain the desired consequence. The implications for the development of appropriate supports, given this scenario, are clear: In order to bring about a decrease in the problem behavior, a socially acceptable replacement behavior must be selected and successfully taught.

Yet, even given that a socially acceptable behavior has been successfully taught, the problem behavior may still persist because the behavior that was taught is not effective in achieving the function-specific outcome served by the problem behavior. For example, a girl who frequently yells out during independent seatwork, resulting in teacher attention, may be taught to read quietly at her desk until the teacher can check in with the student. However, since the function-specific outcome (i.e., teacher attention) is not immediately satisfied by the replacement behavior (i.e., reading quietly), it is unlikely that the student's problem behavior (i.e., yelling out) will decrease.

Similarly, a socially acceptable behavior may be successfully taught, but the environment may remain unresponsive to its use. For example, a girl may be taught to raise her hand, instead of yelling out, to get the attention of the teacher during independent classroom activities. Although hand raising is a socially appropriate behavior in the classroom and would appear to be an effective way to gain the teacher's attention, if the teacher does not acknowledge the student when her hand is raised, it is unlikely that hand raising will replace yelling out. In this case, yelling out remains the only viable option available to the student for effectively recruiting teacher attention. Even if the teacher is able to respond to the student's raised hand after only a short period of time, but continues to respond instantly to the student's outbursts, it is also unlikely that hand raising will replace yelling out, due to the latter's superior efficiency in gaining teacher attention. Thus, in efforts to replace problem behavior with a functionally equivalent alternative, it is of utmost importance that the replacement behavior results in the function-specific outcome, and that it does so (at least initially) more effectively and efficiently than the problem behavior.

In order to develop an understanding of why problem behavior occurs, it is imperative to incorporate the concept of the functionality of behavior into such an understanding. By understanding how consequences follow problem behavior in ways that are beneficial to the individual, we can begin the process of identifying appropriate ways of improving the context, teaching equivalent replacement skills, and more effectively arranging the outcomes for problem and appropriate behavior.

CONSIDERATIONS OF THE INDIVIDUAL AND LIFESTYLE

As indicated throughout this chapter, an understanding of the environmental determinants relevant to the development of behavior support plans is conceptualized most precisely and constructively by examining the components of the four-term contingency. Although imperfect, our knowledge of how these component variables operate is sufficient for us to perform functional assessments and develop effective support plans. Increasingly, however, these are not the only factors we must understand if we are to produce and implement comprehensive support plans that lead to long-term, meaningful outcomes and quality-of-life improvements for people who demonstrate problem behavior. The additional factors we refer to are broader variables involving the characteristics of the individual and his or her lifestyle (see Chapters 3, 6, and 11).

We have noted that problem behaviors serve as an indicator that something is "wrong" in the environment. Problem behaviors are most likely to occur when there is a mismatch between the needs and desires of the individual and the conditions or circumstances in the (internal and/or external) environment. Thus problem behavior may be viewed as a signal that, in some way, conditions of life are unsatisfactory. We have already discussed those setting event conditions (e.g., allergies, exhaustion) that temporarily affect the value of reinforcers (e.g., escape) and thus are entered into the molecular framework of the four-term contingency. Now we are referring to more static conditions that cannot easily be associated with particular instances of problem behavior, but that nevertheless may be related to higher expectancies of problems. The point here is that, overall, problem behaviors are less likely to occur if a person is feeling well, possesses suitable competencies, and is generally satisfied and fulfilled by life's arrangements. In contrast, if the person's health and life circumstances are unsatisfactory and frustrating, and if the person feels unable to effect needed change, then it may be assumed that, in general, the context may be all the more primed to evoke problem behaviors. In short, individual characteristics and lifestyle circumstances are relevant to behavior support, and they should be understood as potential elements of targeted change in comprehensive support plans.

Because we have little empirical evidence regarding the influence that these variables may exert, we also have no developed classification system for them. However, lifestyle variables in general are found within the domains of living environments; leisure, work, and/or school activities; community participation; and social networks, including the range of interpersonal relationships and supports. Variables that are more closely associated with the individual include health, preferences, learning histories, abilities, and other personal characteristics. (See Table 2.4 for a range of examples.) Again, while we cannot assert a documented relationship between these variables and problem behavior (as in the four-term contingency), it is clear that the variables combine to define the quality of an individual's life; as such, it is fully appropriate that they enter into the goals and design of PBS interventions.

One of the critical and extremely far-reaching factors we have mentioned above involves an individual's abilities to interact with the environment in order to satisfy his or her needs. Abilities (competencies) may encompass communication, self-management, locomotion, self-care, social navigation and negotiation, and other skills that are useful for controlling the social environment. Understanding the expectations of the environment, and the match between these expectations and the individual's needs or desires, provides information on the context of challenging behavior. Consider the following example. A 5-year-old boy with severe physical disabilities and limited means of communication is attending a community preschool program. The child is placed in his wheelchair and taken to the playground each day with the other children. The child wants to interact with the other children and join in their play, but is unable to get out of his

---

TABLE 2.4. Examples of Personal and Lifestyle Issues to Consider

- Socially satisfying personal relationships
- Comfortable and safe living environment
- Active engagement in preferred activities
- Freedom of movement
- Ability to express wants, needs, and preferences
- Meaningful daily activities, including employment
- Exercise that is healthful and personally satisfying
- Appropriate medical care and treatment of illness/health concerns
- Pursuit of leisure and recreation interests

wheelchair. If the child could communicate effectively, perhaps he would request assistance from the teacher. Since the child cannot, he bites his wrist; this results in his gaining access to the teacher's attention, and the teacher may then play with him or encourage a peer to come and interact with him. This situation is a "bad fit" for the child. His lack of mobility and communication skills contribute to his frustration and use of problem behavior. If the child is placed in an adapted swing, a chair within the sandbox, or some other piece of adapted equipment that offers him mobility, the use of problem behavior may become irrelevant or unnecessary. Thus understanding the individual's competencies and circumstances can contribute to an understanding of the problem behavior and the strategies that may be used to produce behavioral and lifestyle improvements (Carr et al., 1998).

It is important to understand not only a person's relevant skill competencies (and deficits), but also many other factors related to health, fitness, safety, social/emotional well-being, interest in participating in the social community, environmental enrichment and stimulation, and so on. Personal and lifestyle issues are often very complex and require a deep understanding of the individual's history and of events that have occurred in other environments. For example, consider a girl who has been placed in multiple foster homes because of abuse from her birth parents. This student's social relationships and ability to trust adults and peers are likely to be shaded by these experiences. Intervention to address this student's problem behavior must also consider the student's history and previous experiences, and must include interventions that address those concerns. Examples of lifestyle supports for the student may include fostering the development of a long-term relationship with a caring adult through a Big Sister program; addressing the student's repeated disruptions of foster care placements by placing a priority on placement in a home with a history of stable placements; and providing support to the student to access activities and relationships in the community that can be maintained regardless of residential placement. We cannot delineate all of these variables, and of course the most pertinent will vary from individual to individual, but we wish to emphasize that their breadth and focus are related to quality of life (Goode, 1994; Hughes, Hwang, Kim, Eisenman, & Killian, 1995; Schalock, Keith, Hoffman, & Karan, 1989), with the presumption that a high quality of life is inversely related to the occurrence of problem behaviors. As such, it is important for behavior support team members to appreciate and understand the status of these variables as they affect the lives of individuals, and seek to incorporate supports that will enhance quality of life. Both the assessment and the intervention and support processes should explicitly consider these critical factors.

SUMMARY

In this chapter, we have described the basic kinds of information that are needed to acquire an understanding of problem behavior that is the basis of functional assessment (see Chapter 6) and the PBS process (Chapter 3). We have begun by describing the necessary assumptions and principles that are the foundation for building a functional understanding. These include the notions that human behavior conforms to natural laws; that it is governed by the environmental (internal and external) context in which it occurs; and that it is functional and even sensible from the perspective of an individual's learning history. We have then outlined the four-term contingency and elaborated upon the operations of context, setting events, discriminative (antecedent triggering) stimuli, and maintaining consequences. Finally, we have acknowledged the important roles of individual characteristics and lifestyle considerations, which must be understood in order to develop an optimally comprehensive and effective PBS plan.

A precise and holistic understanding of the variables described in this chapter should lead to behavior supports that are maximally effective, responsive to individual challenges and strengths, and respectful of the person's autonomy and aspirations to a high quality of life. Such an understanding is the hallmark of PBS.

REFERENCES

Aram, D. M., Ekelman, B. L., & Nation, J. E. (1984). Preschoolers with language disorders: 10 years later. *Journal of Speech and Hearing Research, 27,* 232–244.

Baker, L., & Cantwell, D. P. (1982). Developmental, social, and behavioral characteristics of speech and language disordered children. *Child Psychiatry and Human Development, 12,* 195–206.

Bayley, N. (1932). A study of the crying of infants during mental and physical tests. *Journal of Genetic Psychology, 40,* 306–329.

Brownlee, J. R., & Bakeman, R. (1981). Hitting in toddler-peer interaction. *Child Development, 52,* 1076–1079.

Cantwell, D. P., Baker, L., & Mattison, R. E. (1980). Psychiatric disorders in children with speech and language retardation. *Archives of General Psychiatry, 37,* 423–426.

Carr, E. G. (1977). The motivation of self-injurious behavior: A review of some hypotheses. *Psychological Bulletin, 84,* 800–816.

Carr, E. G., Carlson, J. I., Langdon, N. A., Magito-McLaughlin, D., & Yarbrough, S. C. (1998). Two perspectives on antecedent control: Molecular and molar. In J. K. Luiselli & M. J. Cameron (Eds.), *Antecedent control: Innovative approaches to behavioral support* (pp. 3–28). Baltimore: Paul H. Brookes.

Carr, E. G., Dunlap, G., Horner, R. H., Koegel, R. L., Turnbull, A. P., Sailor, W., et al. (2002). Positive behavior support: Evolution of an applied science. *Journal of Positive Behavior Interventions, 4,* 4–16.

Carr, E. G., & Durand, M. (1985). Reducing behavior problems through functional communication training. *Journal of Applied Behavior Analysis, 18,* 111–126.

Carr, E. G., Horner, R. H., Turnbull, A. P., Marquis, J. G., McLaughlin, D. M., McAtee, M. L., et al. (1999). *Positive behavior support for people with developmental disabilities: A research synthesis.* Washington, DC: American Association on Mental Retardation.

Carr, E. G., Levin, L., McConnachie, G., Carlson, J. I., Kemp, D. C., & Smith, C. E. (1994). *Communication-based intervention for problem behavior: A user's guide for producing positive change.* Baltimore: Paul H. Brookes.

Caulfield, M. B., Fischel, J., DeBaryshe, B. D., & Whitehurst, G. J. (1989). Behavioral correlates of developmental expressive language disorder. *Journal of Abnormal Child Psychology, 17,* 187–201.

Durand, V. M. (1990). *Severe behavior problems: A functional communication training approach.* New York: Guilford Press.

Donnellan, A., Mirenda, P., Mesaros, R., & Fassbender, L. (1984). Analyzing the communicative functions of aberrant behavior. *Journal of The Association for Persons with Severe Handicaps, 9,* 201–212.

Gardner, W. I., Cole, C. L., Davidson, D. P., & Karan, O. C. (1986). Reducing aggression in individuals with developmental disabilities: An expanded stimulus control, assessment, and intervention model. *Education and Training of the Mentally Retarded, 21,* 3–12.

Goode, D. (1994), The National Quality of Life for Persons with Disabilities Project: A quality of life agenda for the United States. In D. Goode (Ed.), *Quality of life for persons with disabilities* (pp. 139–161). Cambridge, MA: Brookline Books.

Horner, R. H., & Budd, C. M. (1985). Acquisition of manual sign use: Collateral reduction of maladaptive behavior, and factors limiting generalization. *Education and Training of the Mentally Retarded, 20,* 39–47.

Hughes, C., Hwang, B., Kim, J. H., Eisenman, L. T., & Killiam, D. J. (1995). Quality of life in applied research: A review and analysis of empirical measures. *American Journal on Mental Retardation, 99,* 623–641.

Kaiser, A. P., Cai, X., & Hancock, T. B. (2002). Teacher-reported behavior problems and language delays in boys and girls enrolled in Head Start. *Behavioral Disorders, 28,* 23–39.

Kantor, J. R. (1959). *Interbehavioral psychology.* Granville, OH: Principia Press.

Kincaid, D., & Fox, L. (2002). Person-centered planning and positive behaviors support. In S. Holburn & P. M. Vietze (Eds.), *Person-centered planning: Research, practice, and future directions* (pp. 29–50). Baltimore: Paul H. Brookes.

Koegel, R. L., Dyer, K., & Bell, L. K. (1987). The influence of child-preferred activities on autistic children's social behavior. *Journal of Applied Behavior Analysis, 20,* 243–252.

Maag, J. W., & Kemp, S. E. (2003). Behavioral intent of power and affiliation: Implications for functional analysis. *Remedial and Special Education, 24,* 57–64.

Michael, J. (1993). Establishing operations. *The Behavior Analyst, 16,* 191–206.

O'Neill, R. E., Horner, R. H., Albin, R. W., Sprague, J. R., Storey, K., & Newton, J. S. (1997). *Functional assessment of problem behavior: A practical assessment guide* (2nd ed.). Pacific Grove, CA: Brooks/Cole.

Rincover, A., Cook, R., Peoples, A., & Packard, D. (1979). Sensory extinction and sensory reinforcement principles for programming multiple adaptive behavior change. *Journal of Applied Behavior Analysis, 12,* 221–233.

Risley, T. (1996). Get a life! In L. K. Koegel, R. L. Koegel, & G. Dunlap (Eds.), *Positive behavioral support: Including people with difficult behavior in the community* (pp. 425–437). Baltimore: Paul H. Brookes.

Romanczyk, R. G., & Matthews, A. L. (1998). Physiological state as antecedent: Utilization in functional analysis. In J. K. Luiselli & M. J. Cameron (Eds.), *Antecedent control: Innovative approaches to behavioral support* (pp. 115–138). Baltimore: Paul H. Brookes.

Schalock, R. L., Keith, K. D., Hoffman, K., & Karan, O. C. (1989). Quality of life: Its measurement and use. *Mental Retardation, 27,* 25–31.

Schroeder, S. R., Oster-Granite, M. L., & Thompson, T. (Eds.). (2002). *Self-injurious behavior: Gene–brain–behavior relationships.* Washington, DC: American Psychological Association.

Shodell, M. J., & Reiter, H. H. (1968). Self-mutilative behavior in verbal and nonberbal schizophrenic children. *Archives of General Psychiatry, 19,* 453–455.

Skinner, B. F. (1953). *Science and human behavior.* New York: Macmillan.

Talkington, L. W., Hall, S., & Altman, R. (1971). Communication deficits and aggression in the mentally retarded. *American Journal of Mental Deficiency, 76,* 235–237.

Turnbull, A. P., & Turnbull, H. R. (1990). A tale about lifestyle changes: Comments on "Toward a technology of 'nonaversive' behavioral support." *Journal of The Association for Persons with Severe Handicaps, 15,* 142–144.

Turnbull, A. P., & Turnbull, H. R. (1996). Group action planning as a strategy for planning comprehensive family support. In L. K. Koegel, R. L. Koegel, & G. Dunlap (Eds.), *Positive behavioral support: Including people with difficult behavior in the community* (pp. 99–114). Baltimore, MD: Paul H. Brookes.

Wolff, P. H. (1969). The natural history of crying and other vocalizations in early infancy. In B. M. Foss (Ed.), *Determinants of infant behavior* (Vol. 4, pp. 81–109). London: Methuen.

CHAPTER 3

◆ ◆ ◆

Overview of
the Behavior Support Process

◆

LINDA M. BAMBARA

Currently enrolled in an inclusive second-grade classroom, Derrick is a 9-year-old boy recently diagnosed with learning disabilities and characteristics of a pervasive developmental disorder (PDD). Despite showing early signs of learning problems and having received special education services as a preschooler for speech and language delays, Derrick was not deemed eligible for special education at his elementary school until this year. Previous psychological evaluations failed to reveal a substantial discrepancy between his IQ (85) and his academic achievement, which is needed for a learning disabilities classification. Derrick managed to struggle through kindergarten, but failed and repeated first grade. The building principal believed that Derrick's learning and social problems were due primarily to his immaturity, and encouraged his parents to hold him back a year. Derrick managed to struggle through a second year of first grade, but soon after he started second grade, it became apparent that time alone would not solve his problems. For the third time since kindergarten, Derrick's mother requested another comprehensive evaluation.

Derrick now receives special education services in his second-grade classroom, and meets daily with his special education teacher for intensive instruction in reading and math. However, at midyear, he seems to be mak-

47

ing little progress. In fact, his social behavior appears to be worsening. Derrick's "inability to get along with peers" and his "extremely immature classroom behaviors" have caused his teachers to question whether his current classroom placement is appropriate. In just one recent school day, the following three scenarios occurred.

Scenario 1: Derrick sat alone on the school playground, playing with one of his many miniature toy locomotives. Pushing the train on the ground and swishing it in the air, he seemed oblivious to the running, jumping, and playing of other children who surrounded him. After 20 minutes, he stared at five classmates playing dodgeball. "You're stupid," he shouted. Familiar with Derrick's antics, they ignored him. "You are stupid, stupid, stupid," he shouted again. Just then, the ball escaped and rolled toward Derrick. Derrick quickly scooped it up. Jason attempted to grab the ball, but Derrick pushed back hard, tried to kick Jason, and then ran away with the ball. "Mrs. Nyce," Jason screamed in frustration, "Derrick's at it again."

Scenario 2: Mrs. Nyce told a group of students to get started on their independent math worksheets. Derrick rested his head on his desk, and glided his toy locomotive along the desk's sides. Taking his train away, Mrs. Nyce urged Derrick to get started. He cried. "Do you want help?" she asked. "No, no, no—go away," Derrick sobbed louder, banging his feet on the legs of his desk. "You're a baby," Jason whispered. "Shut up!" Derrick shouted, and threatened to punch Jason by making a fist.

Scenario 3: Later in the day, Mrs. Nyce divided her class into five groups. She instructed the members of each group to paint and decorate a medieval castle, and placed art supplies and a cardboard castle in the center of each group. Derrick's eyes widened with excitement. He eagerly got started on the castle's turret in front of him. Needing black paint and glitter, he grabbed Sue's. "Hey, wait until I'm done," Sue protested. Derrick didn't wait; he continued to grab, placing the materials in front of him. He used his body (pushing, shoving) to block his classmates from using any of his materials. Eventually, Sue cried out in frustration, "Mrs. Nyce, Derrick has all the paint and won't share with us."

There are hundreds of students like Derrick. Some present more severe problem behaviors; others present less problematic concerns. Nevertheless, the question of how to begin designing a positive behavior support (PBS) plan for such a student can be overwhelming—particularly when team members feel pressured to balance the student's needs and family's priorities with the needs and concerns of other students, teachers, parents, and school administrators.

PBS offers a comprehensive, problem-solving approach to understanding reasons for problem behavior and designing effective and long-lasting interventions uniquely tailored to individual students. The problem-solving and ongoing nature of the approach makes the process dynamic and flexible. Team members develop and implement a behavior support plan once they gather sufficient information about a student and potential reasons for problem behaviors. Over time, a number of life changes (e.g., a transition to a new classroom) may require the team to modify these supports to address new concerns.

Although the process for providing PBS is dynamic, it is helpful to conceptualize the entire process—from identifying a problem behavior to evaluating and modifying a behavior support plan—in explicit steps (e.g., Bambara & Knoster, 1985; Janney & Snell, 2000). The purpose of this chapter is to overview five basic process steps for designing PBS interventions for individual students. Specific information on how actually to conduct functional assessments, develop hypotheses, and design and evaluate behavior support plans is described in subsequent chapters. The goal here is to provide an organizing framework for illustrating the entire PBS process.

STEPS IN THE PBS PROCESS

The five-step PBS process is illustrated in Figure 3.1. These five basic steps may be applied effectively across students with various disabilities or diagnoses (e.g., learning disabilities, emotional/behavioral disorders, mental retardation, autism), problem behaviors (e.g., aggression, disruption, self-injury, social withdrawal), and settings (i.e., home, school, community). In this chapter, examples of how the process can be applied are provided for Derrick. Other case illustrations with different students and problem behaviors can be found throughout the text.

Step 1: Prioritize and Define the Problem Behavior

Key Questions: *What is the problem? Is behavior support necessary?*

The first step in the process is to determine what the problem is and whether an individualized behavior support plan is necessary. Not every student who engages in problem behaviors will require a comprehensive behavior support plan as described in this book. Most students are responsive to general schoolwide discipline programs, classroom rules, or informal teacher interventions (see Chapter 13). However, for a student who is

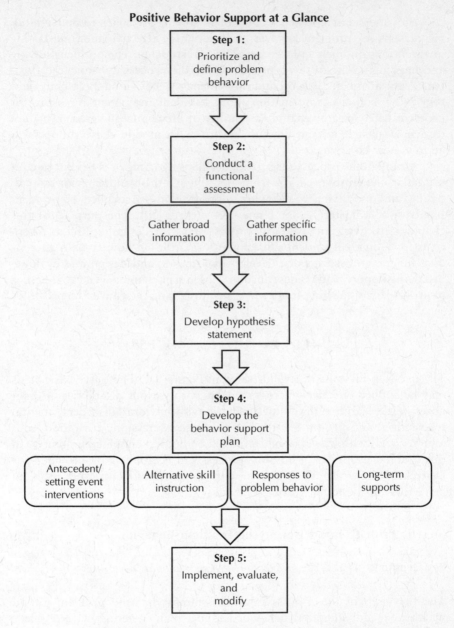

Positive Behavior Support at a Glance

FIGURE 3.1. Five-step process for designing a PBS plan.

unresponsive to general and informal behavior management systems, team members must consider whether an individualized behavior support plan[1] is needed. Furthermore, because most students who engage in persistent problem behaviors present many behavioral challenges, teams must determine which problem behaviors are important to change first, which may be addressed at a later time, and which (relatively speaking) may be unimportant to change or of lesser concern. For the student's and team's sake, it may be simpler not to attempt to intervene in all of the student's problem behaviors at the same time. Also, different behaviors may be responsive to a single support plan, reducing the number of necessary interventions.

Janney and Snell (2000) offer a useful way to prioritize interventions, based upon the seriousness of problem behavior or degree of concern (see also Evans & Meyer, 1985, for a more extensive discussion). They state that a student's behaviors are only problems when they are harmful or threaten the safety of the student or others, have a negative impact on learning, hinder participation in activities, or interfere with the development of positive social relationships and social acceptance by others. In other words, the seriousness of a problem behavior, and whether or not it is a problem to be targeted for intervention, should be judged by its impact on important social and learning outcomes, and not by its general appearance or degree of personal annoyance (e.g., "Her fidgeting is driving me crazy!").

To decide where to start, teams may wish to consider the three levels of priority for intervention shown in Table 3.1. *Destructive behaviors,* or behaviors that are harmful or threaten the safety of the student or others, should receive first priority when team members are considering interventions. Examples of destructive behaviors include head banging, cutting, or other acts of self-injury; hitting other students; kicking during tantrums; refusing to eat; or bringing weapons to school. Destructive behaviors should always be addressed through a comprehensive PBS plan that includes procedures for crisis management to protect the student and others from harm. It is important to note that teams are *required* by IDEA '97 to examine a student's existing behavior management plan and to conduct a functional behavioral assessment when disruptive behaviors prompt a change in educational placement (e.g., suspension from school in excess of 10 days, or alternative school placement due to a weapon or illegal drug violation) (Turnbull, Wilcox, Stowe, & Turnbull, 2001).

---

[1] It should be noted that throughout this book, the terms *intervention* and *behavior support plan* are used interchangeably. However, a behavior support plan usually encompasses a comprehensive collection of supports, while an intervention may be a single strategy.

TABLE 3.1. Priorities for Intervention

First priority: Destructive behaviors

• Is the behavior harmful, health-threatening or life- threatening to the student or others?

Second priority: Disruptive behaviors

• Does the behavior interfere with the student's or other students' learning?
• Does the behavior interfere with or impede social relationships?
• Does the behavior prevent the student from participating in daily school, home, or community activities?
• Does the behavior destroy materials in a dangerous or an interfering way (e.g., shredding clothing, ripping books)
• Is the behavior likely to become destructive without effective intervention?

Third priority: Distracting behaviors

• Does the behavior interfere with social acceptance?
• Does the behavior have a negative impact on the student's image?
• Does the behavior damage (not destroy) materials?
• Is the behavior likely to become disruptive if ignored?

Note. Adapted from Janney and Snell (2000). Copyright by Paul H. Brookes Publishing Co. Adapted by permission.

Disruptive behaviors should receive the next level of priority consideration in a comprehensive support plan. Disruptive behaviors do not immediately endanger the student or others, but do interfere with everyday activities and experiences needed for positive development. Persistent acts of disruptive behaviors can interfere with learning; prevent the student from fully participating in school, home, and community activities; and hinder the student from forming positive social relationships with others. Derrick's team has classified his problem behaviors as disruptive, requiring serious consideration for developing a PBS plan. Crying and refusing to complete independent seatwork not only interfere with Derrick's learning, but also disrupt other students' participation in school activities. Grabbing materials, refusing to share, and threatening to hit others also significantly disrupt typical classroom activities and seriously jeopardize Derrick's opportunities to become an accepted member of his class and to form friendships with his peers. Although Derrick has not yet hurt his classmates, his teachers are very concerned that without intervention, his threats of hitting will soon escalate to destructive behaviors.

Distracting behaviors should receive the lowest priority for intervention. Generally, a distracting behavior deviates from what is typically expected from a student of the same age, but does not substantially interfere with learning and participation in daily activities. Distracting behaviors (such as walking into the classroom and needing to follow the same path every day, flapping hands when excited, or dressing age-inappropriately) may warrant a behavior support plan when a team and family are concerned that the behaviors could develop into disruptive behaviors over time, or interfere with a student's social acceptance. To be clear, not all atypical behaviors are targets for behavior change. Schools should establish a culture of diversity where students, teachers, and parents learn to accept differences in others—especially students with disabilities—even when the differences are atypical. For example, as noted earlier, Derrick is fascinated with locomotives. He owns dozens of miniature toy trains, looks through train books daily, and frequently talks about trains with peers and teachers. This raises some red flags for his parents and teachers, because 9-year-old boys typically have more diverse interests. Although his interest certainly sets him apart from his peers, Derrick's team views his fascination as a "special interest" and not a problem behavior or obsession that requires intervention. It may become a behavior of concern if the team believes that Derrick's special interest in trains prevents him from forming other interests or interferes with his opportunities to play or make friends with his peers.

In addition to determining whether or not there is a problem, another first-step activity is to define the problem clearly. A clear definition of the problem behavior is essential for unambiguous communication, as well as for precise measurement of the problem behavior's frequency during functional assessment and intervention. Rather than using general or lay terms (e.g., "Derrick is noncompliant or aggressive"), a clear definition describes what the student does or what the problem behavior looks like (e.g., "Derrick refuses to work by laying his head on his desk, playing with objects, and/or crying"). Chapter 5 provides more detailed information on how to define problem behaviors in useful ways.

To summarize, team members can justify intervening with a problem behavior and developing a behavior support plan when they can offer a rationale for intervention based upon one of the three levels of priority. Once the team members have identified and defined the problem, they are ready for the next step in the PBS process.

Step 2: Conduct a Functional Assessment

Key Question: *Why is problem behavior occurring?*

Conducting a *functional assessment* (also known as *functional behavioral assessment*) is a critical step in the PBS process. A behavior support plan is most effective when it is informed by assessment information that explains why a student is engaging in problem behaviors. Most educators would not dream of designing a reading intervention without first knowing about a student's strengths, weaknesses, and specific reading difficulties. Just as a thorough assessment is critical for effective academic interventions, so is it vital for effective behavioral interventions.

Before team members ask what can be done to address a student's problem behavior, they must first ask, "Why is problem behavior occurring?" and "What's going on in the student's life and immediate environment?" Although it is often erroneously understood as such, functional assessment is not a single assessment tool or a collection of assessment instruments. Rather, functional assessment is a *process* for gathering information, understanding the reasons for problem behavior, and precisely identifying environmental conditions (both micro-level and macro-level) that lead to and maintain problem behavior. Unlike the medical model, where the focus is on curing or "fixing" a child, PBS emphasizes changing the environment and teaching alternative adaptive skills so that problem behavior is no longer necessary or useful to the student. Thus the primary purpose of functional assessment is not to diagnose the student (e.g., "Problem behaviors are occurring because the individual is autistic or has a behavior disorder"), but to uncover relevant and accurate information needed to change the student's environment, teach alternative skills, and promote a better life—all of which are the aims of behavior support interventions.

Like good detective work, conducting a good functional assessment requires strong diagnostic skills. The process is best guided by team members' knowledge of the many factors that could contribute to problem behavior (as discussed in Chapter 2), information about what questions to ask, and familiarity with what to look for when gathering information and observing a student. Once functional assessment is understood as a diagnostic process, a team can then select from the many available functional assessment tools described in Chapter 6 of this book (e.g., interviews, rating scales, direct observation methods) to assist with information gathering.

A comprehensive functional assessment typically involves gathering two types of information about the student and his or her problem behavior. When gathering *broad information*, team members are interested in learning about the individual's educational background and history; overall health; skills and abilities; and overall quality of life at home and in school (e.g., relationships with family, peer friendships, community and school involvement). Particularly useful when not all team members know the student well, broad information may provide important background information that will help explain how problem behavior developed; provide insight and direction for further, more specific assessment; and suggest broad curricular and lifestyle changes that may be needed. In addition, gathering broad information can help the team learn about student strengths, preferences, and special interests that may be embedded in a support plan to create motivating learning environments for the student and generally enhance a student's quality of life.

An important focal point for Derrick's team is to learn more about how his educational history and current academic abilities affect his ability to work independently. In addition, his team might consider exploring whether his deteriorating social behaviors (i.e., his teachers report that problem behaviors are on the rise) are due to the onset of illness, other physical problems, or changes at home (e.g., "Does he have vision problems?" "Are his allergies worsening?" "Have there been any changes at home?"). Furthermore, Derrick's team might consider learning about his social history, access to peer groups (e.g., "Does he have friends at home, play with neighborhood kids, and participate in after-school clubs and sports?"), and social skills (e.g., "Does he know how to play social games and invite peers to play?" "Is it possible that Derrick is lonely and is attempting, albeit inappropriately, to initiate interactions with his peers?"). Answers to such questions can provide useful, but very general and often speculative, information about potential reasons for problem behavior. To be maximally effective, broad information must be used in conjunction with more specific assessments of problem behavior.

When gathering *specific information*, team members focus their assessment to identify specific environmental events that are more immediately associated with the onset and occurrence of problem behavior. The goals are to reliably predict the precise circumstances that provoke problem behavior, and to determine the function problem behavior serves for the student under the circumstances.

For instance the members of Derrick's team might ask such questions as these: "Does Derrick tease peers and grab materials in all school activities, or only some?" "Does Derrick cry only during math, or all academic activities?" "In situations or activities where problem behavior does occur, what exactly is going on? To answer these questions, team members will observe and record what happens before problem behaviors occur to identify potential antecedent or setting events that trigger or set the stage for problem behavior. Likewise, team members will record what happens after problem behavior occurs, noting how teachers, peers, and others respond and what Derrick seems to get (eventually, if not immediately) from engaging in problem behavior. Noting what happens after problem behavior occurs provides important clues for determining function.

Observation of a student continues over time until the team is able to discern reliable patterns that predict the specific circumstances provoking problem behaviors (i.e., when, where, how, and with whom) and the function(s) served by them. Once a discernible pattern emerges, team members move to the next step of the PBS process—developing hypothesis statements. However, even when a clear pattern emerges, one fascinating aspect of functional assessment is that the process itself may not be complete. There are always more questions to ask about the information gathered that will lead to refinements of the team's hypotheses and improvements in the behavior support plan over time.

Step 3: Develop Hypothesis Statements

Key Questions: *What is the association between specific events and the problem behavior? How may these patterns be summarized?*

The third step of the PBS process is to formulate hypothesis statements that describe why the student is engaging in problem behavior and what function problem behavior serves for the student (this process is described in detail in Chapter 7). Essentially, hypothesis statements concisely summarize the patterns revealed during the functional assessment process. Hypothesis statements are extremely important because, when constructed appropriately, they help team members to link interventions to the assessment information collected. In other words, they identify the exact environmental circumstances that will be addressed through positive supports.

For example, over several days of observation, Derrick's functional assessment reveals two distinct patterns of problem behaviors—one centering around independent seatwork, and the other around social interactions with peers. These patterns are summarized in two hypothesis statements:

> *Hypothesis 1:* When Derrick is given any independent academic assignment to complete in class, he will often lay his head on the side of his desk, cry, and refuse to complete his assignment in order to avoid working independently.
> *Hypothesis 2:* During peer-led activities (play, cooperative learning groups), Derrick grabs materials and/or calls his peers names (teases) in order to get materials and/or initiate peer interaction.

Hypothesis statements are always written in a similar format (as above) to identify specific antecedents and setting events ("when this happens"), describe the problem behavior ("the student does this"), and identify the behavior function ("in order to get or avoid something"). This format parallels the four-term contingency introduced in Chapter 2; as such, it is extremely useful for informing team members what specific aspects of the student's environment need to be changed (e.g., antecedents) and what alternative skills to problem behavior can be taught (e.g., "What else can Derrick do instead of grabbing materials?").

In addition to developing hypothesis statements per se, another important activity in this step is to summarize the broad information gathered during the functional assessment process. When combined with hypotheses for problem behavior, broad information on the student's history, general skills, medical background, preferences, and lifestyle can help the team to make critical decisions about what specific interventions to select and determine what lifestyle changes are needed to promote desired outcomes for the student. In addition, summarizing broad information can help to explain why the patterns of problem behavior developed and what conditions appear to support them.

Based upon their assessment efforts, Derrick's team concludes that independent assignments are a problem for Derrick—not because of actual work difficulty, but because of Derrick's negative work history. Even though Derrick's new curriculum is matched appropriately to his abilities, his history of repeated failure appears to have made working alone unpleasant or aversive to him. He may dread working alone because he remembers frustrating times and thinks that the work will be too hard for him. Combining this understanding with their hypothesis, the members of Derrick's support team will tailor interventions to build Derrick's confidence and help him to experience success when working alone.

With regard to peer interactions, Derrick's team concludes that Derrick's lack of prior social opportunities, lack of social skills, and (more recently) rejection by his classmates all play a role in influencing his problem behavior. This suggests that creating social opportunities for peer interaction, along with social skill training and peer intervention, will be important to consider in Derrick's behavior support plan.

Step 4: Develop a PBS Plan

Key Questions: *Given our hypotheses, what aspects of the student's environment need to be changed? What alternative skills need to be taught?*

Once hypotheses are formulated, the fourth step in the PBS process is to develop a PBS plan. By this stage in the process, team members are often anxious to be rid of problem behavior; despite their well-formulated hypotheses, they may ask, "OK, what can we do to stop it?" Obviously from our discussions thus far, this is the wrong question to ask, because it can lead to highly punitive and ineffective interventions that ignore the conditions contributing to problem behaviors. Rather, when designing a support plan, team members must stay focused on their hypotheses and other relevant assessment information. They must ask, "What conditions should be changed, and what alternative skills can be taught?"

Unlike conventional behavior management plans, which typically employ a single intervention, PBS plans are comprehensive and consist of multiple intervention or support strategies. This is so for several reasons. First, hypotheses and broad assessment information often suggest multiple influences and functions of problem behaviors, as illustrated in Derrick's case. To be maximally effective, support plans will need to address as many of these influences as possible and teach students skills for different situations. Rarely will a single intervention do the job. Second, PBS is aimed at facilitating success in all settings in which a student lives, plays, works, or goes to school. As such, sometimes different supports are needed for different settings. For instance, influences on problem behavior are likely to differ in diverse settings, requiring a different intervention approach for each location. In addition, team members must be concerned with selecting supports that can be realistically carried out by people in different settings. Because people have different values and skills, and have to deal with different setting demands and routines, behavior supports will necessarily need to be adapted to fit these situations. For example, supports aimed at helping Derrick to interact better with his peers on the school playground are likely to differ from the social interaction supports in the classroom.

The third reason for the comprehensive nature of behavior support plans has to do with the purposes of PBS. Whereas conventional behavior management plans focus on stopping problem behavior (usually by punishing it), PBS plans focus on *prevention, teaching,* and facilitating *long-term effectiveness*. Each purpose requires a different intervention approach to achieve and cannot be addressed with a single strategy alone.

Comprehensive behavior support plans are built around four key components. Each component serves a different purpose, and when combined they emphasize prevention, teaching, and long-term effectiveness. As shown in Figure 3.2, these components are (1) *antecedent/setting event interventions*, to change events that evoke problem behaviors; (2) *alternative skill instruction*, to teach socially desired substitutes for problem behaviors; (3) *responses to problem behaviors*, to change (in effective and instructive ways) the reactions of others to problem behaviors; and (4) *long-term supports*, to make broad curricular, social, or lifestyle changes to support desired outcomes over time.

When designing a support plan, team members select support strategies for each component by considering what is most likely to be effective for the student, given hypotheses for problem behavior and other relevant assessment information. In addition, the team selects strategies by consider-

Antecedent/ setting event interventions	Alternative skill instruction	Responses to problem behavior	Long-term supports
• Modify or eliminate problem antecedent and/ or setting events • Introduce positive antecedents/ setting events	• Teach replacement skills that serve the same purpose as the problem behavior • Teach coping and tolerance skills • Teach general skills to expand overall competence	• Reduce outcomes for problem behavior • Provide instructive feedback/ introduce logical consequences • Develop a crisis management plan	• Make lifestyle changes • Implement strategies to sustain support

FIGURE 3.2. Components of a behavior support plan.

ing those that will best fit the settings in which the plan will be implemented. Fortunately, once team members understand the reasons for problem behaviors, there are often numerous support strategies that can address the same problem in different settings.

For most students with persistent and difficult-to-change problem behaviors, all four components will be necessary; however, in some cases, not all components or support strategies may be implemented at the same time. Some teams may decide to focus on antecedent interventions first, and, once problem behavior is prevented, then to direct their attention toward teaching alternative skills and designing long-term supports. Other teams may decide to focus on lifestyle changes (a strategy under long-term supports), and to determine, once the changes have been made, what alternative skills or antecedent interventions are necessary. Although it may be possible to implement less than four components at any one time, *it is never appropriate* for a PBS plan to consist entirely of strategies for responding to problem behavior only. This would make intervention consequence-oriented and reactive, rather than instructive and preventive. The following discussion provides a brief overview of each component and its purpose.

Antecedent/Setting Event Interventions

Antecedent/setting event interventions serve a preventive purpose. Once antecedents or setting events are identified in hypothesis statements, team members can *eliminate or modify* them so that problem behavior is no longer provoked by these troublesome events. In addition to changing problem events, team members may *introduce positive events,* known to promote desired behaviors, into the student's daily routines. When conditions are built in to promote positive behaviors, problem behavior will be less likely.

In Derrick's situation, independent academic assignments trigger Derrick's crying and refusing to work. The members of Derrick's team can prevent this problem behavior by considering how they might change this antecedent event. Depending on what is possible or practical to implement in the classroom, Derrick's team might choose to assign a paraprofessional to work with Derrick during seatwork activities, or have Derrick sit next to his teacher for support and encouragement while she instructs or works with other students. Derrick's team may also consider temporarily not giving Derrick independent academic assignments at all, but rather assign other activities that he can complete successfully alone (e.g., cutting out materials for the class bulletin board, listening to taped stories). The team's selection of intervention or combination of interventions will depend on what makes the most sense for Derrick and what can be practically carried out in he classroom.

Although antecedent/setting event interventions may only provide a temporary solution, their chief advantage is that they quickly prevent problem behaviors, because instigating factors are eliminated or modified. Their quick-acting nature can provide immediate relief for teachers, for parents, and for the student who is troubled by the antecedent or setting events, and in some cases they can result in very powerful outcomes (e.g., placement in a more restrictive setting can be avoided). Just as importantly, antecedent/setting event interventions play an important role in creating positive conditions for learning new or alternative skills. It is extremely difficult to teach students new ways of responding when they are frustrated by troubling events and are engaging in problem behaviors. But when troublesome antecedent conditions or setting events are changed, learning new ways of dealing with difficult situations becomes easier and more enjoyable for the learner. Various antecedent and setting event interventions, along with guidelines for their selection, are presented in Chapter 8.

Alternative Skill Instruction

The purpose of alternative skill instruction is to teach the student socially acceptable substitutes for problem behaviors. Whereas antecedent/setting event interventions are dependent on the actions of others, alternative skill instruction gives the student the power to achieve desired outcomes and change conditions so that problem behaviors are no longer needed. Alternative skill instruction contributes to long-term effectiveness, because the learner is less dependent on teacher or parent interventions and has the ability to control his or her environment in both effective and socially appropriate ways.

Three types of alternative skill interventions may be included in a behavior support plan. The first type, *replacement skills,* teaches the student to use a socially acceptable alternative that achieves *exactly the same purpose or function* as the problem behavior. This intervention is predicated on the assumption that problem behaviors can be effectively eliminated if the learner has another appropriate means of achieving the same outcome as the problem behavior. Simply put, if an alternative skill is as good as or better than the problem behavior at obtaining the desired outcome, the student will use it instead. For example, to replace teasing and name calling, Derrick's team might consider teaching him how to make appropriate initiations (e.g., "Can I play with you?" "Do you wanna play kickball with me?") to gain peer attention and interaction. Similarly, to replace grabbing, Derrick might be taught how to request materials appropriately (e.g., "May I have . . . ?" "Can I borrow . . . ?" "Can I have a turn?").

The second type of alternative skill intervention focuses on teaching *coping and tolerance skills* for dealing with difficult or stressful situations. Like all of us, students with disabilities will need to learn how to cope effectively with difficult situations that cannot or should not be changed or avoided. Targets for intervention might include learning how to wait, relaxing during stressful events, controlling anger, and learning how to problem-solve independently rather than relying on others to generate solutions to problems. An important target for Derrick is learning how to work independently for increasingly longer periods of time. Although antecedent/setting event interventions can reduce some of the burden for Derrick, eventually he will need to learn how to persist through difficult situations without crying in order to be successful in school.

The third type of alternative skill intervention focuses on teaching *general skills* to expand social, communicative, and academic competence. Teaching general skills addresses some of the broad or underlying skill deficits that may be contributing directly or indirectly to problem behavior. The greater students' general competence becomes, the more control they will have to circumvent problems and pursue desired outcomes for themselves through positive means. Team members can target general skills by looking carefully at what outcomes are important for a student and what skills are needed to be successful now and in the future. With regard to

Derrick, it is important not only to teach social initiations to replace name calling, but also to consider what other social skills (e.g., turn taking, learning social games, sharing) he might need to maintain positive interactions with his peers and become a valued member of his class. Strategies for teaching alternative skills are discussed in Chapter 9.

Responses to Problem Behaviors

The third component of a behavior support plan describes how teachers, parents, and others should respond to instances of problem behavior. If the antecedent/setting event modifications and alternative skill training are working, then the frequency of problem behavior should be dramatically reduced. Nevertheless, team members will need to consider how they and others can respond to problem behaviors, if they should occur, in both effective and instructive ways.

Responses to problem behaviors are structured around several goals, although not all may be incorporated in a single support plan. One goal is to *reduce outcomes for problem behavior*. When combined with alternative skill instruction, a critical goal of PBS is to teach the student that only alternative skills work to bring about desired results, and problem behaviors do not. If problem behavior no longer serves a useful purpose for the student (e.g., sobbing does not result in Derrick's avoiding his seatwork, or teasing does not result in peers' responding), then problem behavior will stop.

Another goal is to *provide instructive feedback and introduce natural or logical consequences to problem behavior*. The general objective here is to establish clear social boundaries by communicating what behaviors are acceptable and not acceptable in school, at home, or in the community. Specifically, the goal is to teach students that problem behaviors can violate certain school or societal rules and that negative consequences will follow (e.g., "If you throw food, you will have to clean it up," "If you destroy the tape recorder, you will have to pay for it"). If students are to become good community citizens, then they will need to understand the consequences of their actions. In order to be consistent with the values of PBS, however, negative consequences must be selected and implemented judiciously. Not all natural or logical consequences will be beneficial or appropriate for all students, and the consequences chosen for a particular student should be linked as closely as possible to the team's hypotheses for problem behavior. Furthermore, in order to be maximally instructive, negative consequences must be age-appropriate, respectful, and matched to the student's cognitive understanding.

A third goal is *crisis management*. Despite intervention efforts, some students will engage in very dangerous behaviors that can cause harm to themselves or others, or engage in highly disruptive behaviors that can significantly disrupt school, home, or community activities. In such cases, a crisis intervention plan should be developed. Crisis management plans describe specific steps that teachers, parents, and others should follow to diffuse potentially dangerous or disruptive behaviors, and to keep the student and others safe. It is important to note that unlike the first two strategies described in this section, crisis management is not considered an intervention that reduces problem behavior. Its sole purpose is to protect and deescalate, not to instruct or decrease problem behaviors in the future. Strategies for responding to problem behavior are presented in Chapter 10.

Long-Term Supports

The fourth and last component of a behavior support plan contributes to long-term prevention and maintenance of positive outcomes. One way to ensure that problem behavior is prevented in the long term and that the other intervention components are supported and maintained over time is to make *lifestyle changes* for the student. Problem behavior may continue to persist despite smaller antecedent changes or alternative skill training, because broader issues in the student's life, educational program, or social network impede positive growth and work against the other interventions. For example, despite small instructional adaptations to make schoolwork more interesting, some students may persist in refusing to work and may eventually drop out of school if they believe that their entire educational curriculum is not relevant to their vocational goals. Other students, despite alternative skill instruction, may continue to interact inappropriately with peers if they are routinely excluded from social activities and have limited social outlets. And still others, despite given something to do during some "down periods," may continue to engage in self-stimulation if, overall, their daily school and home routines are boring or repetitive and provide little opportunity for meaningful or enjoyable activities. Unless changes in these broader contexts are considered, interventions that focus only on the immediate conditions that surround problem behaviors are likely to fail. Obviously, team members cannot intervene in all problematic aspects of a student's life, and many problems will be beyond a team's resources and control. However, when professionals and families work together, teams can make very specific lifestyle changes that can support desired outcomes for students. For example, an important lifestyle focus for Derrick is to foster peer friendships and membership in his classroom. One strategy considered by his team is to have Derrick's classmates discuss ways of becoming better friends with Derrick and include him in their play. The team members reason that in order for Derrick to learn new ways of initiating and interacting with his peers, they must nurture peer acceptance and erase the negative perceptions about Derrick that have been built up over time.

Unless Derrick is helped to become an accepted member of his class, the intervention efforts to change teasing and name calling will be futile in the long run.

In addition to making lifestyle changes, this component consists of *strategies to sustain supports* and positive outcomes over time. One of the most frustrating realities, especially for parents, is that problem behavior will resurface year after year, because team members have failed to consider how successful supports can be transferred and adapted to new settings and teachers. When selecting interventions for this component, a team plans longitudinally by considering how supports can be adapted and introduced to new settings or situations, how supports will be communicated and learned by new teachers and other support staff, and what alternative skills the student should learn to apply in new settings. Strategies to sustain support also refer to team needs: What do team members need in order to sustain their efforts to develop and implement PBS interventions? Long-term supports are discussed more completely in Chapter 11.

Step 5: Implement, Evaluate, and Modify the Plan

Key Questions: *Is the behavior support plan working? Is progress being made? If not, what modifications are needed to make it more effective?*

The last step in the PBS process is to implement the behavior support plan—and, just as importantly, to decide whether the support plan is working and, if not, what modifications are necessary to improve effectiveness. Because comprehensive support plans are implemented across settings and involve multiple people (e.g., teachers, support staff, parents), coordination among team members is essential. Effective behavior support will require team members to meet regularly, set specific outcome goals, and based upon the data collected, problem-solve about what to do next. The team will need to make decisions about refining, eliminating, or introducing new interventions and gradually fading out certain interventions over time. Team members may also decide to gather more assessment information and modify their hypotheses based on intervention data and new assessment information. In short, evaluation in the PBS process is ongoing; it begins as soon as the plan is implemented, and continues until desired outcomes are achieved and maintained for reasonable periods of time.

An interesting question to ponder is this: How is *success* or *effectiveness* defined under PBS? Intervention effectiveness is not defined in absolute terms, but rather in terms of the team's satisfaction with the progress being made. For many students with disabilities, especially those who exhibit significant communication deficits or who have difficulty solving problems in stressful or novel situations, 100% elimination of all problem behaviors is not possible. When presented with a problem situation, people in general will respond in ways that they can; if a problem behavior works and no other alternative response is available (or if appropriate alternatives are not responded to by others), it will be used. For most students with disabilities, it is virtually impossible to teach all the skills necessary for every current and future situation, nor is it possible to make modifications in all settings so that problem behavior can be permanently eliminated. By the same token, intervention effectiveness cannot be judged by the complete elimination of a PBS plan. Many students are likely to require some continued adaptations and support to be successful in home, school, or community environments. Continued interventions are often needed to teach new students and teachers how to set up positive learning environments and respond to alternative skills so that positive behaviors are maintained.

Rather than evaluating effectiveness in absolute terms (i.e., the complete elimination of problem behavior or a behavior support plan), team members judge success by their satisfaction with at least three important outcomes. First, is there a satisfactory reduction in problem behavior? Second, has the student learned to use alternative skills? In Derrick's case, has he learned to work more independently without crying? Has he learned to interact with his peers with minimal amounts of teasing and name calling? Third, what impact has PBS had on improving broad social and learning outcomes? This last question addresses broader outcomes expected as a result of implementing a PBS plan. For example, is Derrick a participant in regular classroom activities? Have concerns about the appropriateness of his placement been eliminated? Are peers more accepting of Derrick? Has he formed friendships? Considerations for evaluating and modifying behavior support plans are discussed in Chapter 11.

SUMMARY

The purpose of this chapter has been to overview the five basic steps for designing a PBS plan for an individual student. Specific information on how actually to conduct a functional assessment, develop hypotheses, select interventions for each support plan component, and evaluate the effectiveness of a support plan are described in detail in later chapters of this book. Continuing with our overview of the basic principles and processes of behavior support, the next chapter addresses collaborative teaming. As we will discuss, building a team is just as important as designing a support plan for students. In the next chapter, we discuss how team-building strategies can be infused into the five-step process.

CASE EXAMPLES

To illustrate the complete PBS process, from beginning to end, we offer two student case examples. The stories of Malik and Bethany, and the development of their comprehensive support plans, are described in selected chapters (beginning with the current chapter and ending with Chapter 11). The case information provided at the end of each chapter is intended to demonstrate application of the content within that chapter. In the end, these case illustrations provide examples of fully completed PBS plans, showing how all steps of the PBS process work together.

Background Information for Malik

Ten-year-old Malik is an African American boy diagnosed as having Down syndrome, attention-deficit/hyperactivity disorder (ADHD), and oppositional defiant disorder. Malik was born in a large city in the Northeast. His father died of AIDS when Malik was not yet 2 years old; he never had contact with Malik. The mother, Marina, was 17 when she gave birth. She was living with a friend, did not have a job, and was unable to care for Malik. His maternal grandparents obtained temporary custody. When Malik was 18 months old, Marina obtained a job with a regional newspaper. She worked the 11:00 P.M. to 7:00 A.M. shift, inserting flyers into newspapers in preparation for delivery. At that time, she took custody of Malik. However, she was fired from her job after 1 month because of drug involvement, and her parents once again obtained temporary custody of Malik. During the years that followed, Marina entered various drug rehabilitation programs. Although she sometimes experienced brief success, she was unable to remain drug-free for longer than a month or two. When Malik was 4 years old, Marina was arrested for prostitution. At that time, Malik's grandparents were awarded permanent custody. At this point in Malik's life, Marina has only infrequent contact with Malik, and he does not appear to have a close relationship with her.

Malik lives in a small, well-kept single home. In addition to Malik, his grandparents cared for their son's children, 19-year-old Jenna and 17-year-old Thomas. Malik's family members were very devoted to his care and well-being. Although Malik's grandparents asserted that they sometimes felt the lack of energy needed to care for a young boy, they were very grateful for the support and assistance of Jenna and Thomas. In fact, Malik often treated Jenna as a mother, which Jenna enjoyed. Malik was eager to please Jenna and took pleasure in assisting her with household routines. Thomas was active in sports; he was often busy with practice or games, which kept him away from home during the evenings and weekends. However, when he was home he played a "big brother" role, teaching Malik to throw and catch and to operate the DVD player. Periodically, his grandparents expressed concern that Jenna and Thomas would soon be moving out on their own, and that they themselves might not be able to meet all of Malik's needs.

At 6 years old, Malik first attended public school in an inclusive kindergarten classroom. At that time, Malik appeared to understand simple requests and questions, and would respond affirmatively or negatively by shaking his head. He began to develop spoken language, but his speech was very difficult to understand. For his academic and language difficulties, he received support services from the special education teacher and language therapist several times a week. However, he had difficulty making friends, due to his lack of spoken language. During the school year, his teacher noticed that Malik began to push and shove his peers when they would not let him play or did not understand him. He also began to refuse engaging in activities that were difficult for him, such as cutting, identifying letters, and tracing objects. Because of concerns about Malik's failure to progress academically and socially, the following school year he was placed in a special education resource room for most of the school day, with the exception of recess, lunch, art, and physical education. He remained in that classroom for 2 years.

Because Malik had begun to develop a verbal repertoire, his special education teacher felt it was important to promote verbal language as his mode of communication. Thus she encouraged him to respond verbally, often using prompts or requiring him to imitate her. In addition, Malik could discriminate objects and a few letters by pointing to them. Therefore, she determined that a traditional academic program was appropriate. She vigorously and enthusiastically worked on letter and number discrimination and identification, as well as other early academic skills. However, Malik's challenging behavior began to escalate. He began to engage in disruptive and aggressive behaviors that included destroying materials, throwing objects, hitting and kicking his teacher, and (on two occasions) biting her. Not knowing what to do, she consulted the district behavior specialist. The behavior specialist hypothesized that Malik's teacher was allowing him to get out of his assigned work, and encouraged her to ignore Malik's behavior problems and "work through" tasks, even if this required physically guiding him to complete the task. In addition, despite Malik's reluctance to speak at times, the behavior specialist encouraged the teacher to continue prompting him to speak and not let him "get away with" nonverbal communication. Malik's teacher consented to these recommendations, but saw no improvements in Malik's behavior. In fact, she noted that Malik became more aggressive when she physically guided him through task completion or repeatedly prompted him to respond. Furthermore, she was beginning to see aggression occurring outside of the classroom, directed toward peers and other school staff. This resulted in phone calls to the principal by a number of parents who believed that their children were at risk of being injured. A meeting was held in which the principal stated that Malik "could not stay in this school and put the other students in harm's way." His special education teacher agreed that her classroom was not an appropriate placement for Malik, because he had made little progress in academics and his behavior had deteriorated. Thus, in third grade Malik was moved to a private school serving students with behavior problems.

Malik's new school offered services to approximately 100 students, all of whom had been removed from their public school setting. He was placed in a classroom with seven other students, a teacher, and two teaching assistants. There was a schoolwide behavior system in place that encouraged good behavior. After the proverbial "honeymoon" at his new school, Malik began to engage in very high rates of aggressive and destructive behavior, similar to those of the previous school year. An additional teaching assistant was hired to work on a one-to-one basis just with Malik. However, throughout the first half of the school year, no progress was made toward reducing his behavior problems. Malik's grandparents had heard of a new approach called PBS through a support group they attended. They made a plea to the school to try this approach with their grandson. With nothing effective in their armory to date, the school agreed to work with the family to approach Malik's behavior problems in a systematic and comprehensive way.

Background Information for Bethany

Bethany, a 12-year-old European American girl, attends an elementary school in a suburban area that serves students in kindergarten through sixth grade. Bethany was currently labeled as having ADHD and an emotional/behavioral disorder. Bethany's parents had separated several times in her first few years of life. They worked hard at reconciliation, but were unable to work out their differences and live compatibly. They divorced when Bethany was 4. Bethany was an only child and had lived with her mother since the divorce. Her father had had difficulty maintaining employment since high school, due to mental health issues (he experienced bipolar disorder, for which medication had limited effectiveness). Shortly after his divorce, he moved back in with his parents to save expenses. Unfortunately, his parents lived almost 300 miles from Bethany, so he was unable to spend time with her on a regular basis. Bethany did, however, visit him on weekends whenever it could be arranged, and for a month every summer.

Bethany's mother, Ms. DeLope, worked for a cleaning agency, making slightly over minimum wage. She received very little financial support from Bethany's father, who sent money only sporadically even when he was employed. Ms. DeLope had a very difficult time making ends meet and described this as a constant source of stress for her. She felt compelled to work extra hours whenever she had the opportunity, to improve the family's financial situation, but did not enjoy doing so because she missed out on time with Bethany. Also, when she worked late, Bethany was home alone until early evening, and Ms. DeLope was worried that her daughter did not have ample supervision.

Bethany and her mother had moved several times, because they were unable to afford rent increases. They currently lived in a two-bedroom apartment in an area of town with a relatively high crime rate. Ms. DeLope has always tried to make sure that Bethany is inside by dark, but this had become a serious problem in the past few years. Bethany preferred hanging out with her friends in the neighborhood. Bethany often failed to inform her mother of her whereabouts and often did not return home until past midnight. After staying out late at night, Bethany did not want to get up the next morning for school. Ms. DeLope also worried because she thought that Bethany's friends were a bad influence on her. She suspected that they might drink alcohol and do drugs.

Bethany had difficulty with preacademic skills beginning in kindergarten. Although she was quite verbal and articulate, she had a hard time paying attention and completing tasks. An intelligence test indicated that her IQ was above average. Bethany's mother requested advice from her pediatrician, but was told that Bethany was just "immature" and would catch up. School personnel attributed her school difficulties to adjustment problems resulting from her parents' breakup. They also assured Bethany's mother that she would do just fine, once she got used to the school environment. Because of these assurances, Ms. DeLope did not seek additional assistance for Bethany.

Bethany's academic problems persisted into elementary school. Because of her strong verbal skills, she was able to compensate and get by. But she gradually fell further and further behind. Her academic difficulties caused her a great deal of frustration in school. In third grade, Bethany's behavior problems accelerated. Her teacher was determined that Bethany was capable of doing the assigned work, but was not trying. She was also convinced that Bethany's previous teachers had failed to be stern enough, and was sure that her no-nonsense approach to schoolwork would solve the problem. She constantly stayed on top of Bethany, reminding her to get to work or reprimanding her for not finishing. Bethany found this very embarrassing. In an attempt to redeem herself, she began refusing to do her work by saying "No" or "Make me" to her teachers when they gave her work assignments that seemed overwhelming. Unwilling to tolerate this behavior, Bethany's teacher kept her inside the classroom during recess and free time to complete her assignments. She also punished her by giving her after-school detention. In addition to her problems with classwork, Bethany began to have difficulties with her peers. As her classmates were making friends and enjoying socializing together, she was overlooked. On the few occasions she was permitted to join them in play, she felt like an outsider. She began to lash out at them by verbally criticizing them and ordering them to stay away from her. She grew to hate going to school.

By the end of third grade, Bethany's behavior and academic performance had deteriorated. She was completing fewer academic assignments, had become disruptive in the classroom, and was aggressive with her peers. At the end of the school year, Bethany's' teacher referred her for a special education evaluation. Bethany was tested during the beginning of her fourth-grade school year, and it was determined that she had an emotional/behavioral disorder. Her pediatrician also diagnosed her as having ADHD.

Convinced that Bethany's problems were rooted in poor motivation, her fourth-grade teacher believed she would respond positively to a structured point and level system. However, as the year passed, the teacher and staff were very surprised to find that her problem behaviors not only continued, but in fact increased. She appeared to be uninterested in earning points for tangible rewards and weekly activities. Bethany regularly failed to complete her assigned work, and was required to remain in the classroom almost every Friday afternoon while her classmates enjoyed weekly activities (free time, movies, swimming excursions, etc.).

Bethany's mother and teachers were very surprised when triennial testing revealed that Bethany was only slightly behind grade level in all academic areas. During the past 2 school years, Bethany had never received a grade in any academic area that surpassed a C. Although Bethany continued to be in general education, with support from the special education, her team determined that her current supports were not adequate. The team decided to attempt additional and more individualized supports so that she could be maintained in general education. They decided that a functional assessment was the most parsimonious way to specify individualized supports that were likely to be effective.

The stories of Malik and Bethany continue at the end of Chapter 4 with a discussion of their support teams.

REFERENCES

Bambara, L. M., & Knoster, T. (1998). *Designing positive behavior support plans* (Innovations No. 13). Washington, DC: American Association on Mental Retardation.

Evans, I. H., & Meyer, L. H. (1985). *An educative approach to problem behaviors: A practical decision model for interventions with severely handicapped learners.* Baltimore: Paul H. Brookes.

Janney, R., & Snell, M. E. (2000). *Teachers' guides to inclusive practices: Behavioral support.* Baltimore: Paul H. Brookes.

Turnbull, R. H., Wilcox, B. L., Stowe, M., & Turnbull, A. (2001). IDEA requirements for use of PBS: Guidelines for responsible agencies. *Journal of Positive Behavior Interventions, 3,* 11–18.

CHAPTER 4

◆ ◆ ◆

Teaming

◆

LINDA M. BAMBARA
STACY NONNEMACHER
FREYA KOGER

Throughout this book, we advocate a collaborative team-based approach for designing positive behavior support (PBS) plans. This chapter is about *teaming*, or how school personnel, other professionals, and families can work together to design individualized supports for students who engage in challenging behaviors. We begin by providing a definition and rationale for collaborative teaming, followed by a discussion of essential elements of a good team. The remainder of the chapter illustrates how team-building strategies can be infused into the five-step PBS process introduced in Chapter 3.

WHAT IS A COLLABORATIVE TEAM?

In its simplest form, a *collaborative team* consists of two or more people working together to meet a common goal (Snell & Janney, 2000; Robbins & Finley, 2000; Thousand & Villa, 2000). A team may consist of a parent and teacher working together to design supports for the home; in the case of more comprehensive supports across settings, a team may involve many people, such as parents, teachers, school administrators, behavior specialists, social workers, paraprofessionals, and the student with disabilities. When applied to PBS, collaboration takes on added meaning. A collaborative team:

- Is committed to using person-centered values and the PBS process to establish common goals and to direct the team's activities.
- Uses an agreed-upon process that is respectful of each team member's contribution.
- Coordinates activities to produce outcomes that are satisfactory to all team members, especially the student with disabilities and his or her family.

Successful collaboration requires a commitment both to designing effective PBS interventions for the student and to building a teaming environment where positive, ongoing collaborative interactions among team members can occur (Bambara, Gomez, Koger, Lohrmann-O'Rourke, & Xin, 2001).

Collaborative teams differ from other school-based multidisciplinary teams. Although both collaborative teams and multidisciplinary teams may consist of parents and an array of professionals who are committed to making improvements for the student, each member of a multidisciplinary team works independently to address student objectives. For example, after writing separate individualized education program (IEP) goals, a speech therapist, special education teacher, and general education teacher are responsible for implementing and monitoring instructional interventions for their distinct goals. Team members do not necessarily need to share the same values, agree upon common goals, or work together to achieve improvements. Each member works independently. By contrast, collaborative teams are defined as people working *together* to achieve a *common goal*. Collaborative teams take *joint action* (Snell & Janney, 2000) to make things happen. Given the complexity of most problem behaviors, collaboration among all stakeholders (e.g., parents, teachers, support specialists) is essential to ensure consistent supports and meaningful outcomes in all settings in which the student with disabilities participates.

WHY IS TEAMING IMPORTANT?

Collaborative teaming serves two important purposes. The first is *student-centered*. That is, a team's first goal is to design effective supports that are responsive to a student's current and long-term needs, and that will result in meaningful outcomes for the student and his or her family. The second purpose is *team-centered*. That is, a team's second objective is to build the capacity of team members to work collaboratively in order to carry out positive supports for the student (Bambara et al., 2001; Snell & Janney, 2000).

Student-Centered

By definition, the PBS process mandates the active participation of the people who are integrally involved with the student, whether at home, in school, or in the community. Team involvement contributes to the overall effectiveness and meaningfulness of a support plan in several important ways. First, team involvement is needed to obtain a valid, comprehensive functional assessment. During the functional assessment process, information about the student and potential reasons for problem behavior are gathered from all the people who are significant players in the student's life (e.g., parents, teachers, school support specialists). Rich assessments involving multiple people will result in a more comprehensive understanding of the reasons for problem behavior, which in turn will result in more effective supports. Family input is especially needed for conducting valid, rich assessments (Dunlap, Newton, Fox, Benito, & Vaughn, 2001; Schwartz, Boulware, McBride, & Sandall, 2001). Family members almost always provide a deep understanding of and insight into a student's strength's, needs, interests, and problem behavior, because they know their child the best, have spent the most time with him or her, and have interacted with the child across settings (Dunlap et al., 2001). The information provided by family members is invaluable to the design of effective supports.

Second, team involvement is needed to ensure a good *contextual fit* between the support plan and (1) the settings in which the plan will be carried out; and (2) the values, culture, and skills of the team members responsible for carrying out the plan (Albin, Lucyshyn, Horner, & Flannery, 1996). Even the best-designed support plan will be rendered ineffective if it is not used by parents, teachers, or other school personnel. And a plan will not be implemented if it is viewed as too difficult: as unrealistic, or as a poor match for home or school values and culture. To be effective, support plans must meet two criteria. They must be *technically adequate,* that is, assessment-based and comprehensive, and *contextually* fit, that is, matched to the targeted settings and values of the people who will carry out the plan. To achieve a good contextual fit, consideration is given to many factors, including *setting demands* (e.g., "Can the interventions be reasonably carried out, given the hectic routines of busy teachers and family members?"), *skills of the plan implementers* (e.g., "Do teachers and parents know what to do? Do they need additional education, training, or support?"), *setting resources* (e.g., "What sources are available for support? Are additional resources needed?"), and *home and school culture* (e.g., "Do teachers and parents see the interventions as fitting in with their beliefs? Do they see the interventions as being appropriate in terms of the student's age or cultural and religious practices? Do interventions fit in with teachers' and parents' personal values? Does the student feel comfortable with how he or she is supported?"). A support plan that fits its context well can only occur when team members actively collaborate to inform the planning process.

The third student-centered reason for team involvement is to ensure that meaningful changes or differences do indeed occur for the student. Team members who are most invested in the student are most likely to insist that positive outcomes are realized. Because of their emotional attachment to their child, family member can play a tremendous role in this regard—often pushing other team members to ensure that intervention plans are appropriate, carried out, and maximally beneficial for the student. However, other team members also may play this vital role. Many teachers, community support staff, and behavior support specialists who have worked with the student over time make personal and professional commitments to see that PBS interventions are carried out to fruition and meaningful outcomes are achieved. The teaming approach capitalizes on team members' personal and professional commitments to make a difference in the life of a student with disabilities.

Team-Centered

Teaming is essential also for building the capacity of each team member to carry out the PBS process, to apply person-centered values, and to make a difference in the student's life. Traditionally, behavioral interventions focused on changing the person with the problem behavior. However, in reality, effective interventions *require the behavior change of others*. Teachers, parents, and other interventionists change environments that will result in lifestyle improvements for the focus student, teach alternative skills, and respond to instances of problem behavior in ways that reduce their future occurrence. Without changes made by others, behavior change for the student with disabilities is not possible. Logically, then, intervention efforts should also focus on helping team members to change their own behaviors, so that positive outcomes for the student can be achieved.

Teaming offers a process for ongoing behavior change and support for team members. First, teaming can help team members acquire the necessary values, beliefs, and skills for implementing positive, person-centered interventions. Many team members will lack PBS experience and knowledge; in fact, they may be initially resistant to the approach, because it differs from the behavior management strategies they have used in the past. By enabling such individuals to work with others who understand PBS, the teaming process can help all team members develop needed expertise and positive values. Second, teaming can provide ongoing emotional support for team members as they implement supports for the student. Working or living with a student who engages in challenging behaviors is not easy; it is often fraught with anxiety and uncertainty about what is best, what to do, or whether interventions will work. Furthermore, challenging behaviors may cause parents and teachers to become fearful or angry. The teaming process can help team members cope and develop confidence to work with the student through trying times. Finally, teaming helps team members develop effective communication and interpersonal skills for working with other team members, professionals, or family members. Because comprehensive supports require the cooperation of many people, learning how to communicate with others in nonthreatening, collaborative ways is essential for achieving successful outcomes.

ESSENTIAL CHARACTERISTICS OF A COLLABORATIVE TEAM

What makes a team collaborative? What elements or characteristics are necessary for team success? Based upon a review of the professional literature in educational leadership and business management, we describe five essential characteristics that make up successful collaborative teams (see Figure 4.1).

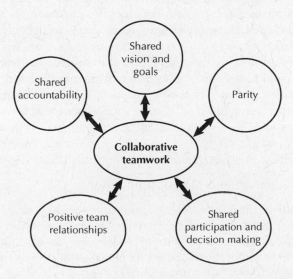

FIGURE 4.1. Essential characteristics of a collaborative team.

Shared Vision and Goals

Teams that agree upon and articulate a common purpose and goals are teams that are likely to be successful in their collaborative efforts (Fleming & Monda-Amaya, 2001; Straka & Bricker, 1996). Mutually agreed-upon goals build team commitment and provide a sense of purpose and direction from the beginning (DeBoer & Fister, 1994). In addition to agreeing upon student-centered goals, team members must agree on a set of common values that will guide a team's activities. This means agreeing to use the PBS process and accepting person-centered and collaborative team values, such as "We are in this together," "We are here for Janice [the student with disabilities]," "We are willing to make changes to make things happen for Janice," "If this doesn't work, we'll try another way," and "Janice's happiness is important." To establish mutual goals, team members must move beyond their individual agendas to embrace the goals and values established by the team. This is not an easy process; it often requires a "letting go" and commitment to working with others for the greater good of the team or the student with disabilities (LaFasto & Larson, 2001).

Parity

Effective collaborative teams establish *parity* among team members. Parity involves the basic belief that all team members have unique expertise, which is needed in helping the team meet its goals (Snell & Janney, 2000; Thousand & Villa, 2000). When a team demonstrates parity, there is a sense of equality among team members, despite each member's position or role (as parent, teacher, administrator, team leader or behavior specialist). In other words, everyone on the team has something to learn from and offer others. Parity helps team members feel valued, knowing that their contributions add to team outcomes. When team members feel valued, they are more likely to be vested in the PBS process, make contributions to team discussions, and "hang in there" during difficult times, because they know that what they have to say is important and can make a meaningful difference (Bambara et al., 2001).

Shared Participation and Decision Making

For collaborative teams to be effective, all team members actively engage in deliberations and decision making around essential components of the PBS process (e.g., conducting a functional assessment, developing hypotheses about problem behavior, developing PBS plans). While all members participate, the type of contribution may differ, depending on the expertise or knowledge of individual team players. Nonetheless, participation and decision making are valued and shared by all. Shared decision making along with parity leads to better decisions, greater collaboration and commitment among team members, and eventually better team outcomes (DeBoer & Fister, 1994; Harrington-Mackin, 1994; LaFasto & Larson, 2001).

Positive Team Relationships

Successful collaboration depends upon the establishment of good interpersonal relationships among team members. Obviously, team goals cannot be met if team members do not get along or cannot work together. Teams work best when they have created an atmosphere of *openness* and *supportiveness* (LaFasto & Larson, 2001). Openness refers to the capacity of teams to raise critical (and often delicate) issues and deal with them objectively, without making any team members feel defensive, unintelligent, or inferior. Supportiveness refers to the capacity of teams to help all team members transcend their limitations and do their best to succeed. Both openness and supportiveness require effective communication and positive interpersonal skills, such as listening to understand others' perspectives, honest communication, blameless conflict resolution, and the sincere desire to help others understand new concepts and learn new skills. Effective teams take the time to foster positive team relationships as part of the teaming process (e.g., Friend & Cook, 2000).

Shared Accountability

Effective teams assume responsibility by having team members carry out actions jointly (DeBoer & Fister, 1994; LaFasto & Larson, 2001; Thousand & Villa, 2000). All team members agree to do their part. Moreover, *shared accountability* means that the collective team is responsible for team success or failure, and that no one person is credited for success when things go right or blamed if things go wrong. Effective teams constantly work to make improvements by examining outcomes for the student ("Did we make a difference?") and procedures for teaming ("Are we really working as a team?").

BUILDING COLLABORATIVE PBS TEAMS

Thus far, we have discussed why teams are important and the essential elements of effective collaborative teams. In this section, we illustrate how collaborative teaming can be established within a PBS framework.

Teams move through three basic collaborative phases: (1) *initiating;* (2) *assessment and planning;* and (3) *implementing, evaluating, and revis-*

ing. As discussed, effective PBS teams must be concerned with achieving both student-centered outcomes and team-centered outcomes in each phase of collaborative teamwork. Figure 4.2 illustrates PBS student-centered and team-centered activities for each of the three phases of collaboration. As shown, the student-centered activities consist of the five steps for designing PBS plans for individual students. These steps, introduced in Chapter 3, are detailed in chapters throughout the book. The team-centered activities listed in the same figure consist of strategies for building good teaming and collaboration among team members. The remainder of this chapter focuses on these important team-building strategies. One word of caution before we begin: Although the teaming strategies are presented in sequence, teaming, like PBS itself, is ongoing in real life; therefore, many of the strategies may be used flexibly as needed.

Initiating

A student in crisis; a single episode of problem behavior that significantly threatens the student's or others' health or safety; or persistent challenging behaviors that are unresponsive to classwide or schoolwide behavior management practices—any of these can create the impetus for forming a PBS team for an individual student. During the initiating phase, the team will carry out Step 1 of the PBS process. This step includes defining the problem behavior of concern, prioritizing problem behavior for assessment and intervention, and providing a rationale for why a PBS plan is necessary. In some cases, the team may need to consider developing an emergency crisis intervention plan to keep the student and others safe, or to keep the student in his or her current educational placement, while the team conducts a functional assessment and designs a PBS plan.

Although PBS student-centered activities are often the team's first concern, joint priority must also be given to team-centered activities. Team-centered activities during the initiating phase lay the critical foundation for building team structure and collaboration during the entire PBS process.

Identify Team Membership

Who should serve on a student's PBS team? Obviously, answering this question is the first order of business when a PBS team is being established. PBS teams are individually constructed around student needs; however, they may draw from and share membership with other, already formed student-based, program-centered, or school-based teams. For example, members of the PBS team may also serve as members of the student's IEP team or may be derived from a schoolwide teacher assistance team that provides behavioral or instructional consultation to teachers. Membership

Collaborative phases	PBS steps	Student-centered activities	Team-centered activities
Initiating	**Step 1: Prioritize and define problem behavior.**	**Team comes to consensus on:** • Goals, outcomes, and values. • Priority for behavior change. • Definition of problem behavior.	• Identify team membership. • Define team members' roles and responsibilities. • Agree on team purpose and goals. • Set ground rules for collaboration. • Schedule and structure team meetings.
Assessment and planning	**Step 2: Conduct a functional assessment.**	**Team decides on:** • What information should be gathered. • How information will be gathered. • Who gathers information and summarizes for the team.	• Enhance capacity for understanding. • Use collaborative problem-solving strategies for team decision making. • Create an atmosphere of openness and honesty.
	Step 3: Develop a hypothesis.	**Team will:** • Analyze and interpret gathered information. • Agree on hypothesis statement (which will guide team planning efforts).	
	Step 4: Develop the support plan.	**Team will:** • Develop a mutually agreed-upon PBS plan. • Develop action steps for carrying out plan.	
Implementing, evaluating, and revising	**Step 5: Implement, monitor, and evaluate support plan.**	**Team will:** • Determine important outcomes. • Decide on ways to measure progress and outcomes. • Determine whether the intervention plan is working. • Modify plan.	• Provide support for team members. • Apply problem-solving strategies to make decisions about modifications. • Celebrate. • Reflect on team process.

FIGURE 4.2. PBS collaborative teaming: Student- and team-centered activities.

may also be derived from a student's community-based service team, which may consist of community mental health professionals (e.g., county case managers, social workers) in addition to school personnel.

Regardless of whether a team is formed initially to develop a PBS plan for a student or is derived from an already existing team, several considerations should be addressed to determine the best composition for collaboration. Thousand and Villa (2000) offer three questions for consideration.

• *Who has the expertise needed to help a team make the best decisions for a student?* This first question focuses on effectiveness. In order to make informed decisions and develop an effective behavior support plan, a team needs to engage as members the people who have the greatest expertise or knowledge regarding specific student concerns. This may include professional content area expertise, such as that of a behavior support specialist, a speech pathologist, a school psychologist, or a special educator. It must also include the personal knowledge expertise gained by the people who interact with the student daily and know the student the best, such as family members, teachers, and paraprofessionals. And, it may include team leadership expertise—the expertise of people who have learned specific skills in helping team members to stay organized, focus on their agenda, and work collaboratively with others.

• *Who will be affected by the team's decisions?* According to Thousand and Villa (2000), this question pertains to democracy and fairness by involving those who are affected by the team decisions, but it also reflects the concept of contextual fit (Albin et al., 1996). That is, a PBS plan is more likely to be used and accepted by the people who are integrally involved in the planning process. The people who are most likely to be affected by the team's decisions are teachers, parents, and paraprofessionals who interact with the student on a daily basis. But team members should also consider including school administrators and other program leaders (e.g., the special education supervisor, the elementary education coordinator) who have the power to influence and educate others about the team's decisions, and who can provide resources and opportunities for the team. Finally, team members should consider including the student with disabilities, especially as the student nears the high school years and should make critical decisions about his or her educational program.

• *Who has a vested interest in participating?* Moving beyond the first two questions, this question asks simply who *wants* to be involved. People who have a vested or personal interest in the student or the PBS process may energize the team with their motivation and commitment to make things work. Some examples include a former teacher who has formed a personal relationship with the student; a building principal who is interested in learning how to apply the PBS process with other students; and a student teacher who, as part of a school requirement, is interested in learning how to conduct functional assessment interviews and collect student observation data. Of course, family members (including siblings and other relatives, as well as parents) may have a strong interest in lending support.

By answering these questions, a team will consider a broad membership. In many cases, the same people are likely to emerge as answers to all three questions. For example, parents are needed for their expertise, are likely to be affected by the team's decisions, and have the highest vested interest in seeing that the student succeeds. Despite the potential for overlap, the questions are likely to yield a large number of team members—particularly for students who require support in school, home, and community settings; who have many teachers, related services personnel, and paraprofessionals working with them; and who are recipients of other community-based services (e.g., mental health, community case management, juvenile justice).

Because a group of 15 or more can make scheduling and coordination difficult, several professionals suggest organizing membership around a *core team* and an *extended team* (Thousand & Villa, 2000; Snell & Janney, 2000). A core team consists of a small group of people who are most immediately and directly involved with the student and the problem situation at hand. An extended team includes the core team, plus other experts or professionals who are called upon as needed to address specific issues on the core team's agenda.

The core team functions as the "working group," meeting regularly to coordinate the entire PBS process, including conducting assessments and designing the support plan. Core team members generally consist of one or more special education and general education teachers (if the student participates in inclusive classrooms); paraprofessionals (e.g., teacher assistants, job coaches, therapeutic support staff); the student with disabilities, as appropriate; and a behavior support specialist or equivalent who can lend technical expertise to the group. Parents are always considered members of the core team, even though they may not be able to attend all team meetings. In contrast, the extended team may meet at least annually, if it constitutes part or all of the student's IEP team, or may enter into the collaborative process a few times a year as determined by the core team's needs. It is also possible for the extended team never to meet as an entire group; rather, individual members may only participate in core team decisions when it is appropriate to lend their particular expertise. Figure 4.3 provides examples of core and extended team membership.

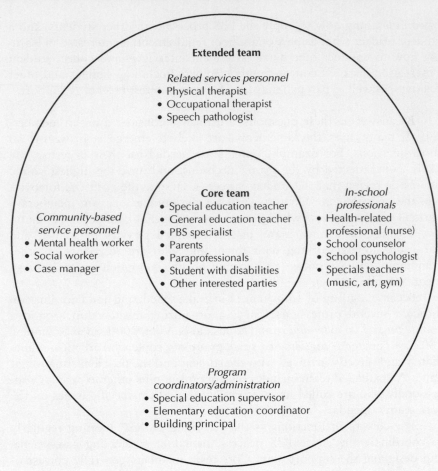

Extended team

Related services personnel
• Physical therapist
• Occupational therapist
• Speech pathologist

Community-based service personnel
• Mental health worker
• Social worker
• Case manager

Core team
• Special education teacher
• General education teacher
• PBS specialist
• Parents
• Paraprofessionals
• Student with disabilities
• Other interested parties

In-school professionals
• Health-related professional (nurse)
• School counselor
• School psychologist
• Specials teachers (music, art, gym)

Program coordinators/administration
• Special education supervisor
• Elementary education coordinator
• Building principal

FIGURE 4.3. Extended and core team membership. Adapted from Snell and Janney (2000). Copyright by Paul H. Brookes Publishing Co. Adapted by permission.

Define Team Members' Roles and Responsibilities

In order for a team to function well, team members will need to know what is expected of them and how the work of the team will be facilitated and divided up among team members. Defining key roles should occur as soon as the team forms and may influence decisions about team membership if gaps are evident. Three key roles vital to the PBS process are the *team leader or facilitator*; the *PBS expert* (i.e., someone with expertise in PBS); and the *general team member*. Figure 4.4 lists sample responsibilities for each of these essential roles.

PRIMARY TEAM MEMBER ROLES

Team leader/facilitator	PBS specialist	General team member
• Guides team to articulate and work within stated values, purposes, and expectations.	• Guides team decisions in PBS values and practices.	• Works within team values, goals, and expectations.
• Keeps the team moving and focused on the team's agenda and goals.	• Ensures the technical adequacy of the functional assessment and the behavior support plans.	• Actively participates in team discussions; offers opinions and shares expertise and information.
• Encourages all team members to participate.	• Serves as a resource to the team; shares knowledge/materials on functional assessments, PBS plans, and specific interventions.	• Listens to other team members' suggestions and opinions; accepts alternative ways of doing things that meets the team's purpose or goals.
• Coaches the team members to demonstrate good teaming skills. For example:		
• Models excellent interpersonal skills.	• Guides team to adapt PBS practices to settings, cultures, and resources of the team.	• Communicates openly and respectfully with other team members.
• Acknowledges the contributions of team members	• Helps team members to develop skills in assessment, planning, and implementation.	• Accepts and supports team consensus decisions.
• Protects the right of all members to be heard.	• Serves as a general team member.	• Serves in other team roles as needed.
• Guides team to resolve conflict.		
• Ensures that team functions are assigned and carried out.		
• Serves as the contact point for communicating with extended team members.		
• Takes care of logistics during team meetings.		
• Serves as a general team member.		

OTHER ROLES

Recorder	Observer	Time keeper
• Records minutes and decisions for team.	• Monitors team's progress (are team members doing what they said they would?).	• Monitors time spent on team discussions.
• Reports at the beginning of each meeting.	• Helps facilitator keep track of team discussions.	• Alerts team when time is running out.

FIGURE 4.4. Roles and responsibilities of team members. Sources: Harrington-Mackin (1994); LaFasto and Larson (2001); and *Team Memory Jogger* (1995).

A skilled team leader or facilitator keeps the team moving and focused on achieving student-centered objectives (e.g., designing a PBS plan), while promoting positive, collaborative interactions among team members. Skilled team leaders are well organized and action-oriented, but also model and facilitate effective communication skills to keep team discussions open and respectful. For example, a team leader helps the team to clarify its agenda, encourages communication and participation by all members, paraphrases so that all team members may understand one another, asks team members to express their feelings and concerns to resolve conflict, guides team members to communicate in nonthreatening ways, and helps the team to move to action once team decisions are made (Harrington-Mackin, 1994). Being a team facilitator requires considerable skill, but it is a role that team members can take turns sharing. When team facilitation is shared, team members are less likely to be critical of others in this position (Harrington-Mackin, 1994).

Because the PBS process is likely to be unfamiliar to most school teams, at least one member who can serve as the PBS expert is needed on a team. A PBS expert shares technical know-how on conducting functional assessments, interpreting data, and designing a PBS plan; he or she can also facilitate team problem solving by offering suggestions for interventions. Increasingly, school districts are employing behavior support specialists to provide itinerant technical assistance to student-centered teams across district schools. However, it is more likely that special education teachers or school psychologists trained in PBS will assume this role. If they have not received prior training, then it is important for schools to facilitate training through inservice education and workshops.

The role of the general team member is the backbone of the team. All team members assume responsibility for contributing to team discussions, carrying out team activities and other assignments, and interacting with other team members in respectful ways. Consistent with the concept of parity, the team facilitator and the PBS expert are also team members, and take on the additional role of the general team member during the course of team activities. Likewise, a general team member can take on the role of facilitator or PBS expert as knowledge and skill are acquired.

In addition to these three key roles, teams may assign other team roles to keep team members on track during team discussions. Because these meeting roles require little technical expertise, they can be easily rotated across team members. A *team observer* can help the facilitator keep track of team discussion and evaluate how well the team is following agreed-upon procedures. A *team recorder* takes team minutes and records team activities and decisions. A *team timekeeper* monitors team discussion time and alerts the team as it nears the end of an agreed-upon time period. See Figure 4.4 for more complete descriptions.

Agree on Team Purpose and Goals

Establishing and agreeing upon the team's purpose and goals bind the team's commitment to a central agenda—namely, providing PBS for one student. Clearly articulated student-centered goals help everyone on the team to understand what the team is supposed to do and why; just as importantly, they can help to establish boundaries as what the team will not be doing (*Team Memory Jogger*, 1995). If team members come to the table with different agendas, the team will be pulled in different directions, making it impossible to achieve any single objective. Furthermore, team members can become easily dissatisfied if they believe that their pet agendas are not being addressed. Competing agendas can be eliminated at the onset if the team can agree upon a few central goals.

Although the process takes time, one way of establishing team purpose and goals is to have team members develop goal statements jointly, using a problem-solving or brainstorming strategy as described later in this chapter. In this way, each team member will have the opportunity to provide input into the team's ultimate purpose and reflect upon what the goals mean to him or her. An important role of the facilitator during this process is to establish parameters for goal setting that are consistent with PBS values and processes. For example, goal statements that focus on removing the student from his or her classroom, "stopping" a student from engaging in problem behavior, seeking behavior-suppressive medication, or placing the student in an alternative school are inconsistent with the values of PBS.

Good goal statements are brief, are understood and agreed upon by all, and (importantly) are consistent with PBS assumptions and values. Team members may choose to write one or two broad, overarching long-term goals that are reflective of the team's desired long-term outcomes for the student, or several more immediate short-term goals that are reflective of the PBS steps for designing support plans (Snell & Janney, 2000). Some examples of goal statements are shown in Table 4.1.

Set Ground Rules for Collaboration

Just as important as team goals are *ground rules* for collaboration (Schwarz, 1994). Ground rules are informal guidelines that reflect team members' views on how they should operate to (1) stay action-oriented and focused on the team's agenda, (2) implement the PBS process, and (3) interact among themselves in positive and productive ways. By specifying expectations for team conduct, ground rules can help minimize disruptions and team conflict, while enhancing team effectiveness.

One way to establish ground rules for collaboration is to encourage team members to write down rules that reflect their individual concerns

TABLE 4.1. Sample Goal Statements

Our goal is to . . .

- Understand what Leroy may be communicating by his challenging behaviors.
- Implement effective supports that will maintain Eric's participation in the general education classroom.
- Identify and implement strategies that can be used to prevent Calvin's challenging behaviors from happening.
- Identify and teach Tiffany alternative communication and coping strategies.
- Teach Al to use self-management strategies that he can use to schedule his daily activities.
- Create opportunities for Dawn to develop friendships with her peers who do not have disabilities.
- Design a support plan that works for Aisha at both school and home.

about team conduct, and then to compile the rules into one list for team discussion and agreement. To facilitate this process, Snell and Janney (2000) suggest using "trigger questions" to spark team discussion. Here are some sample questions appropriate for PBS teams:

"What will it take for us to get our work done?"
"What PBS assumptions are central to accomplishing our work?"
"How should we behave to ensure that our interactions are respectful of one another?"

Examples of ground rules for each of these questions are shown in Figure 4.5. Once ground rules are established, the team should revisit them periodically to determine whether all team members are following the rules. If rules are broken repeatedly, the team may need to consider addressing the problem at a team meeting, speaking to individual team members, or changing a ground rule if it is impractical or no longer relevant to the team's activities.

Schedule and Structure Team Meetings

The last consideration for establishing team structure during the initial stages of collaboration involves establishing regular meeting times and deciding on a format for conducting team meetings. When scheduling, teams will need to address the following questions and considerations.

- *How often will we meet?* There are no hard and fast rules for the ideal frequency of team meetings; however, regular meetings matched to a

What will it take to get our work done?	• We will come to meetings prepared and focused. • We will adhere to the meeting agenda. • We will remain team-oriented during all meetings. • We will adhere to the ground rules set by the team.
What PBS assumptions are central to accomplishing our work?	• We will be data-based in identifying the function(s) of the problem behavior. • We will develop support plans based on functional assessment data. • We will develop interventions that respect student and family preferences. • We will use data to guide our decision making.
How should we behave to ensure that our interactions are respectful of one another?	• We will each have an opportunity to voice our opinions. • We will listen and try to understand one another. • We will make important decisions by reaching consensus. • We will attempt to communicate effectively and constructively.

FIGURE 4.5. Examples of ground rules.

team's purpose or agenda are key. The core team should meet regularly enough to (1) address student-centered goals in a timely way, (2) keep team members actively engaged and productive in carrying out team responsibilities, (3) keep team activities coordinated, and (4) address individual team members' concerns and help the members feel confident and supported. How often a team meets is influenced by a number of factors, including the team's experience (i.e., generally the more inexperienced the team, the more frequently it should meet to establish a critical foundation for success); the phase of the collaboration process (i.e., the assessment and planning phase generally requires more frequent meetings than the implementing, evaluating, and revising phase); and the particular student problem at hand (e.g., frequent crisis situations require prompt and frequent responses from the team).

• *Where should we meet?* Generally, teams are most productive when members work in a meeting place that is free from distractions and interruptions from their other daily responsibilities. Teams may also wish to consider privacy, so that team deliberations will not be overheard by other staff or students.

• *How long should meetings last?* Problem solving and planning are time-consuming activities, particularly when multiple people are involved. Although meeting length can be adjusted flexibly to fit the task, some experts (e.g., Thousand & Villa, 2000) recommend keeping meeting times to 1 hour or less. It may be more efficient in the long run to have short, frequent meetings where team concentration is focused on a small task, rather than long meetings that require sustained attention. Logistically, it may be easier to get busy team members to commit to time blocks of 1 hour or less than to longer meeting times.

• *How can we accommodate people with different schedules?* Given the diverse schedules of school personnel and families, this may be the most challenging question. The goal is to identify a standard time that is predictable (e.g., "We will meet every other Tuesday at 2:30") and protected (i.e., "We will attend and not let other obligations interfere with this time"). Because teachers' schedules are not completely under their control, the support of the building principal is usually needed to explore existing opportunities for team collaboration, and to create opportunities if none exist (e.g., rearranging teacher preparation periods, using already established program meetings to plan for individual students, using paraprofessionals or substitutes for short time periods, creating work–study periods for students where teachers can more easily be released from instruction) (Thousand & Villa, 2000; Weigle, 1997). Ideally, the commitment to teaming is a schoolwide initiative. Team members may also consider rotating or changing schedules if it is impossible for all to meet in the same room or to accommodate extended team membership. A rotating schedule (e.g., every third meeting at 3:15 instead of 2:00) may work best for accommodating family participation. Many parents will find it impossible to attend every meeting; nor is it necessary when the team's agenda focuses on internal logistics (e.g., scheduling student observations, figuring out how to implement a teaching strategy).

• *How will we communicate between meetings?* With today's technology, numerous ways to maintain communication exist. Simple progress reports or updates (e.g., "I just finished interviewing Mrs. Glasco and Mrs. Hernandez, and am ready to share what I learned," "I tried changing Joey's work assignment, and it seems to be working!") can be provided via telephone calls, short notes, e-mail, or even text messaging to other team members. Between-meeting updates can create team trust, since team members know that agreed-upon activities are being completed. And, just as importantly for busy people, such updates can clear valuable meeting time for other purposes.

In addition to scheduling, team members will need to establish a standard meeting format to structure how the team conducts its business. A standard format can greatly enhance team efficiency and effectiveness. The facilitator is responsible for assuring that all team members participate and adhere to the meeting format. A sample meeting format is shown in Figure 4.6.

	What do you do?	What do you say?
Opening	Review agenda items.	• Does anyone have anything to add to the agenda? • What did we decide on in our last meeting?
	Prioritize items if necessary; set time limits.	• What is most important? • How much time should we spend?
	Assign meeting roles.	• Who will facilitate, keep time, record, etc.? • Who has not played a primary team role?
Define outcome and process	State desired outcome.	• What do we want to accomplish in this meeting?
	Decide on process for meeting goal(s).	• How can we best meet the meeting goals? • Does anyone have other suggestions as to how to proceed?
Conduct meeting	Engage in whole-group discussion.	• Does anyone else have something to contribute regarding the desired outcome?
	Participate in brainstorming (if problem solving).	• What are some ideas that we can generate?
	Evaluate solutions.	• What solution best meets our criteria?
	Come to consensus during decision making.	• How can we negotiate so that we all agree on what to do?
Closing	Summarize team discussion.	• What were the ideas that were brought to the table? • What conclusion was reached through team consensus?
	Agree on next steps.	• What needs to be done next? • What steps will we take?
	Assign tasks/responsibilities.	• Who will best be able to complete each step?

FIGURE 4.6. Sample meeting format.

Assessment and Planning

The assessment and planning phase is the core of PBS teamwork. With regard to student-centered outcomes, teams focus on Steps 2–4 of the PBS process. These steps include conducting and coordinating a functional assessment, developing and agreeing upon hypotheses for problem behaviors, and designing a comprehensive behavior support plan with a good contextual fit. This is a tall order! However, equally important during this phase are team-centered processes that foster PBS values, collaboration, and good teaming skills. In this section, we discuss three team-centered activities essential to assessment and planning.

Enhance Capacity for Understanding

During the assessment and planning phase, the PBS expert lends technical expertise. However, it is not just a simple matter of the PBS expert telling the team what to do. Success will depend on the entire team's "buying into" and understanding PBS processes and values (Hieneman & Dunlap, 2000, 2001; Ruef, Turnbull, Turnbull, & Poston, 1999). Unfortunately, because some team members lack exposure to PBS or have had negative experiences interacting with difficult students, they may come to the table wearing biased "glasses" that will prevent them from seeing legitimate reasons for problem behavior. These team members may try to explain problem behavior by blaming the student or applying their pet theories without any consideration of environmental determinants (e.g., "He's doing it on purpose!" "He's doing it for attention!" "She's trying to irk me!"). When it comes time to intervene, the same team members will select interventions based on their own preferences or experience without consideration to assessment data or team hypotheses (e.g., "I refuse to put up with that nonsense; he will make up his school work during recess").

Helping such team members to "see" or understand core PBS assumptions is an essential and ongoing part of the teaming process. Traditional inservice workshops on conducting functional assessments or designing PBS plans can open team members to new perspectives, but often such workshops are not enough. Without continual guidance and reflection on how to apply PBS assumptions to specific situations, novice PBS team members will revert to old ways of thinking when faced with challenges. Perhaps one of the best ways of bringing people along is to make PBS assumptions explicit during team meetings, so that team members will see for themselves and therefore understand.

Person-centered planning (PCP; described in more detail in Chapter 11) is one example of an explicit process that can be used. In PCP, team members who know the student best come together to create an action plan for achieving a desirable future or life for the student. Although PCP has a clear student-focused agenda (i.e., the creation of an action plan), the PCP process of having team members discuss and illustrate through wall charts the student's history, personal strengths/positive characteristics, personal challenges (including specific disabilities), and personal preferences/interests has a way of helping team members to develop empathy for the student and his or her current situation (Bambara et al., 2001). According to attribution theory (Kando, 1977), when people empathize, they are more likely to seek external explanations for problem behavior than to blame the student for the problem. In other words, the PCP process can help team members remove their biased glasses by opening them up to alternative, previously unconsidered perspectives. One goal of PCP is to guide all team members to view the student as a person first with unique strengths and interests, and not as a collection of problem behaviors.

Illustrative wall charts can also be applied to hypothesis development, to help all team members see and understand specific environmental influences of problem behavior. The *initial line of inquiry* (Lohrmann-O'Rourke, Knoster, & Llewellyn, 1999), is an example of a group process for formulating an initial hypothesis. Using a wall chart divided into columns for "slow triggers" (setting events, lifestyle factors), "fast triggers" (antecedent events), problem behaviors, and perceived functions, a team facilitator guides team members to discuss potential variables based upon their observations and data collection. Through a discussion of potential variables, team members come to consensus on a single hypothesis for the targeted problem behavior. Similar to PCP, the initial line of inquiry has both a student-centered (i.e., formulating a hypothesis) and a team-centered agenda. The team-centered agenda is to make the hypothesis development process explicit, so that all team members can come to a common understanding of the specific factors that influence problem behaviors for the student.

In our experience, explicit group discussions about team observations and data collection not only are helpful for establishing initial hypotheses, but can be useful throughout the teaming process whenever team members begin to stray from environmental explanations. During periods of stress and high rates of challenging behaviors, it is not uncommon for team members to put on their biased glasses again and blame the student or seek medication as the sole answer to intervention. When team members begin to stray in this manner, it is important for the entire team to reflect upon its data collection and assessments to make decisions about what is happening and why. Similarly, group processing of student progress data can make disbelievers (e.g., "That will never work") into believers, once they can see for themselves how interventions result in improvements (e.g., "Wow, that really works"). Ongoing, explicit discussions and team processing of data can serve to reframe biased perceptions by opening team members to alternative perspectives and new ways of thinking.

Use Collaborative Problem-Solving Strategies

Choosing the most appropriate assessments, formulating hypotheses about problem behaviors, and designing support plans can be conceptualized as a series of problem-solving activities requiring collective team decision making. Regardless of the type of problem, members of an effective team approach problems optimistically ("What can we do to figure this out?") and systematically, using a process that helps the members to carefully consider and analyze potential solutions (LaFasto & Larson, 2001). Team members can choose from a number of problem-solving strategies to help them with the process. Fortunately, research suggests that it does not really matter which particular strategy a team uses, as long as the problem is approached systematically (LaFasto & Larson, 2001) and the collective wisdom of the team is utilized. Below is a generic five-step problem-solving framework described by Snell and Janney (2000) that can be applied across a variety of team activities requiring decision making.

• *Step 1: Identify the problem.* In this first step, team members agree on the single most important issue or problem that the team needs to resolve now. To keep from feeling overwhelmed, it is important to focus on a single issue at a time. Problem identification can cluster around (1) planning for assessment and intervention (e.g., deciding how to conduct a functional assessment, selecting assessment-based interventions) or (2) troubleshooting to uncover solutions to unanticipated problems (e.g., "Our plan is not working; what do we do next?"). Problem definitions can be expressed as questions or statements, but are always worded to focus on finding a solution as an outcome. Here are some examples:

"How should we conduct a functional assessment for Michael?"
"Now that we know that Natasha screams when the work is difficult, what can we do to prevent screaming in the classroom?"
"The support plan for Josh is not working—what might be going on, and what should we do next?"
"Our objective is to develop a practical way of monitoring student progress."

• *Step 2: Brainstorm potential solutions to the problem.* In this step, the team generates as many potential solutions to the posed problem as possible without critiquing or evaluating. The goal is to hear from many team members and to gather a wide variety of ideas.

• *Step 3: Evaluate the solutions.* In this step, team members analyze and then narrow down ideas to potential solutions that will work the best. To evaluate solutions, team members compare each idea to a set of criteria that is used to judge acceptability along the lines of technical adequacy (e.g., "Is the idea consistent with PBS assumptions?") and contextual fit (e.g., "Does the idea match the values, skills, and resources of the team?"). We encourage teams to generate their own specific criteria for evaluating ideas. Table 4.2 provides some examples for evaluating "good-fit" solutions consistent with PBS values and assumptions.

• *Step 4: Choose a solution.* After evaluating the solutions, the team selects the most desirable one or ones. In PBS problem solving, team members are likely to generate more than one acceptable solution to a problem and can either elect to try one solution or combine several solutions into a more comprehensive plan. For example, for Natasha (see above), it is possible for the team to agree on several strategies to prevent her screaming, all of which can be combined into one support plan. Regardless of whether the team settles on one or more solutions to a problem, it is important to view all solutions as tentative until they are proven workable and effective.

• *Step 5: Develop an action plan.* In the last step, the team writes an action plan to carry out solutions; if this is not done, even the best ideas may never be realized. Key elements of an action plan include the following:

TABLE 4.2. Criteria for Evaluating "Good-Fit" Solutions

• Is it doable?
• Is it time-efficient?
• Does it fit the setting?
• Does it address hypotheses for problem behavior?
• Is it data-based?
• Does it address team members' priorities and concerns?
• Is it acceptable to the plan implementers (teachers, family members)?
• Is it acceptable to the student?
• Is it consistent with PBS values and procedures?
• Is it best practice?
• Is it team-generated?
• Is it age-appropriate and respectful of the student?
• Does it acknowledge the student's and family's cultural background?

Note. Adapted from Snell and Janney (2000). Copyright by Paul H. Brookes Publishing Co. Adapted by permission. (Originally adapted from Giangreco, M. F., Cloninger, C. J., Dennis, R. E., & Edelman, S. W. [1994]. Problem-solving methods to facilitate inclusive education. In J. S. Thousand, R. A. Villa, & A. I. Nevin [Eds.], *Creativity and collaborative learning: A practical guide to empowering students and teachers* [pp. 321–346]. Baltimore: Paul H. Brookes Publishing Co.)

Summary: "What key issue was decided?"

Action: "What action steps did we decide to take to address this issue?"

Who is responsible: "Who will carry out the action steps?"

By when: "When will the action steps be implemented?"

When team members use a problem-solving strategy to plan or to troubleshoot problems, they build team commitment by coming to consensus. Formulating team consensus does not necessarily mean that all team members agree with every idea or solution; it means that they are willing to support and go along with team decisions to make things happen.

Create an Atmosphere of Openness and Honesty

"A hallmark of an excellent team is its members' ability to say what they think or feel, without putting other people down or being put down themselves" (Willcocks & Morris, 1997, p. 18). To be effective, a team must create an atmosphere of open communication, where members feel free to express their thoughts without becoming or causing others to feel defensive. Most of the teaming strategies discussed thus far contribute to an open climate. For example, the processes inherent in agreeing on team goals, establishing ground rules for collaboration, and engaging in team problem solving can make team members feel valued and listened to, even if they do not always get their way (Willcocks & Morris, 1997). However, teams are made up of people, and people are not always respectful of others—especially when they are stressed, are concerned, or disagree with others. We've all seen that team problem behaviors, such as personal attacks, angry statements, finger pointing, and sneering at ideas, can cause resentment, counterattacks, and withdrawal. Who would want to participate in team discussions after being put down? Unfortunately, when team members stop communicating and collaborating with one another, the student, who is dependent on team action, suffers the most. Nothing can be accomplished for the student when team members feel hurt and angry.

To maintain open and honest communication, the team facilitator plays an important role in managing and resolving team conflict. There are several things that a team facilitator can do to keep communication open (LaFasto & Larson, 2001; Harrington-Mackin, 1994; Willcocks & Morris, 1997):

- Keep ground rules for fair play in the forefront of team discussions, and encourage team members to follow them (e.g., "Just a minute, Fred, Suzanna isn't finished speaking yet").
- Guide team members to really listen to what others have to say.

Encourage them to understand others' perspectives and walk in their shoes to understand. PBS is for team members, too (e.g., "Fred, you feel very strongly about this. Help us understand why this issue is important to you").

- Help team members see the value in what others are saying, even if it differs from their own beliefs (e.g., "That's interesting. I would have never thought of that. Great idea!").
- When conflicts arise, help team members to uncover issues and deal with the facts. Use problem-solving strategies to resolve problems, rather than blame others for failure (e.g., "It seems like we have not completed the functional assessment for Leroy as planned. What is causing the problem? What can we do to address the problem?").
- Model and encourage effective communication skills. Good communication depersonalizes issues and avoids putting people on the defensive (e.g., say, "That idea may not work because . . . ," not "That's a stupid suggestion").

The bottom line is that creating an atmosphere of openness and honesty requires good team manners and effective communication skills. All team members are responsible for being open to different perspectives and communicating in ways that do not discourage people from contributing. The team facilitator is responsible for ensuring that team members honor their commitment to good communication. Table 4.3 illustrates effective and ineffective communication statements in four team scenarios. As shown in the second column, ineffective statements are "difficult to hear" because they blame others or put other team members on the defensive, which in turn shuts down collaboration. The third column illustrates how a team facilitator or another team member can respond to or defuse difficult statements, should they occur in a team meeting. The last column illustrates alternative or effective ways of communicating (easy-to-hear statements) that do not belittle or attack others, but rather communicate openness and respect.

Implementing, Evaluating, and Revising

In this last collaborative phase, team members continue to meet regularly to ensure that the behavior support plan is implemented as planned, is working, and (if necessary) is revised to improve student and family outcomes (Step 5 of the PBS process). By this point, team members are well on their way to working collaboratively; however, team-centered activities are still important to maintain good teamwork and realize student-centered outcomes. In this section, we discuss four team-building activities that are especially important during this last phase.

TABLE 4.3. Examples of Ineffective and Effective Communication Statements

Team scenario	Ineffective statements (difficult to hear)	How to respond to ineffective statements	Effective statements (easy to hear)
An emergency team meeting is convened. Justin's problem behaviors have increased significantly during the past 2 weeks. Members are struggling to identify reasons for the increase. Justin's teacher appears to be taking the increase in challenging behaviors personally.	*Justin's teacher says:* "He's doing it on purpose because he knows it bothers me." "I've tried everything, and there is no reason why—he's psychotic and needs to have his medication changed."	*A team member responds:* "You seem very frustrated. Let's take a look at the data to see if we can figure out what's going on."	*Justin's teacher might have said:* "I'm having a hard time understanding why he's been so disruptive lately."
Team members are brainstorming to identify alternative strategies to resolve a problem. A frustrated special education teacher thinks she has all the answers.	*The special education teacher says:* "I know that idea won't work—what you need to do is . . ." "I tried all these things—they don't work—nothing works."	*A team member responds:* "You seem frustrated. But remember, we're brainstorming—the idea is to generate as many solutions as possible without critiquing." *or* "We just have to try again, and that's why we're here—to come up with new ideas and support one another."	*The teacher might have said:* "These ideas are all great and ones we've suggested in the past. I was thinking we could try . . ."

96

| During a meeting, a member raises an issue that was discussed and resolved in a previous meeting. A busy administrator, eager to move on, is frustrated. | *The administrator says:*

"That issue has already been discussed and resolved. We have other things to address."

"If you had been at the last meeting you would know that we talked about that issue and resolved it." | *A team member responds:*

"Yes, we discussed this at the last meeting. To quickly update you, I'll summarize what we decided."

or

"Can you meet later today, and one of us will update you?" | *The administrator might have said:*

"At the last meeting, we discussed this issue. We have several other things to cover today; can we meet at another time? I'd be happy to update you."

or

"I realize you weren't able to attend the last meeting. Perhaps we can set up a time to meet to update you and hear your concerns." |
| A frustrated mother expresses that she feels as if nothing is being done to address her son's problem behavior. | *An equally frustrated behavior specialist says:*

"No, that's not the case, and there's no reason for you to feel that way."

"Of course things have been done to address the situation." | *A team member responds:*

"I'm worried about Mrs. Cruz's concern. Can we take a few minutes to discuss this issue?" | *The behavior specialist might have said:*

"Can you help me understand why you feel as though nothing has been done?" |

Provide Support for Team Members

Just as behavior support plans contain specific strategies for helping students avoid or cope with difficult problem situations, strategies for team support are essential for helping team members feel confident and secure as they support the student. Helping team members maintain their commitment to using PBS strategies can be very difficult when they are scared, frustrated, or uncertain. For example, some team members may lack skills for carrying out specific interventions, causing them to become frustrated and give up easily. Other team members may worry about whether they are doing the right thing when applying strategies to new situations, and consequently may fail to respond appropriately to challenges. Others may experience high degrees of stress when faced with frequent or high-intensity episodes of challenging behaviors, making it difficult for them to maintain positive future interactions with the student. And still others might fear being blamed for the student's problem behavior, particularly during public or high-risk situations (e.g., a student's threatening to break ceramics in a museum gift shop), causing them to back away during times of crisis. Left unaddressed, issues such as these can erode the best-laid plans for PBS. Intervention failure can be caused by the team's failure to support its members.

Designing team supports is much like designing support plans for students. Team members may ask, "What do *we need* in order to carry out the support plan for [student's name]?" Or "What are our fears and worries about carrying out the support plan? What can we do to address them?" Like supports for individual students, support for team members can take a variety of forms, depending the needs of individual members. One simple but helpful strategy is to provide opportunities for team members to share and process their experiences during meetings. In this way, team members may be comforted by knowing that they are implementing strategies correctly, that other team members are sometimes worried or stressed just as they are, and that other members are there to help them problem-solve through difficult situations. Support for team members can be provided both inside and outside of team meetings. Other ways of supporting team members include the following:

- Provide ongoing encouragement and praise for team members' efforts to try new approaches or overcome their fear.
- Have team members "buddy up" or observe one another as they learn specific interventions.
- Provide team training in areas that reflect team concerns (e.g., specific interventions, crisis management).

- Create opportunities for teachers and other plan implementers to take a short break after a crisis or a highly stressful experience.
- Build in informal supports by having team members check in with one another during the day, or call or e-mail one another for immediate problem solving between meetings.

Apply Problem-Solving Strategies to Make Decisions about Modifications

After a behavior support plan is implemented, team members regularly review data on student progress to determine whether modifications are needed. Decisions about what to do next are made by using the same problem-solving strategy described in the "Assessment and Planning" section of this chapter. Continued input from all team members is necessary to maintain good decision making and team ownership. During this last phase of collaborative teamwork, problem solving is applied to resolve issues of accountability ("Are we doing what we said we should be doing?"), feasibility ("Can our plan be realistically carried out over the long term?"), and effectiveness ("Is the plan making a difference for the student?"). It is important to point out that when evaluating and revising, the entire team is held accountable for the team's success or failure. Praising just a few individuals for their efforts, or blaming a few individuals for the lack of progress, can easily undermine teamwork. As long as team members are making an honest effort to honor their responsibilities, no matter how big or small, then all team members are acknowledged for making equal contributions to the team. Likewise, if problems are encountered, then it is the team's responsibility to uncover issues and resolve them. If a behavior support plan is not working, the team is held accountable; no one person is ever blamed.

Celebrate

"Recognizing and celebrating the team's achievements [help] to reinforce the positive feelings that come from working together to solve problems" (*Team Memory Jogger*, 1995, p. 132). Celebration boosts team morale and inspires a sense of pride and accomplishment during long and difficult work. Although we introduce it in the last phase of collaborative teamwork, a team should find ways of celebrating contributions and successes along the way. Team members may easily lose sight of the fact that they are making progress, and therefore lose motivation, if celebrations are reserved for final successes at the end. (This is analogous to good teaching. We do not withhold praise until a student has learned a new skill; we praise learning along the way.) Teams may celebrate any number of events: agreeing on team purpose and goals, completing a functional assessment, designing a support plan, decreasing a problem behaviors, and finding a solution to a problem once considered insurmountable. Team celebrations can be rather simple: a round of applause, a checklist marking off accomplishments, doughnuts and coffee, thank-you notes to team members. Periodic recognition of team efforts can go a long way toward keeping the team motivated and working together to resolve problems.

Reflect on Team Process

By reviewing student data and team accomplishments, team members regularly evaluate their progress toward achieving student-centered outcomes. An equally important evaluation is to reflect regularly on team process. Here team members ask, "Are we really a team?" (Thousand & Villa, 2000) or "How are we doing as a team?" (Willcocks & Morris, 1997). Throughout this chapter, we have discussed a number of team-building activities essential for establishing collaboration and good working relationships among team members. As a final reflection, and as way to summarize our key points, we offer a checklist (Figure 4.7) that team members may use to evaluate healthy team functioning. As with all evaluations, it is best to reflect on these questions as the team moves through the PBS process.

SUMMARY

Collaborative teaming is essential for designing and carrying out comprehensive support plans for individual students. Because team members are the instruments of change, their learning, their support, and their ability to communicate and work effectively with others are prerequisites for creating positive student outcomes. A team is created not just to address student concerns, but also to enhance the capacity of team members to carry out its work. In addition to describing why teaming is important, we have highlighted several important team-building strategies designed to enhance collaboration within a PBS framework. These strategies should provide team members with a starting place to understand the value and complexity of teamwork. However, we recognize that we are addressing only the tip of the iceberg. Readers are strongly encouraged to read the excellent sources on teaming in this chapter's reference list for more detailed discussions of how to build and maintain collaborative teams.

Are We Working as a Team?

Instructions: Evaluate each area as it relates to your team's overall performance. Place a checkmark in the box if you believe that the team could improve in this area. For each area in need of improvement, identify barriers that may be preventing effective teaming. Lastly, identify one or more solutions that may eliminate the identified barrier. Discuss solutions with your team.

Rating for team	Evaluation area	Barriers preventing effective teaming	Solutions to improve
√	Before our meetings, we have an agenda, time, location and assigned roles.	At times, we get the agenda when we arrive at the meeting, so it's hard to plan ahead.	Agenda could be sent by e-mail a day or two in advance.
	Before our meetings, each member knows his or her responsibilities to the team and what he or she should prepare.		
	During our meetings, each team member has the opportunity and feels safe to express his or her opinion.		
√	During our meetings, our team takes the opportunity to highlight our accomplishments.	If we are in crisis, we may skip over what we've accomplished and just start working on the problem.	We could make a commitment to always celebrate especially during crisis times.
	During our meetings, we are able to develop a plan to address problem situations that all team members agree with.		
	During our meetings, communication is respectful among team members.		

FIGURE 4.7. Example of a team evaluation checklist.

COMMONLY ASKED QUESTIONS

Is a team always needed to design behavior support plans? Couldn't I just do it alone? With time and experience, the five-step process for designing a support plan (see Chapter 3) will become intuitive for many school personnel and parents. In limited circumstances, it may be possible for a single person with experience in PBS to design and implement an intervention plan alone, particularly when problem behavior occurs in only one setting (e.g., in only one class or in just the home). However, in our experience, persistent and difficult problem behaviors typically occur across settings and people, necessitating a comprehensive approach to intervention. The more comprehensive the assessment and intervention, the more advantageous it will be to involve the people who are most affected by the individual's problem behavior and who are invested and involved in the person's life. Although it may be possible to design PBS plans without the involvement of others, long-term success is questionable.

How will we (and other busy professionals and parents) find the time to meet? No doubt, finding time to meet regularly will be a big challenge for most school personnel and parents, largely because schools are not typically structured for collaboration. Besides core team members' searching for common times to meet, administrative support is often necessary to create opportunities that may not typically exist. Such support is most likely when the entire school "buys into" the importance of teaming to make things happen. Although finding time is often difficult, one of the biggest mistakes that professionals can make is believing that creating time for teaming is unnecessary. As we have stressed throughout the chapter, teaming serves many important functions; without it, long-term success is threatened.

What if some team members resist changing their ways of doing things? In answering this question, extend PBS principles to understanding team members' behavior. Before asking what to do, ask, "Why are certain team members resistant to change?" Various reasons will yield different solutions. For example, is a team member resistant because he doesn't know how to implement the procedures or is fearful of making a mistake? If so, the answer might be to provide more training or support. Is a team member resistant because the intervention strategies are too difficult to implement? If so, the answer might be to change the intervention so it better fits the setting. Is a team member resistant because she doesn't believe the intervention will be effective? If so, then use team meetings to review student progress data and share team success stories. Helping team members to overcome their initial hesitation or resistance to new ways of doing things is part of the teaming process. Be patient and provide time for growth and learning.

How can team conflict be resolved? Conflict is inherent in all teaming. Healthy conflict, characterized by respectful disagreement and a commitment by all to find an agreeable solution to a problem, can move the team forward. Unhealthy conflict, characterized by stubborn and disrespectful arguments, can cripple a team. If team conflict becomes unhealthy, the first course of action is to remind all team members about the ground rules for good communication. In some cases, it may be necessary for the team facilitator to speak with certain team members individually and privately about their behavior and team concerns. In rare cases, a team member will just refuse to yield to others' ideas, despite attempts at implementing these suggestions. In this circumstance, the rest of the team may consider dismissing the disagreeable team member or working around him or her.

CASE EXAMPLES

Malik's Team

To initiate the behavior support process, Malik's core team, which would be responsible for carrying out all PBS activities, was established. Core team members included Malik's grandmother and grandfather, who were his primary care providers; his classroom teacher, Mrs. Nelson; his teaching assistant; and the building principal. The school's behavior support specialist, Mr. Rodriguez, who had previous experience developing PBS plans, was also included as a core team member and served as the team facilitator. Extended team members were identified as well. Because Malik's young Aunt Jenna and Uncle Thomas played an active role in Malik's life, they wished to be included in core team activities; however, as a result of their busy school and work schedules, they could only attend an occasional meeting. Malik's grandparents agreed that they would update Jenna and Thomas about new developments and bring back to the team any suggestions or concerns that Jenna and Thomas raised. Malik's grandparents also suggested inviting his mother to participate, because of the possibility that she might become more involved in his life in the future. The level of Malik's mother's involvement was left up to her discretion. Finally, although Malik was not currently prescribed any medications, his family members wanted their pediatrician, Dr. White, to be a part of the extended team. They deemed this important because she had been Malik's pediatrician since birth and had prescribed and monitored his medications in the past. Because of her busy schedule, Dr. White was unable to attend team meetings regularly. Instead, she participated by way of conference calls at her own or any team member's request, or when the team was discussing issues that needed her input.

Once a core team was established, the team scheduled a regular time to meet, which was arranged for every other Wednesday at 2:30. This worked out perfectly for the school staff, because students were dismissed early on Wednesday afternoons to allow for teacher planning and parent conferences. The building principal arranged for after-school child care on Wednesdays, should parents or other family members need someone to look after their children while they met with teachers. Because Malik's grandmother worked part-time with flexible job hours, she could attend most meetings. On days when she could not attend, the team promised to update her and her husband through e-mail and telephone calls, and would postpone critical decision making until she or her husband could attend a team meeting. Malik's grandfather would need to take time off from work to attend meetings. Confident that his wife would represent him at meetings, Malik's grandfather felt comfortable with attending meetings only a few times during the year.

A critical first-step activity of any team is agreeing on the team's purpose and goals. All team members entered with an understanding that they would use PBS strategies to address Malik's problem behaviors. At the first meeting, Mr. Rodriguez briefly explained the PBS process and philosophy so that all members would understand the steps they would take in developing a support plan for Malik. To establish team goals, Mr. Rodriquez asked Malik's grandmother to state what she wanted the team to accomplish. After expressing her worry and deep concern that Malik's problems were growing worse each year, she said with a sigh, "All I want is for Malik to be happy and enjoy school." After some discussion, the team quickly decided on two goals to guide the team's initial activities:

- To figure out why Malik was having problems in school (i.e., why was he engaging in problem behaviors?).
- To develop a support plan that would reduce Malik's problem behaviors and increase his participation in and happiness with school activities.

Malik's grandmother quickly added that she wanted to see him back in his neighborhood school with his friends and cousins, but for now, she was comfortable with more the immediate goals of putting an end to Malik's "downward cycle" of school failure.

Bethany's Team

As with Malik, a core team was identified for Bethany. Her team included her mother, her general education teacher, her special education teacher, her physical education teacher, the school psychologist, and the building principal. Bethany's mother felt strongly that Bethany herself should also be a core team member. She discussed the idea with Bethany; although Bethany was reluctant at first, she agreed to participate primarily in areas involving review of her support plan. In addition,

Ms. DeLope requested that her next-door neighbor, Mrs. Lane, be included as an extended team member. She was a constant source of support to Ms. DeLope and had become very close to Bethany. Because of his unavailability for regular meetings, Bethany's father requested to be a part of her extended team. It was agreed that he would participate by being regularly informed of decisions by Bethany's mother, and by receiving, from the school, documents that were produced during team meetings.

Because of Ms. DeLope's work schedule, regular meetings were not feasible. Ms. DeLope did, however, want to be an integral part of the planning process. Thus it was decided that school-based team members would meet regularly during the support-planning process, and would communicate by e-mail and phone with Ms. DeLope. When adequate information was gathered, Ms. DeLope would schedule a few hours off work to attend the meeting to develop Bethany's support plan. Thereafter, meetings would be scheduled on an as-needed basis.

Because Bethany's mother was unable to meet regularly, goals were established and problem behaviors identified via a conference call. As with Malik, the team set out to determine why Bethany was engaging in problem behavior and to develop a support plan. The team members agreed that their primary goal at the current time was to identify the supports needed to be able to maintain Bethany in general education and to improve social interactions with her peers. At Ms. DeLope's suggestion, the team concurred that it was important to improve her overall quality of life; this meant providing additional structure outside of school, identifying enjoyable activities for Bethany, and providing time for her to develop friendships.

REFERENCES

Albin, R. W., Lucyshyn, J. M., Horner, R. H., & Flannery, K. B. (1996). Contextual fit for behavioral support plans: A model for "goodness of fit." In L. K. Koegel, R. L. Koegel, & G. Dunlap (Eds.), *Positive behavioral support: Including people with difficult behavior in the community* (pp. 81–98). Baltimore: Paul H. Brookes.

Bambara, L. M., Gomez, O., Koger, F., Lohrmann-O'Rourke, S., & Xin, Y. P. (2001). More than techniques: Team members' perspectives on implementing positive supports for adults with severe challenging behaviors. *Journal of The Association for Persons with Severe Handicaps, 26,* 213–228.

DeBoer, A., & Fister, S. (1994). *Strategies and tools for collaborative teaching.* Longmont, CO: Sopris West.

Dunlap, G., Newton, J. S., Fox, L., Benito, N., & Vaughn, B. (2001). Family involvement in functional assessment and positive behavior support. *Focus on Autism and Other Developmental Disabilities, 16,* 215–221.

Fleming, J., & Monda-Amaya, L. E. (2001). Process variables critical for team effectiveness. *Remedial and Special Education, 22,* 158–171.

Friend, M., & Cook, L. (2000). *Interactions: Collaboration skills for school professionals* (3rd ed.). White Plains, NY: Longman.

Harrington-Mackin, D. (1994). *The team building tool kit: Tips, tactics, and rules for effective workplace teams.* New York: American Management Association.

Hieneman, M., & Dunlap, G. (2000). Factors affecting the outcomes of community-based behavioral support: I. Identification and description of factor categories. *Journal of Positive Behavior Interventions, 2,* 161–169, 178.

Hieneman, M., & Dunlap, G. (2001). Factors affecting the outcomes of community-based behavioral support: II. Factor category importance. *Journal of Positive Behavior Interventions, 3,* 67–74.

Kando, T. M. (1977). *Social interaction.* St. Louis, MO: Mosby.

LaFasto, F., & Larson, C. (2001). *When teams work best: 6000 team members and leaders tell what it takes to succeed.* Thousand Oaks, CA: Sage.

Lohrmann-O'Rourke, S., Knoster, T., & Llewellyn, G. (1999). Screening for understanding: An initial line of inquiry for school-based settings. *Journal of Positive Behavior Interventions, 1,* 35–42.

Robbins, H., & Finley, M. (2000). *The new why teams don't work: What goes wrong and how to make it right.* San Francisco: Berrett-Koehler.

Ruef, M. B., Turnbull, A., Turnbull, H. R., & Poston, D. (1999). Perspectives of five stakeholder groups: Challenging behavior of individuals with mental retardation and/or autism. *Journal of Positive Behavior Interventions, 1,* 43–58.

Schwartz, I. S., Boulware, G., McBride, B. J., & Sandall, S. R. (2001). Functional assessment strategies for young children with autism. *Focus on Autism and Other Developmental Disabilities, 16,* 222–227, 231.

Schwarz, R. M. (1994). *The skilled facilitator: Practical wisdom for developing effective groups.* San Francisco: Jossey-Bass.

Snell, M. E., & Janney, R (2000). *Collaborative teaming.* Baltimore: Paul H. Brookes.

Straka, E., & Bricker, D. (1996). Building a collaborative team. In D. Bricker & A. Winderstrom (Eds.), *Preparing personnel to work with infants and young children and their families: A team approach* (pp. 321–345). Baltimore: Paul H. Brookes.

Team memory jogger. (1995). Salem, NH: GOAL/QPC.

Thousand, J. S., & Villa, R. A. (2000). Collaborative teaming: A powerful tool in school restructuring. In R. A. Villa & J. S. Thousand (Eds.), *Restructuring for caring and effective education* (pp. 254–291). Baltimore: Paul H. Brookes.

Weigle, K. L. (1997). Positive behavior support as a model for promoting educational inclusion. *Journal of The Association for Persons with Severe Handicaps, 22,* 36–38.

Willcocks, G., & Morris, S. (1997). *Successful team building.* Hauppauge, NY: Barron's Educational Series.

CHAPTER 5

◆◆◆

Strategies for Measuring Behavior Change

◆

RAYMOND G. MILTENBERGER

In order to evaluate whether a student is making progress when a positive behavior support (PBS) plan is implemented, there must be some measurement of the behaviors targeted for change. The target behaviors should include one or more problem behaviors to be decreased, and one or more desirable alternative behaviors or skills to be increased to replace the problem behaviors. Measurement of the target behaviors (also called *behavioral assessment*) should occur before a support plan is implemented, to establish the baseline level of the behavior, and during implementation, to determine whether the support plan is producing the desired changes in the target behaviors (Miltenberger, 2004). Assessment of the target behaviors also should continue for a period of time after the support plan is in place, to establish whether behavior changes endure over time.

Measurement of the target behaviors before the support plan is implemented is important for a number of reasons. First, it will help determine the seriousness of the problem. Preintervention behavioral assessment can establish the need for intervention by documenting that the problem behaviors occur frequently, occur for long durations of time, or occur with sufficient intensity to be problematic, and that the desirable behaviors occur too infrequently or not at all. It is also possible, however, that objective measurement of target behaviors prior to intervention may lead to the conclusion that a support plan is not warranted because the problem behaviors do not occur with sufficient frequency, duration, or intensity, or the desirable behaviors do occur with sufficient frequency. Second, behavioral assessment will establish the preintervention or baseline level of the problem behavior and desirable behaviors, so that the effects of the support plan can be evaluated. Third, carrying out behavioral assessment procedures requires that teachers, parents, and/or staff get actively involved in the process—something that will be essential for the success of PBS, as these same individuals will be responsible for carrying out the intervention procedures.

There are two categories of behavioral assessment: *direct assessment* and *indirect assessment* approaches (Iwata, Vollmer, Zarcone, & Rodgers, 1993; O'Neill et al., 1997). Direct assessment involves directly observing and recording the target behaviors as they occur in the natural setting. Indirect assessment involves gathering information retrospectively (e.g., through interviews, questionnaires, or rating scales) or using product measures (e.g., schoolwork completed, incident reports). Although the process of behavioral assessment typically gets started with interviews of the teachers, parents, staff, and student to identify possible target behaviors and obtain preliminary information on their level of occurrence, direct assessment information is used to establish the baseline levels of the target behaviors and to evaluate levels after the behavior support plan is in place. Given the importance of direct observation assessment in the process of designing and implementing a support plan, this chapter focuses on recording procedures involving direct observation of the target behaviors. This chapter also briefly discusses the use of permanent product measures and social validity assessments to evaluate progress when a PBS program is implemented.

Although this chapter focuses on the measurement of specific target behaviors to evaluate the success of a PBS plan, it must be noted that the plan should also produce meaningful lifestyle changes. Chapter 11 discusses ways to evaluate broader and long-term outcomes (lifestyle changes) associated with the implementation of PBS.

DIRECT OBSERVATION

To record the target behaviors successfully as part of a behavior support plan, team members must consider each of the following five steps: (1) Define the target behaviors, (2) decide when and where recording will occur, (3) decide who will record the target behaviors, (4) choose the most appropriate recording method, and (5) choose the most appropriate recording instrument (Miltenberger, 2004). The following sections detail these steps.

Defining the Target Behaviors

The first step in developing a plan for recording behavior is to define the target behaviors objectively. This is also the first step of the entire PBS process (see Chapter 3). To define the target behaviors, the team must identify exactly what the student says and does that constitute the problem and the desirable behavior.

1. A good behavioral definition will include active verbs that describe the observable actions of the student.

2. A label for the behavior does not define the behavior. For example, defining Nolan's problem behavior as "aggressive behavior" is simply labeling the behavior. On the other hand, defining Nolan's problem behavior as "slapping another student on the head" is identifying the behavior that has been labeled "aggressive."

3. A behavioral definition is clear and unambiguous; it does not make references to internal states or infer motivation. For example, saying that "Nolan slaps another student on the head when he is frustrated" is making an inference about an internal state. Likewise, saying that "Nolan slaps another student on the head when he wants a toy" is making an inference about the motivation for the behavior. In either case, reference to an internal state or an inference about motivation is superfluous to a good behavior definition. However, information about motivating events will be assessed in the course of a functional behavioral assessment (see Chapter 6), to try to determine what factors are influencing the behavior (e.g., Carr, McConnachie, Carlson, Kemp, & Smith, 1994; Chandler & Dahlquist, 2002; O'Neill et al., 1997).

4. A behavioral definition should be thorough; that is, it should include all of the different responses involved in the behavior being defined. If any of the responses that constitute the behavior are not included, then the person recording the behavior may fail to record each instance of the behavior.

5. One measure of a good behavioral definition is that two independent observers can observe the student at the same time and, based on the behavioral definition, agree whether or not the behavior is occurring (Bailey & Burch, 2002).

Table 5.1 lists some behavioral definitions for Nolan's behavior problems and desirable alternative behaviors. It is important to note that there is

TABLE 5.1. Behavioral Definitions for Nolan's Problem and Alternative Behaviors

---

Disruptive behavior

- Calling other students names (e.g., "You're stupid") or yelling at other students (e.g., "Shut up")
- Grabbing toys or materials from other students, running away with toys or materials, and/or blocking other students from accessing toys or materials
- Crying or sobbing
- Banging hands or feet on desks or other surfaces

Aggressive behavior

- Making a fist and threatening to punch or hit another student
- Punching, pushing, shoving, or kicking (or attempting to punch, shove, push, or kick) another student

Off-task behavior

- Looking around the room or out the window, putting head on desk or face in hands, getting out of seat, or playing with a toy when the teacher is providing group instruction to the class
- Engaging in any other activity except assigned seatwork when independent work is assigned
- Engaging in any other activity except assigned group work when group activities are assigned

Sharing

- Offering a toy or material to another student, providing a toy or material to another student upon request, or politely asking another student for a turn to use a toy or material

Cooperative play

- Engaging in a play activity with another student that involves interacting with the other student in the context of the activity

---

no such thing as a standard behavioral definition for a particular class of problem behavior or desirable behavior. Instead, target behaviors must be specifically defined for the individual in question, because it is unlikely that any two individuals will present with exactly the same behaviors.

Deciding When and Where Recording Will Take Place

Once the target behaviors are defined, the team must decide when and where observation and recording of the behavior will take place. Recording should occur at the times when the problem behavior is most likely to occur (and the desirable behavior is needed), so that representative samples of the behavior can be obtained. If the problem behavior occurs across the day in multiple settings, then recording should occur across the day in multiple settings. If the problem behavior occurs only in particular classes or at particular times, then recording should occur primarily at those times and places, with occasional recording in other settings to determine whether the behavior has generalized to other settings. Although the team wants to record the behavior wherever it occurs, the team should not burden teachers or paraprofessionals with data collection procedures if the behavior does not occur in their classes. One characteristic of a good behavior-recording plan is that it is practical or efficient, requiring the least amount of time or effort to carry out. In this way, it is more likely that the individuals responsible for recording the behavior will conduct the recording successfully.

Deciding Who Will Carry Out Behavior Recording

In most cases, a team of individuals will be involved in the development and implementation of a behavior support plan. These individuals may include a behavior support specialist, teachers, paraprofessionals, parents, support staff, administrators, and possibly others. Because several individuals are involved in the process, it is important to identify which individual(s) will be responsible for data collection (and intervention implementation) at any particular time. If the individual responsible for recording the behavior at a particular time is not clearly specified, one person may incorrectly assume that another person is recording the behavior. For example, a teacher may assume that a paraprofessional is recording the student's behavior in the class period, while the paraprofessional believes that the teacher is recording the behavior. As a result, recording may not be carried out in the class period, and valuable information about the behavior may therefore be lost. The person responsible for recording the behavior in a particular observation period should (1) be in a position to directly observe the student throughout the observation period, (2) have the necessary time available for observation and recording in the observation period, and (3) have the training necessary to carry out the observation and recording procedures.

Choosing a Recording Method

Once it has been established where and when recording will take place, and who will record the behavior, the next step is to choose a recording method. Choice of a recording method will be based on the characteristics of the behavior to be recorded, as well as practical considerations related to the observer and the setting. There are two types of recording procedures: *event recording*, in which every instance of the target behavior is recorded in the observation period, and *sampling procedures*, in which the target behavior is recorded as occurring or not occurring within specified intervals of time.

Event Recording

When an observer is conducting event recording, different dimensions or aspects of the behavior can be recorded so it is important to choose a recording method that captures the most relevant aspect(s) of the behavior. The dimensions of behavior that can be measured include frequency, duration, intensity, and latency.

Frequency is measured when the number of times the behavior occurs is the most important aspect of the behavior. For example, frequency recording can be used to record the number of times a student pushes other students in the observation period. If one goal is to decrease the number of times the student pushes other students, then a frequency measure will provide the best information to judge whether the student is achieving this goal.

Duration is measured when the most important aspect of the behavior is how long it lasts when it occurs. If one goal is to increase the total time of occurrence of a desirable behavior, then a duration measure will allow the team to assess progress toward this goal. For example, if increasing the time a student spends engaged in cooperative play is a goal, then the duration of cooperative play will be an appropriate dimension of the behavior to measure. In the process of recording duration, the observer may also generate a measure of frequency because he or she records the time when each occurrence of the behavior starts and stops.

Intensity is measured when the force or magnitude of the behavior is the most important aspect of the behavior or the aspect of the behavior that is targeted for change. Intensity can be measured with a rating scale or specific instruments. For example, if the loudness of a student's screaming during a tantrum is being targeted for change, an observer may use a rating scale to measure the intensity of a student's behaviors during a tantrum (e.g., loudness of screaming). Intensity ratings are sometimes used to assess emotional responding or mood states by rating overt behaviors as an indication of the particular emotion or mood. If a rating scale is used, the points on the scale should have descriptive anchors to facilitate reliable recording. For example, Carr, McLaughlin, Giacobbe-Grieco, and Smith (2003) investigated the relationship between individuals' moods and subsequent problem behaviors, and used a rating scale to assess the intensity of the individuals' moods. Carr et al. (2003, p. 55) included the following descriptive anchors on their 0–5 rating scale:

Yelling, pouting. Appears to be irritable, angry, or frustrated. This person does not seem to be enjoying things (score 0 or 1 depending on the extent of unhappiness).

Does not appear to be decidedly happy or particularly unhappy. May smile or frown occasionally, but overall seems rather neutral (score 2 or 3 depending on extent of happiness).

Smiles, laughs appropriately; seems to be enjoying things (score 4 or 5 depending on extent of enjoyment).

Latency is measured when the most important aspect of the behavior is how long it takes the student to initiate the behavior following some event. For example, if the goal is to get a student to start working immediately upon request, an observer may record the number of seconds it takes for a student to begin working on a task after the request to begin working is made.

In some cases, more than one dimension of the target behavior may be recorded if the goal is to change multiple aspects of the behavior. For example, the team may wish to increase the frequency and duration of appropriate social interaction, or to decrease the frequency and intensity of tantrums. If more than one dimension of the behavior is relevant, then multiple dimensions of the behavior should be recorded.

Percentage of trials or percent correct is one final way in which event recording may be conducted. In this method, an observer records the occurrence of a behavior in relation to some other event, such as a learning trial or a response opportunity. To say that a student complies with a teacher's requests 11 times during the observation period or gets 13 words correct on a spelling test is inadequate information, because there is no mention of response opportunities. Reporting the results in terms of the number of times the behavior occurs divided by the number of opportunities provides more useful information. If the teacher makes 12 requests and the student complies with the teachers' requests 11 times, the percentage of compliance is 11/12, or 92%. However, if the teachers made 25 requests and the student complies 11 times, the percentage is only 44%—a much less acceptable level of the behavior.

Sampling Methods

When sampling methods are used for behavior recording, the observer does not record each instance of the behavior. Rather, the observation period is divided into periods of time or intervals, and the observer records whether the behavior occurred or not in each interval. Sampling methods may be best when behaviors that occur at a high rate are being recorded, or when the observer has competing responsibilities that make event recording more difficult. There are two types of sampling procedures: *interval recording* and *time sample recording*.

In interval recording, the observer records the presence or absence of the behavior in consecutive intervals of time. For example, a class period may be divided into consecutive 10-minute intervals, and the observer records whether a student's problem behavior or appropriate behavior occurs within each 10-minute interval. The observer does not record each instance of the behavior in the interval, but rather simply notes whether the behavior occurs or not. The behavior is scored once in an interval if it occurs one or more times.

In time sample recording, the observer records the occurrence or non-occurrence of the behavior in nonconsecutive intervals of time. The recording intervals are separated by periods of time without recording. For example, an observer may observe and record a student's disruptive behavior or task-related behavior in the classroom for 10 seconds every 1 minute. In the 10-second observation period, the student's behavior is recorded as occurring or not occurring. No observation or recording occurs in the 50 seconds between observation intervals.

In both interval and time sample recording, the results of recording in the observation period will be reported as the percentage of intervals scored. The percentage of intervals scored is calculated by dividing the number of intervals in which the target behavior is observed by the total number of intervals in the observation period.

Choosing a Recording Instrument

The final step in the process of developing a plan for recording behavior is to choose a recording instrument. In most cases, paper-and-pencil instruments are used to record the behavior. The observer is given a data sheet on which to record each occurrence of the behavior (for event recording), or to record the intervals in which the behavior occurred (for sampling methods). Data sheets are typically structured to make it easy for the observer to record the behavior.

Figure 5.1 shows an example of a data sheet that can be used for recording the frequency of a target behavior. Note that there is a space to indicate the day in which observation is taking place, followed by spaces to indicate each occurrence of the behavior on that day. The data sheet also has a space for the name of the student and the definition of the target behavior, so it is clear who is being observed and what behavior is being recorded. With this data sheet (or a similar one), the observer puts an × or a check mark in a box to record an occurrence of the behavior. Alternatively, the observer can write the time of occurrence of the behavior in the

Frequency Data Sheet

Name _____

Definition of behavior being recorded _____

_____

_____

Obs. initials	Date/ time	Frequency										Daily total
		1	2	3	4	5	6	7	8	9	10	

FIGURE 5.1. This frequency data sheet is used to record each instance of the target behavior. Each time the behavior occurs, the observer puts an × or check mark in a box for that day.

box, to generate information on the frequency and the times of day that the behavior occurs. If the observer is recording more than one behavior, the observer can write a code in the box to indicate which behavior occurs. For example, if recording aggressive behavior and noncompliance, the observer can use an A and N to indicate the respective behaviors.

Figure 5.2 shows a data sheet that can be used for recording the duration of a target behavior. The data sheet has spaces to record the times that each instance of the behavior starts (onset) and stops (offset). By recording the onset and offset of each instance of the behavior each day, the team will be able to determine the total duration of the behavior each day (daily total), as well as the average duration of each occurrence of the behavior (average duration = total duration divided by the frequency of the behavior). The team will also be able to see the times that the behavior occurs each day.

Duration Data Sheet

Name _____

Definition of behavior being recorded _____

_____

_____

Duration

Obs. initials	Date/ time	Start	Stop	Start	Stop	Start	Stop	Start	Stop	Start	Stop	Daily total

FIGURE 5.2. This duration data sheet is used to record the time of onset and offset of each instance of the target behavior.

Figure 5.3 shows a data sheet that can be used for interval or time sample recording. This data sheet is structured for using 10-minute interval recording across different class periods of the day. A similar data sheet can be developed for shorter observation intervals, such as 10-second interval recording in a 15-minute observation period; longer observation intervals, such as 30-minute interval recording across the day; or any other interval arrangement that is desired. To use an interval data sheet, the observer puts an × or a check mark in a box if the target behavior occurs in that interval of time. If the target behavior does not occur in that interval, the interval box is left blank. The observer must have a way to time the intervals, so that he or she knows in which interval box to record the behavior. For 10-second interval recording, the observer can use an audiotape recording to indicate the consecutive observation intervals. For longer observation intervals (e.g., 10- or 15-minute intervals), a teacher can use a watch or a timer to signal the consecutive intervals.

Interval Data Sheet

Name _____

Definition of behavior being recorded _____

_____

_____

Obs.	Date/	Ten-minute intervals					
initials	time	1	2	3	4	5	6

FIGURE 5.3. This interval data sheet is used to record the occurrence or nonoccurrence of the target behavior in consecutive 10-minute intervals in an observation period.

In addition to data sheets for recording behavior, other recording instruments are available. For example, an observer can use a hand-held counter or a wrist counter (such as a golf stroke counter) to record the frequency of a target behavior. If a teacher is the observer, he or she can place small check marks in the corner of a chalkboard or white board to record occurrences of a target behavior (this will have to be done without other students' knowledge that a fellow student's behavior is being recorded). An observer can use a wristwatch with a stopwatch function to record the duration of a target behavior. A personal digital assistant (PDA) or hand-held computer (Kahng & Iwata, 1998) can also be programmed to permit recording of the frequency or duration of behavior. Other creative recording instruments can be devised as well. The main consideration is that, whatever recording instrument is used, it must permit the observer to record the target behavior immediately as it occurs. The observer also must write down the results of recording on a data summary sheet or plot the data on a graph immediately after the observation period, so there is a permanent record of the results. If a PDA or computer is used, the observer must download or store the data soon after an observation session, so that the data are not lost.

GRAPHING AND EVALUATING BEHAVIOR CHANGE

Members of a team implementing a support plan will record the target behavior to determine whether the plan has produced a beneficial change in the behavior. The graph is a valuable tool for evaluating behavior change resulting from an intervention. A graph shows the level of the target behavior across time (days or observation periods). Each data point on a graph gives the team two types of information: the level of the target behavior, and the day or session during which the target behavior was observed.

Graphing Behavior

Six steps are necessary to construct a graph (Miltenberger, 2004). First, a vertical line (called the *vertical axis*) and a horizontal line (the *horizontal axis*) are drawn on a sheet of graph paper, with the intersection in the lower left corner.

Second, each axis is labeled. The behavior is labeled on the vertical axis, and the time period of observations is labeled on the horizontal axis. For example, the vertical axis can be labeled "Number of head hits" and the horizontal axis can be labeled "Days" when a student's self-injurious behavior is being recorded over time.

Third, the units on the vertical and horizontal axes are numbered to correspond to the expected level of the behavior and the time frame of observations, respectively. For example, if the student hits her head up to 20 times per day, then the vertical axis will be numbered from 0 to 20. If the behavior is to be recorded at school over a 2-month period, then the horizontal axis will be numbered from 1 to 40 or 45.

Fourth, a data point is plotted on the graph each day or after each observation session (or as soon after as possible). To plot a data point, the observer locates the coordinate on the graph that corresponds to the level of the behavior (on the vertical axis) and the day of the observation (on the horizontal axis).

Fifth, a phase line is inserted in the graph to indicate a change from the baseline phase to the intervention phase. A *phase line* is a vertical line that separates the two phases and allows the viewer to better judge the level of the behavior in each phase.

Sixth, each phase is labeled so that the person viewing the graph can see whether the data points reflect baseline or intervention observations. For example, the word "Baseline" is written at the top of the baseline phase, and a descriptive label for the intervention (e.g., "Choice of academic task") is written at the top of the intervention phase.

Evaluating Level and Trend

Once data points are plotted on a graph across baseline and intervention phases, the team can look at the graph to evaluate the nature of the behavior change resulting from the support plan (Parsonson & Baer, 1986). Two aspects of the data are evaluated to judge the effects of an intervention: the level of the behavior in each phase, and any trend in the data.

Level

The *level* of the behavior refers to how much the behavior is occurring in observation sessions in baseline and intervention phases, as judged by its frequency, duration, or intensity, or by the percentage of intervals of its occurrence. If a goal of the support plan is to decrease occurrences of a problem behavior, then the graph should show a lower level of the behavior in the intervention phase than in the baseline phase. If a goal is to increase a desirable behavior, the graph should show a higher level of the behavior in the intervention phase than in the baseline phase. If there is a specified goal level for the behavior, then evaluation of the graph will indicate whether the behavior has decreased or increased to this particular level. Changes in the level of the behavior across phases can be quickly and easily determined through visual inspection of the data in graphic form.

Trend

A *trend* in the data refers to whether the level of the behavior is increasing or decreasing within the baseline or intervention phase. In many cases, the effects of a behavior support plan take time to develop. Therefore, there may not be an immediate difference in the level of the behavior from the baseline phase to the beginning of the intervention phase. However, a trend in the level of the behavior in the expected direction in the intervention phase suggests that the support plan is producing the desired change in the behavior. It is important to continue recording the behavior over time to determine the ultimate level of the behavior when a trend occurs in an intervention phase. Figure 5.4 shows an effective support plan for a problem behavior (cursing) in which the changes in the levels of the problem behavior and the desirable alternative behavior (requesting assistance) are immediate (there is no trend in the data for either behavior). Figure 5.5 shows an effective support plan in which the changes in the target behaviors are more gradual (there is a downward trend in the problem behavior and an upward trend in the desirable behavior).

If the behavior is already trending in the desired direction during the baseline phase, it may be prudent to delay introducing the support plan for a period of time to see where the behavior will stabilize (i.e., where there is no more trend for a period of time). After the behavior stabilizes, the team should determine whether additional behavior support is still warranted. Sometimes a target behavior will change in the desired direction before a support plan is implemented, simply because someone is recording the behavior or because some other events have influenced the behavior. In either case, it is important to continue recording and graphing the behavior to determine whether the behavior change is maintained or whether behavior support becomes necessary in the future.

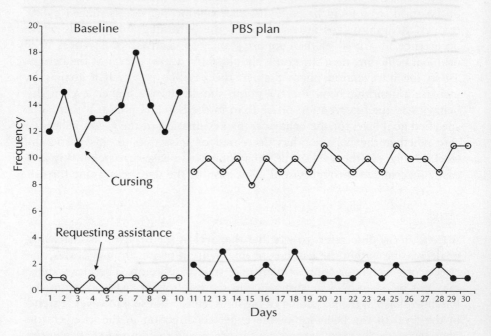

FIGURE 5.4. This graph shows the frequency of cursing and of requesting assistance each day in baseline and intervention phases. The levels of cursing and of requesting assistance both change immediately once the PBS plan is implemented.

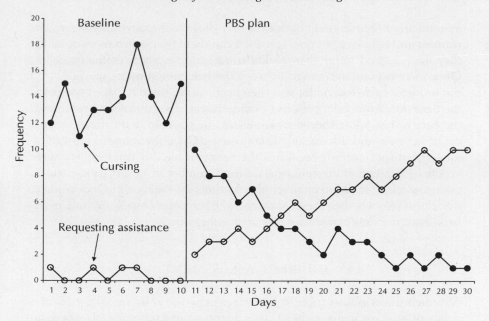

FIGURE 5.5. This graph shows the frequency of cursing and of requesting assistance each day in baseline and intervention phases. There is a downward trend in the level of cursing and an upward trend in the level of requesting assistance in the intervention phase, showing that the intervention is changing the behaviors more gradually.

OBSERVER TRAINING

Once the behavior-recording plan is developed and ready for use, individuals must be trained to carry out observations before beginning to observe and record the target behavior. At a minimum, observer training consists of a review of the target behavior definition; discussion of who is to record the behavior, where, and when; and instructions in how to use the data sheet to record instances of the behavior. Although this level of instruction may be sufficient for some individuals with prior experience in carrying out behavior-recording procedures, other individuals may need further training to carry out the procedures reliably. For these individuals, a behavior support specialist or other individual with behavior-recording experience will arrange one or more practice sessions of recording.

The first practice session begins with the behavior support specialist and the trainees (teachers, paraprofessionals, support staff, or others) unobtrusively observing the student from the same location and simply announcing to one another each time they observe the target behavior. The trainees and behavior support specialist can then discuss instances in which they disagree and refine their ability to identify instances of the behavior. Once there is good agreement between the behavior support specialist and the trainees, each individual will then begin using the data sheet to record the behavior. After brief periods of independent observation and recording, the behavior support specialist will check the trainees' data sheets against his or her own and discuss any discrepancies. Once the trainees and behavior support specialist are recording the behavior reliably (they largely agree on the occurrence of the behavior) across a number of observation periods, the trainees are ready to conduct observations on their own. Once trained, the observers (whether they are teachers, paraprofessionals, or staff members) may then take an active role in training others.

INDIRECT ASSESSMENT

Although direct observation of the target behavior is an integral part of a behavior support plan, indirect assessment procedures may also be conducted to supplement the data collected through direct observation. Collecting information from memory through interviews or questionnaires is one form of indirect assessment. Another form of indirect assessment involves recording permanent products of the behavior. Still another form of indirect assessment is the collection of individuals' perceptions or subjective evaluations of changes in the target behavior resulting from intervention, often referred to as *social validation*. A brief description of the use of product measures and social validity assessment follows.

Product Measures

Product measures are useful when the target behavior results in permanent products or changes in the physical environment that can be counted or evaluated later as an indication of the occurrence of the target behavior. Product measures are particularly useful when the observer cannot be present continuously to observe the target behavior, such as when a teacher must work with all of the students in a classroom and cannot observe a particular student's academic work continuously throughout the class period. In such cases, the teacher can evaluate the products of the student's work (number of addition problems completed correctly, number of questions answered correctly on an assignment, etc.). Completed academic work is a useful product measure because of its one-to-one correspondence to academic behavior.

Not all target behaviors result in permanent products, however, so the use of product recording is necessarily limited. Many, if not most, problem behaviors do not result in permanent products; once the behavior has occurred, there is no lasting effect on the physical environment to record. Therefore, product measures are of limited utility with many problem behaviors. In cases where problem behaviors do produce physical products, there may not be a one-to-one relationship between the behavior and the product. For example, scratches, bruises, or cuts resulting from self-injurious behavior are physical products of the behavior, but there is no indication how much behavior the individual has engaged in to produce the physical damage. Likewise, hair pulling may produce bald spots on the scalp, but one cannot determine the frequency or duration of hair pulling from examination of the size of the bald area or the thickness of the hair in the affected area. Nonetheless, using rating scales or other physical indices to measure the damage from self-injurious behavior can be a valuable complement to direct observation of the behavior that has produced the damage (Iwata, Pace, Kissel, Nau, & Farber, 1990; Rapp, Miltenberger, Long, Elliott, & Lumley, 1998).

Other types of product measures that might be useful in an academic setting are school records, which are broad indications of the occurrence of desirable academic behaviors or interfering problem behaviors. Such records may include attendance records, injury reports, incidence reports, or grades. Although such records do not have the same utility as product measures that bear a one-to-one relationship to the behavior, school records can be useful adjuncts to other behavior-recording procedures. One can expect that changes in the behavior documented through direct observation or other product measures will correspond to changes in these broad product measures. Therefore, these broad product measures, when available, can be used to validate the results of a behavior support plan.

Social Validity

One other way to validate the results of an intervention is through the use of subjective ratings of improvement in the target behavior or improvement in the student's life more generally, called *social validation* (Kazdin, 1977; Wolf, 1978). It is not only important for the objective results of data collection to show an improvement in the target behavior; it is also important for the changes in behavior to be noticeable and meaningful to significant individuals in the student's life (parents, support staff, teachers, etc.). Assessing the social validity of the results of a support plan will determine whether significant individuals judge the student's behavior to be improved and whether they are pleased with the improvement in the behavior. Furthermore, assessing the social validity of an intervention may help determine whether the intervention has resulted in other important outcomes for the student. For example, is the student engaging in more activities with peers, forming new friendships, or working more independently?

Social validity of the results of an intervention can be assessed with a brief questionnaire in which significant individuals use a rating scale to answer a small number of questions. Individuals can provide their ratings at some point when the support plan has been implemented or after it has been faded. Alternatively, individuals can provide ratings after watching videotapes of the student before and after the intervention to evaluate improvement resulting from the intervention. Examples of questions that can be included in social validity questionnaires are presented in Figure 5.6.

To what extent are you pleased with the improvement in Nolan's behavior?				
1	2	3	4	5
Very displeased	Somewhat displeased	Neutral	Somewhat pleased	Very pleased
How would you judge Nolan's ability to stay on task since the intervention?				
1	2	3	4	5
Much worse	Somewhat worse	The same	Somewhat improved	Much improved
How well does Nolan interact with his peers?				
1	2	3	4	5
Very poorly	Poorly	Neutral	Well	Very well
How appropriate is Nolan's behavior in comparison to his classmates?				
1	2	3	4	5
Very inappropriate	Somewhat inappropriate	Neutral	Somewhat appropriate	Very appropriate
How satisfied are you with the changes in Nolan's behavior as a result of the plan?				
1	2	3	4	5
Very dissatisfied	Somewhat dissatisfied	Neutral	Somewhat satisfied	Very satisfied
Overall, how has the quality of Nolan's life changed as a result of the plan?				
1	2	3	4	5
Much worse	Somewhat worse	No change	Somewhat improved	Much improved

FIGURE 5.6. Examples of social validation questions.

SUMMARY

Behavioral assessment is an integral step in the process of implementing a PBS plan. By directly observing, recording, and graphing the target behaviors before and after the plan is implemented, the team can assess changes in the behavior and evaluate the student's progress. This chapter has discussed the steps involved in developing a behavior-recording plan: (1) defining the target behaviors, (2) deciding when and where recording will take place, (3) deciding who will record the target behaviors, (4) deciding what recording method to use, and (5) deciding what recording instrument to use. The chapter has also described the process of graphing behavior and evaluating behavior change. Finally, the chapter has discussed two indirect assessment methods, product recording and social validity assessment, that can complement the use of direct assessment to help determine the effectiveness of a behavior support plan.

CASE EXAMPLES

Defining and Measuring Malik's Behavior

Malik's team knew that in order to begin the functional assessment process, and also to determine whether the support plan they were about to develop was effective, they needed to have a way to measure Malik's problem behaviors. The first step was to prioritize and define the behaviors the team wanted to decrease. The team agreed on two priorities and definitions. The first was *aggression*, which they defined as Malik's pushing, hitting, or biting others, and/or throwing or destroying materials. The second priority was *refusal*, which was defined as Malik's physically or verbally expressing "no," failing to follow directions, and/or flopping on the floor.

The second step was to determine who would carry out the recording. Malik's team decided to attempt to collect data across the entire day. They believed they could deveop a simple form of data collection that would be easy to use, but it would have to be carried out by more than one person. Mr. Rodriguez, the behavior specialist, Mrs. Nelson, the classroom teacher, and the classroom aide all agreed to pitch in with data collection. Mrs. Nelson and the classroom aide suggested they could collect data in the classroom. Mr. Rodriquez offered to collect data at times when the classroom staff was not with Malik, such as during cafeteria activities.

The third step was to come up with a way of measuring these behaviors. Electing to use a simple frequency count, Mrs. Nelson, the teaching assistant, and Mr. Rodriguez would record, throughout the school day, each time an episode of aggression and refusal occurred by keeping a tally of each. An episode was defined by the onset and offset of a problem behavior associated with a particular task or activity. Thus, if Malik refused to make the transition from art to reading, this would be counted as one episode, regardless of the number of times he said "no." Later, if he refused to make the transition to a second activity, that would be counted as a second episode. Because neither problem behavior occurred at a rate too numerous to count, Mrs. Nelson and the teaching assistant felt confident that they could keep an accurate record without too much trouble.

The final step was to choose a recording instrument. The team elected to use a simple pencil-and-paper approach whereby both target behaviors could be recorded with a single instrument. At the same time, they could also note occurences of appropriate replacement behaviors, such as requests for a break. Mr. Rodriguez constructed a data collection sheet so that the frequency of inappropriate and appropriate behaviors could be noted in columns corresponding to each class period and the transitions between. Armed with a clear definition of problem behaviors and a way to measure them, Malik's team was ready to begin the functional assessment process.

Defining and Measuring Bethany's Behavior

The members of Bethany's team also first set out to define the behaviors they wanted to focus on during the functional assessment. The team unilaterally agreed that Bethany had two primary problem behaviors. The first was that she failed to engage in class assignments. The team termed this *off-task behavior* and defined it as failing to engage in assigned work or to follow teacher instructions. Bethany's teachers noted that this usually took the form of wandering about the classroom, putting her head on her desk (and sometimes sleeping), and talking with peers.

The second problematic behavior, generally observed outside the classroom, was *poor peer relations*. This was defined as making inappropriate or derogatory comments to peers.

After defining the problem behaviors, the team discussed who would collect data. The team members thought it was important to document as many incidents of problem behavior as they could during the functional assessment. Therefore, Bethany's general education teacher agreed to conduct observations whenever she was not directly teaching or when a volunteer was in the classroom. Bethany's special education teacher and the school psychologist also agreed to complete some observations. In addition, the school psychologist agreed to conduct some observations outside the classroom.

The team members believed that it was well worth their time and effort to conduct direct observations to determine whether the support plan was effective after it was developed. But they knew that such intensive efforts were not feasible on an ongoing basis. Brittany's general education teacher needed a simpler strategy that would not distract her from teaching a class full of students. She remembered learning about an approach called *time sampling*. Using this approach, she would set a timer to sound periodically, then briefly look at Bethany and note whether she was on task or off task. She thought it would be feasible to do this once every 10 minutes, at least until the team could get an idea of whether the support plan was working. The school purchased a vibrating watch that would cue her at the end of each 10-minute interval, without distracting her students. The special education teacher photocopied an event-recording data sheet from a textbook she had used in a prior class. The team felt that this measurement strategy would provide a good enough representation of Bethany's behavior, while still being feasible for the teacher.

Next, a process for data collection was needed for interactions outside the classroom, including where data would be collected, who would collect the data, and what instrument and method of recording would be used. Because the cafeteria was staffed with a number of volunteer monitors, the team solicited their assistance. One of the volunteers agreed to collect data on Bethany's interactions. She did, however, need to monitor other students in the cafeteria; still, she felt that she could collect data for two 5-minute intervals during the lunch period while tending to her other responsibilities. The team concluded that the best way to measure interactions was to use a frequency count, noting each time inappropriate or derogatory comments to peers occurred. The volunteer suggested that an easy way to do this would be to use her husband's golf counter, which she could keep in her pocket, out of sight of the students. With behaviors defined and a strategy for measurement, the team was ready to begin the functional assessment process, described at the end of Chapter 6. In addition, they had a strategy for collecting data during baseline and after the support plan was implemented.

REFERENCES

Bailey, J. S., & Burch, M. R. (2002). *Research methods in applied behavior analysis*. Thousand Oaks, CA: Sage.

Carr, E. G., McConnachie, G., Carlson, J. I., Kemp, D. C., & Smith, C. E. (1994). *Communication-based interventions for problem behavior: A user's guide for producing positive change*. Baltimore: Brookes.

Carr, E. G., McLaughlin, D. M., Giacobbe-Grieco, T., & Smith, C. E. (2003). Using mood ratings and mood induction is assessment and intervention for severe problem behavior. *American Journal on Mental Retardation, 108,* 32–55.

Chandler, L. K., & Dahlquist, C. M. (2002). *Functional assessment: Strategies to prevent and remediate challenging behavior in school settings*. Upper Saddle River, NJ: Merrill/Prentice Hall.

Iwata, B. A., Pace, G. M., Kissel, R. C., Nau, P. A., & Farber, J. M. (1990). The Self-Injury Trauma (SIT) Scale: A method for quantifying surface tissue damage caused by self-injurious behavior. *Journal of Applied Behavior Analysis, 23,* 99–110.

Iwata, B. A., Vollmer, T. R., Zarcone, J. R., & Rodgers, T. A. (1993). Treatment classification and selection based on behavioral function. In R. Van Houten & S. Axelrod (Eds.), *Behavior analysis and treatment* (pp. 101–125). New York: Plenum Press.

Kahng, S., & Iwata, B. A. (1998). Computerized systems for collecting real-time observational data. *Journal of Applied Behavior Analysis, 31,* 253–261.

Kazdin, A. E. (1977). Assessing the clinical and applied significance of behavior change through social validation. *Behavior Modification, 1,* 427–452.

Miltenberger, R. G. (2004). *Behavior modification: Principles and procedures* (3rd ed.). Pacific Grove, CA: Wadsworth.

O'Neill, R. E., Horner, R. H., Albin, R. W., Sprague, J., Storey, K., & Newton, J. S. (1997). *Functional assessment and program development for problem behavior: A practical handbook* (2nd ed.). Pacific Grove, CA: Brooks/Cole.

Parsonson, B. S., & Baer, D. M. (1986). The graphic analysis of data. In A. Poling & R. W. Fuqua (Eds.), *Research methods in applied behavior analysis* (pp. 157–186). New York: Plenum Press.

Rapp, J. T., Miltenberger, R. G., Long, E. S., Elliott, A. J., & Lumley, V. A. (1998). Simplified habit reversal treatment for chronic hair pulling in three adolescents: A clinical replication with direct observation. *Journal of Applied Behavior Analysis, 31,* 299–302.

Wolf, M. M. (1978). Social validity: The case for subjective measurement, or how applied behavior analysis is finding its heart. *Journal of Applied Behavior Analysis, 11,* 203–214.

CHAPTER 6

♦ ♦ ♦

Gathering Functional
Assessment Information

♦

LEE KERN
ROBERT E. O'NEILL
KRISTIN STAROSTA

The foundation of every positive behavior support (PBS) plan is a *functional assessment* (also referred to as a *functional behavioral assessment*). Functional assessment defines a process of gathering a collection of information about an individual and his or her environment. The outcome of a functional assessment is a documentation of events related to problem behavior, as described in the four-term contingency model introduced in Chapter 2. That is, it will define setting events, antecedents, and maintaining consequences related to problem behavior. In addition, it will reveal broad lifestyle issues that need to be enhanced to improve an individual's life in general. This information is essential for identifying effective and efficient ways to reduce undesirable behavior, increase desirable behavior, and ensure a good quality of life.

Because effective and enduring behavior support plans include multiple components and address all areas of an individual's life, the assessment information must be comprehensive. Specifically, it should document both historical and current events, and should reveal issues both immediately and peripherally related to challenging behavior. In addition, information that is derived in various ways (e.g., through interviews, record reviews, and direct observation) and from multiple informants (e.g., family members, teachers, mental health workers) engenders a richer, more multifaceted understanding of the individual.

When a team is beginning the assessment process, it is important to keep in mind that the information gathered should be useful for developing a support plan for behavior improvement. There are multitudes of assessments that are routinely administered to children and adults, especially those with disabilities, but that do not provide the types of information needed to build a support plan. For instance, tests of intelligence do not specify the skills that an individual possesses, nor do they indicate events in the environment that are associated with desirable and undesirable behavior. Information pertinent to support plan development focuses on understanding the issues and variables related to challenging behavior, as well as strategies to eliminate it. Ultimately, the information gathered during this process should allow the support team to formulate summary statements or hypotheses about why the challenging behavior occurs and what changes can be made so that it will not occur in the future, as described in Chapter 7.

As discussed in Chapter 3, the first step for designing a PBS plan is to prioritize and define the problem behavior. Chapters 3 and 5 offer detailed procedures and considerations for completing Step 1. This chapter will guide readers through Step 2 of the PBS process: conducting a functional assessment.

GATHERING RELEVANT INFORMATION

Conducting a functional assessment primarily involves information gathering. Although information that will contribute to developing a support plan comes in many forms, it can be grouped generally into two broad categories. The first category is *broad information*. Broad information may include relevant history and quality-of-life variables. This type of information paints a "big picture" of the individual and his or her life. That is, it creates an understanding of general lifestyle arrangements and of how prior events an individual has experienced may affect current and future behavior and learning. Knowledge of these issues also aids in understanding how and why challenging behavior has developed, and in identifying aspects of an individual's lifestyle and general well-being that are objectionable and may indirectly contribute to problem behavior. In addition, broad information assists in determining long-term supports that will produce meaningful outcomes over time, as described in Chapter 11.

The second type of information that is essential for support plan development is *specific information*. Specific information pertains directly to those events that are immediate to the problem behavior. In other words, this type of information details antecedent events that evoke problem behavior, setting events that combine with antecedents to cause problem behavior, and maintaining consequences that reinforce or encourage the behavior to continue; together with the behavior itself, these phenomena are defined as the *four-term contingency*. Chapter 2 offers a detailed description of the framework underlying the four-term contingency. The importance of information about antecedents and setting events identified to cause problem behavior is that they can be modified or eliminated, while antecedents identified to result in desirable behavior can be increased. Similarly, consequences that reinforce problem behavior can be eliminated, while consequences that discourage problem behavior can be increased. The following sections further define the many forms of broad and specific information that may be useful for support plan development.

TYPES OF BROAD INFORMATION

Various types of broad information are relevant to the PBS process (see Table 6.1). The first type is *major life events*. Major life events often provide insight into why challenging behavior began or continues, and can shed light on intervention components that need to be included in the support plan. Important life events may include traumatic experiences, such as the death of someone close, parental divorce, a pattern of frequent moves, or serious illness. For example, information obtained about major life events helped team members to understand Jeanette's problem behaviors at school. Soon after Jeanette entered her first year of middle school, several teachers referred her to the school counselor because she appeared to be withdrawn and depressed. They indicated that she failed to participate in class or to complete assignments, and she rarely interacted with her peers. Historical information revealed that her mother and only sister had been killed in an automobile accident the previous school year. Her father had difficulty coping with the loss and decided that relocation to a different state would help him to move on with his life. As a sixth grader, Jeanette was just entering middle school, so her teachers were not aware of her relocation. This historical information allowed them to support her in coping with her loss, ease the transition to a new school and neighborhood, and formulate a peer support network.

The next type of broad information that will facilitate development of a support plan is *health factors and physical issues*. Health factors can influence both the occurrence of problem behavior and the effectiveness of a support plan. Mental health issues, such as depression and anxiety disorders, have a significant influence on an individual's general functioning and

TABLE 6.1. Types of Broad Information and Key Questions/Examples

Types of broad information	Key questions and examples
Major life events	Did the individual experience a traumatic event? • Death • Major illness Did a major life change occur? • Move • Parental divorce • School transfer
Health factors and physical issues	Are there mental health concerns? • Depression • Anxiety Is the individual healthy? • Allergy-free • Gets adequate sleep • Gets sufficient nutrition • Free of infections/illnesses
History of problem behavior	When did problem behavior begin? • Association with specific event How have others responded to problem behavior? • Reinforced or punished
Past interventions	What interventions showed signs of success? • Reductions in problem behavior • Increases in alternative behavior • Improvements in overall happiness What interventions were ineffective? • Increases in undesirable behavior • No change in undesirable behavior • Disliked • Difficult to implement
Academic skills/task performance	What key skills/tasks are critical? • Communication • Academic (reading, math, writing) • Organization • Activities of daily living • Social interactions
Strengths and weaknesses	What strengths can be capitalized upon? • Social skills • Motor skills What weaknesses need to be accommodated? • Cognitive limitations • Communication deficits • Physical limitations

(continued)

TABLE 6.1. *(continued)*

Types of broad informations	Key questions and examples
Preferences	What does the individual prefer or enjoy? • Learning approaches • People to be with • Recreation/leisure activities
Overall quality of life	Does the individual have regular access to meaningful events? • Preferred activities • Friends • Role models • Inclusive environments

also define situations that he or she may avoid or escape in some way. Spring allergies may cause an individual to feel physical discomfort, which can result in higher rates of challenging behaviors. An ear infection or an abscessed tooth can cause an individual without spoken language to engage in self-injurious behavior in an attempt to express pain. Difficulty with ambulation may cause a person to engage in problematic behaviors when asked to engage in activities that require walking or standing. Sleep problems may cause disruptive behaviors when strenuous or demanding tasks are requested.

Danielle provides an example of the relationship between health factors/physical issues and challenging behavior. Danielle, a high school student, spent part of her school day participating in a training program at the Salvation Army in preparation for future employment. She was observed to engage in frequent self-injury while at her worksite. Careful examination of her patterns of self-injury indicated that it occurred during physically demanding tasks, such as hanging heavy clothes on elevated racks. Her support staff noticed that during these activities she would sweat profusely and breathe heavily. Danielle's physician suggested that because of her obesity, she might not have the physical endurance to complete strenuous activities. When these activities were removed from her job tasks, her self-injury decreased.

An understanding of the *history of the problem behavior*, which includes how others have responded to the behavior, is also pertinent broad information. Historical information of this nature may help to determine why it began, why it continues, and perhaps what degree of support is needed to reduce it and teach new behaviors. For example, Elias was a boy who had experienced severe abuse and neglect in his early years. He had a great deal of difficulty trusting others, let alone making and maintaining friendships. Elias periodically engaged in extensive bouts of destruction, where he selectively demolished expensive classroom property, such as computers and televisions. In efforts to address these destructive episodes, Elias was moved to several different and increasingly restrictive classrooms and school programs. He finally ended up in a self-contained special education classroom with Ms. Chandler, who was determined to develop a trusting relationship with Elias and identify effective supports. At the end of one very difficult day, Elias engaged in a serious episode of destruction, ruining Ms. Chandler's laptop computer and several pieces of furniture. Following the incident, Ms. Chandler set out to collect as much information as she could to identify additional supports Elias needed so this would not happen again. Surprised by this response, Elias asked Ms. Chandler, "Aren't you going to send me to a different classroom now?" Through examining Elias's records, Ms. Chandler determined that each time a serious destructive incident occcurred, Elias had been moved to a different classroom. Because he believed that a different classroom would solve his problems, from Elias's perspective he was gainfully engaging in destructive episodes when he felt he could not cope with his current environment. Understanding how serious behavioral episodes had been shaped in the past helped Ms. Chandler to build a support plan that focused on building the skills necessary for Elias to deal appropriately with stressful situations, as well as to develop trust and friendships.

In addition to understanding the history of problem behavior, it is important to be aware of *past interventions*. Often a past intervention has resulted in some success. Conversely, knowledge of an unsuccessful past intervention can save a great deal of time. In our work with Eddie (Kern, Childs, Dunlap, Clarke, & Falk, 1994), a sixth-grade boy with poor attention skills, a previous teacher reported that she had sometimes used a kitchen timer with him to remind him when his task had to be completed. She indicated that this was partially successful. We relied upon this information when developing his support plan by including a self-management procedure in which a timer was set at 5-minute intervals. When the timer sounded, Eddie monitored whether or not he was engaged in the task. This cueing and monitoring procedure helped with his timely completion of tasks.

Academic skill/task performance is another important piece of broad information. It is unmistakable that there is a direct relationship between the ease with which students can perform a task and the occurrence of problem behavior. Consider the example of Enzo, a fourth-grade student. Enzo routinely antagonized the students sitting next to him in math class. As a result, his teacher often asked him to leave the classroom. However, she began to notice that inappropriate comments to his peers almost always occurred a few minutes before review of the previous night's homework.

His teacher discovered that Enzo did not complete his homework because he did not understand the assignments. Thus a complete picture of the state of a student's academic functioning or skill performance is important for interventions in the school setting. In addition to a complete understanding of an individual's skill level, it is important to be aware of whether the student has had a history of failure with activities or tasks. Many students with long histories of failure require very intensive interventions implemented over long periods of time to overcome feelings of inability or learned helplessness.

An additional and critical category of broad information is an individual's *strengths and weaknesses*. A well-designed behavior support plan will capitalize on a student's strengths and tackle his or her weaknesses. For example, Laticia's mother was concerned about her daughter's lack of communication. For nearly a year, Laticia had been learning to use a communication system that required her to remove one of several small 1-inch-square pictures with Velcro from a board and hand it to another person in order to indicate her wants and needs. Laticia wanted to communicate with others. She often walked toward other girls who were conversing in a group and tried to join them. However, because of her poor fine motor skills, she usually fumbled for several minutes attempting to remove a picture from the board, and frequently dropped the picture on the floor while she was handing it to a peer. In order to capitalize on her strong desire to communicate with her peers, Laticia's mother and teacher decided to teach her to use a voice output device for communication. This device only required her to touch a larger box lightly in order to communicate. This system compensated for Laticia's poor fine motor skills, while giving her the ability to talk with her friends as she had always wanted to do.

It is also important to know about the student's *preferences*. Preferences should be considered in the development of a support plan. This will assure that interventions are meaningful and valued, and it will increase the likelihood that the support plan will be successful. For instance, information about Stuart's preferences was used to craft an effective support plan. Stuart's test results indicated that he was gifted; however, he frequently engaged in disruptive classroom behavior. Assessment information indicated that he was bored with his classwork. His teacher identified several preferences and incorporated them into his assignments. During reading, he was allowed to select books about space or other topics of interest. Math assignments were modified so that required problems were interspersed with the opportunity for Stuart to create his own problems requiring calculations about distances between the planets. During writing, Stuart was permitted to choose a topic, rather than to write about the teacher-generated topic.

The final facet of broad information pertains to *overall quality of life.* When individuals have a less than adequate quality of life, problem behaviors are much more likely. It is important to identify issues that interfere with a reasonable or, better yet, rich quality of life. Considering quality-of-life issues requires an examination of features of a student's personal life that make it meaningful, are enjoyable, and prepare him or her for a successful future, as well as those features that create stress, unhappiness, or dependency. Among the many important lifestyle variables that should be available to individuals with disabilities are opportunities to engage in preferred leisure activities, to share time with friends, to access attention and assistance, to participate in inclusive environments, and to be exposed to role models or mentors. For individuals who are unable to communicate via spoken language, it is critical that they have an alternative means for communicating their needs, preferences, and desires.

Many barriers that can interfere with an individual's quality of life can contribute to problem behavior. These barriers range from the systemic (e.g., lack of resources to provide needed support for a student to enjoy inclusive situations, such as lunch in the cafeteria) to the personal (e.g., parental depression so severe that it interferes with the parent's ability to provide the student with adequate attention). During the assessment process, it is important to attempt to identify barriers so that strategies for overcoming them can be generated as part of the support plan. Lifestyle issues are discussed in much more detail in Chapter 11. In addition, Chapter 11 describes person-centered planning activities—a process to facilitate an understanding of the student, including gathering broad information. The remainder of this chapter focuses primarily on specific information.

TYPES OF SPECIFIC INFORMATION

Specific information details *antecedents*, or events in the immediate environment that occur before a problem behavior; *setting events*, or events that indirectly influence the role of antecedents and consequences associated with problem behavior; and *maintaining consequences*, or events in the immediate environment that occur after a problem behavior and are thought to contribute to continuance of the behavior. It is likewise important to identify antecedents, maintaining consequences, and setting events that result in desirable behavior.

Although it is often tempting to attribute problem behavior to internal or physiological states or to an individual's upbringing, specific information about antecedents and consequences must identify environmental events that can be both observed and modified. For example, teachers often state that students engage in problem behavior because they have attention-deficit/hyperactivity disorder (ADHD), a physiological imbalance, or a bad home. These attributions involve circular logic because they merely describe a constellation of behaviors, ungrounded assumptions, or presumed explanations that cannot be substantiated. They are not precise and do not offer specific information about events that are subject to modifications useful for support plan development. Although information such as a diagnosis of ADHD (or some other disorder) may serve a purpose, it does not implicate specific ways to intervene to reduce behavioral challenges. Useful information will specify variables or environmental features that are subject to direct observation and can be modified to create an intervention. Figure 6.1 offers key questions to guide the assessment of antecedents, setting events, and maintaining consequences of problem behavior. Each of these assessment areas is discussed below.

Information about Antecedents

Many different events can precede problem behavior. In the process of narrowing down the specific antecedents that incite problem behaviors, it may be helpful to focus on a few key pieces of information. First, it is useful to determine the time of day when the behavior usually occurs. Information about time of day may be useful for two reasons. First, it can streamline the assessment process by specifying when it would be most prudent to conduct additional direct observations. That is, it can serve as a starting point for determining when to collect more detailed information to isolate the specific antecedents for problem behavior. For example, Natalie's team was concerned with her disruptive classroom behavior. Her teachers began to document when the behaviors occurred. After 1 week of documentation, the data indicated that disruptions always occurred between 8:30 and 9:15. This happened to coincide with reading class. The information allowed Natalie's team to focus further information gathering on identifying aspects of reading or reading class that might be causing her problems.

Second, when problem behavior occurs throughout the day, patterns of higher and lower frequencies of challenging behaviors may be detectable. Thus it may be possible to detect commonalities across problematic and nonproblematic times. For example, an evaluation of the times when Chyna's disruptive behaviors occurred indicated that academic subjects that routinely required group work (e.g., science, social studies) were associated with higher frequencies of disruption, while academic subjects that only required independent activities (e.g., math, spelling) were associated with lower frequencies of disruption.

A second type of important specific information is the activity in which the individual is engaged. It is helpful to be as precise as possible when documenting the activity. For example, to identify the antecedents to

Types of specific information	Key questions to guide assessment		
Antecedents	**Does problem behavior occur:**	Yes	No
	At specific times? If yes, when? _____	☐	☐
	More often during some times of the day than others? If yes, when? _____	☐	☐
	During certain activities? If yes, what? _____	☐	☐
	With particular people? If yes, with whom? _____	☐	☐
	When certain environmental features are present? If yes, what? _____	☐	☐
Setting events	**When problem behavior occurs inconsistently:**	Yes	No
	Did an event out of the ordinary occur? If yes, what? _____	☐	☐
	Did an event occur that may influence an antecedent? If yes, what? _____	☐	☐
	Did an event occur that may influence a consequence? If yes, what? _____	☐	☐
Maintaining consequences	**When problem behavior occurs:**	Yes	No
	Does a specific type of response follow? If yes, what? _____	☐	☐
	Does a specific response intermittently follow? If yes, what? _____	☐	☐
	Does response provide a desirable outcome? If yes, what? _____	☐	☐
	Could past responses still be maintaining behavior? If yes, what were they? _____	☐	☐

FIGURE 6.1. Types of specific information and key questions.

Shane's off-task behavior, Ms. Yin noted not only the subject matter, but also the specific assignment. This helped her determine that worksheets with more than 10 problems were likely to cause off-task behavior and failure to complete the assignment. Data on antecedents to Samantha's target behavior revealed that problem behaviors occurred during transitions, but only when a transition was from a preferred to a nonpreferred activity.

The people in the environment, and the types of interaction they have with the individual (including the absence of any interaction), are also important to document. Often problem behaviors occur more frequently with a specific person, for any of a number of reasons. The specific manner in which an instruction or request is provided can also lead to problem behavior. For example, Mr. Scott collected detailed information about Harrison and his interactions with the three instructional assistants surrounding episodes of self-injury. The data revealed that Harrison engaged in self-injurious behavior during tasks only with a specific teaching assistant. Furthermore, the data indicated that this assistant issued stern directives in a harsh tone, provided demeaning reprimands whenever Harrison made an error, and rarely provided praise or encouragement. When this assistant changed her style of interactions, this resulted in immediate decreases in problem behavior.

Finally, features of the environmental structure also may be informative. For example, bright lights or noisy environments have been found to be associated with increases in problem behaviors. Also, group activities are problematic for some students, while independent seatwork is problematic for others.

In addition to collecting specific information in the areas described above as they pertain to occurrences of problem behavior, team members should collect similar data as it relates to appropriate or problem-free behavior. Information of this nature is useful in two ways. First, it can help the team to understand variables related to problem behavior. For example, observations indicated that Heather never engaged in problem behavior during vocational training class. Further observations determined that the activities in vocational training class required only gross motor skills. In addition, these tasks were brief, with frequent activity changes. This contrasted with the requirements and structure of Heather's other classes, in which problem behaviors were frequently observed. With this information, modifications were made in all of Heather's classes so that several brief tasks were presented rather than a single long task, and activities requiring fine motor skills were reduced.

The second way that information about appropriate behavior can be useful is for identifying the types of situations that may make desired behavior more likely. Students generally exhibit appropriate behavior when they are engaged in activities or situations that they enjoy. Once activities, individuals, or classroom structures associated with desirable behavior are identified, they can be infused throughout the curriculum.

Information about Setting Events

It is sometimes the case that particular antecedents are inconsistently associated with problem behavior. This can happen when setting events are present and exert an influence on the student. When problem behavior is clearly associated with a particular antecedent, but does not consistently occur in the presence of that antecedent or consequence, this should serve as a trigger for a support team to examine the potential presence of a setting event. When team members are attempting to identify a setting event, incidents out of the ordinary should be considered. For example, in Stuart's eighth-grade homeroom, the morning routine involved a peer's calling the roll and collecting lunch money. Stuart's teacher noted that on occasion, Stuart refused to respond when his name was called and made rude comments to the peer who was collecting lunch money. Because this did not happen consistently, his support team suspected the presence of a setting event. Indeed, interviews indicated that a group of students sometimes teased Stuart on the bus ride to school. This angered Stuart and subsequently made interactions with peers during homeroom particularly punishing. In other words, teasing on the bus, followed by a peer interaction, resulted in Stuart's problem behavior to escape further uninvited peer interactions.

Setting events also can be mediated by internal states. For instance, Anna's daily schedule was structured so that less preferred tasks were interspersed among highly preferred tasks. This schedule generally worked well, because Anna was motivated to complete her less preferred tasks in order to engage in highly reinforcing preferred tasks. Upon her arrival at school, her daily schedule required her to complete a hygiene routine first thing (e.g., toileting, washing her face and hands, and brushing her hair), which was nonpreferred. This was followed by breakfast, a highly preferred activity. Anna usually followed her schedule uneventfully. However, she periodically engaged in severe problem behavior during the morning routine. After gathering additional information, Anna's support team was able to identify the source of the problem. Anna's mother worked rotating shifts. When she had not worked late the previous evening, she arose early and prepared breakfast for Anna. Anna's mother began to record days when Anna ate breakfast at home on her home–school communication log. These days coincided exactly with the days that problem behaviors occurred during hygiene. In Anna's case, school breakfast was generally reinforcing as a result of hunger, and she readily completed the hygiene routine to obtain the reinforcer. However, when she did not experience the internal state of hunger, food no longer functioned as a reinforcer. Thus the request to complete hygiene activities prior to breakfast resulted in problem behavior on days when she had already eaten.

Although setting events are usually more difficult to isolate than antecedents and consequences, many have been documented in the literature. These include lack of sleep, a long bus ride, difficulties with peers, an argument at home, allergies, and illness.

Information about Maintaining Consequences

When team members are collecting assessment information, it is also important to identify the type of interaction, as well as any resulting activity or environmental changes, that occurred following problem behavior. Specifically, some type of adult or peer interaction usually follows a problem behavior. It can range from a reprimand, to a consoling comment by a teacher, to a derisive peer reaction (e.g., laughing). The interaction may be accompanied by other consequences, such as assistance with a task, assignment of an easier activity, change in seat assignments, a point loss, time out, an office referral, or a peer giving up a toy or activity.

Information about consequences is important, because it often suggests events that may be reinforcing the behavior. For example, Brianna's job coach noticed that her screaming had increased in volume and frequency over the past 6 months. The coach was concerned, because the screaming was very disruptive in the workplace. She knew that Brianna's work expectations had increased rapidly and was attempting to provide her with assistance to complete these new work demands whenever possible. A closer look revealed that the job coach usually provided help after Brianna screamed. Although her intentions were good, the job coach had inadvertently reinforced Brianna's screaming. Brianna had learned that if she needed help, she could get it by screaming.

In Benji's case, when problem behavior occurred, he was required to complete a problem-solving process prior to returning to the classroom activity. Problem solving was intended to help Benji self-identify alternative and more appropriate classroom behavior. However, problem solving did not lead to reductions in his problem behaviors. Benji's support team noted that problem solving was a lengthy process with Benji, rather than being brief as originally designed. Eventually, it was determined that Benji enjoyed the one-to-one attention the process provided him, and that he was intentionally engaging in problem behavior during times when he did not have ready access to teacher attention. This illustrates the importance of documenting the specific type of interaction following problem behavior, to permit a determination of whether it may be unintentionally reinforcing the behavior.

When the team is considering consequences, it is important to keep in mind that an event need not occur after every incident of behavior in order to maintain a behavior. Reinforcement that is intermittent, even if it is very infrequent, can cause behavior to continue. A very simple example is the slot machine. The intermittent payoff keeps gamblers persisting, even to the point of addiction. When team members are determining potential consequences maintaining problem behavior, intermittent and infrequent responses should also be considered. In addition, problem behavior sometimes continues for long periods of time even when there is no longer a desirable consequence in place. This is particularly true after behavior has been subject to reinforcement for a very long time. This possibility likewise should be considered when a maintaining consequence cannot be readily identified.

A final point is that consequences need not be proximal to behavior. Events that occur at a much later time can also maintain behavior. For instance, a high school student may engage in disruptive classroom behavior if he believes it will heighten his standing with a deviant or antisocial peer group. Although the regard is not immediate, it occurs over time via an established reputation.

METHODOLOGIES FOR GATHERING INFORMATION

There are two primary methodologies used to gather broad and specific information. *Indirect methods* are those approaches that rely on existing records or the reports of knowledgeable individuals. These approaches are referred to as indirect because information is obtained at a time other than when the behavior of interest is actually occurring. *Direct methods*, on the other hand, are used to obtain information at the time the behavior occurs. Information regarding behavior is recorded immediately after it occurs by someone who has directly observed it.

Indirect Methods

There are several different types of indirect methods of assessment. One type is record review. A student's school file generally contains a wealth of pertinent information; this includes information about medical history and status, past academic performance, current level of functioning, disciplinary referrals, and previous support plans. When team members are reviewing records, it is useful to summarize information in a format that will directly assist with support plan development. For example, rather than collecting an abundance of disordered information about every past intervention used with a student, it may be prudent to focus on strategies that were particularly effective and those that were ineffective. The School Archival Record Search (SARS) provides a format to collect information on a variety of services received by the student, disciplinary contacts, and other relevant information (Walker, Block-Pedego, Todis, & Severson, 1991).

Interviews offer another indirect method of information gathering. Interviews are most commonly administered to individuals who know the target person well. Family members and teachers should always be interviewed, in addition to any support personnel who work closely with the student. The primary purpose of an interview is to seek as much information as possible about the student and the problem behavior. At a minimum, most interviews obtain information about the range or topography of problem behaviors; the history of problem behavior; broad factors that might contribute to problem behavior (e.g., medications, health issues, major life events); specific antecedents to the problem behavior; specific consequences that follow the problem behavior; and the student's preferences, strengths, and limitations. Several interviews are commercially available. For example, the Functional Assessment Interview (FAI; O'Neill et al., 1997) is a multiple-section interview that solicits information about the topography of problem behavior, broad and specific factors that may influence problem behavior, and possible behavior functions. Although completing the FAI can take a fair amount of time (45–90 minutes), the resulting detailed information is worth the effort. Similar interview formats have been provided by Dunlap, Kern, Clarke, and Robbins (1991), Fad, Patton, and Polloway (2000), and Nelson, Roberts, and Smith (1998). The ultimate outcomes of such interviews should be summary statements or hypotheses (see Chapter 7) that succinctly pull together the information and describe the behaviors of concern, potential setting events, and specific antecedents and consequences, as well as the functions or motivations that appear to be maintaining them.

Interviews may also be administered directly to the student. There are several advantages of soliciting information from students themselves. Their firsthand knowledge of situations that cause them difficulty has the potential to be much more accurate and insightful than information provided by others. In addition, certain behaviors are not subject to observation by others. For example, stealing, drug use, and anxious feelings are often covert or undetected. Information provided by students themselves may be the only way to obtain an understanding of ecological variables related to occurrence of the behavior. Student interviews acquire information similar to that obtained in adult interviews. Specifically, students are asked about variables they think are related to their problem behavior, such as task difficulty, insufficient attention, or lack of adequate rewards. They are also asked to suggest changes that could be made to reduce or prevent their behavior problems. Furthermore, student interviews may attempt to identify preferred activities or items that can be incorporated into activities or used as reinforcers.

One example is the Student-Assisted Functional Assessment Interview (Kern, Dunlap, Clarke, & Childs, 1994). This interview is divided into four sections. The first section consists of 12 questions designed to assist in identifying potential antecedents and functions of problem behavior (e.g., "In general, is your work too hard for you?" "Do you think people notice when you do a good job?"). Students are asked to respond "always," "sometimes," or "never." The second section, consisting of 7 open-ended questions, solicits direct information about the target behavior and potential interventions—for example, "When do you have the most problems with (target behavior)?" and "What changes could be made so you would have fewer problems with (target behavior)?" The third section asks students to rate, on a 1–5 Likert scale ranging from "not at all" to "very much," how much they like each school subject. The final open-ended section queries what students like or do not like about each school subject. The interview generally takes approximately 30 minutes to complete. Some students prefer to respond in written format, while others would rather dictate their responses. O'Neill et al. (1997) offer an alternative student interview, the Student-Completed Functional Assessment Interview, that focuses on ratings indicating the extent to which students perceive they have difficulties in each subject. Using this format, students also participate in developing support strategies.

Indirect methods may also come in a checklist format. For example, the Motivation Assessment Scale (MAS; Durand & Crimmins, 1988) is a 16-item questionnaire designed to determine the functions of problem behaviors (i.e., escape, attention, tangible, sensory). Using a Likert-type scale, respondents record the extent to which they agree that a specific problem behavior occurs under conditions described. Sample questions include "Does the behavior occur following a request to perform a difficult task?" and "Does the behavior occur whenever you stop attending to this person?" Responses to various questions are summed to yield a numerical score corresponding to the escape, attention, tangible, and sensory functions. The final result is a hierarchical order of functions, with the highest score suggesting the most likely function. The MAS is brief and simple to complete; however, it is recommended that it be used in conjunction with other assessments, to substantiate the accuracy and reliability of the outcomes.

Indirect methods have advantages and disadvantages. Record reviews, interviews, and checklists can quickly obtain information from knowledgeable people in the student's life that can be put to use in conducting further assessment. Student interviews are also the only way to access a student's perspective. Although indirect methods can therefore collect valuable information, it may not be enough information for developing interventions. Also, these methods may be subject to bias because people's recollections are not always accurate. Indirect methods should thus be paired with direct methods to gather comprehensive information.

Direct Methods

Direct methods of information gathering document behaviors at the time they occur. There are various methods for direct observations, ranging from very informal to quite structured. An example of an informal method is an anecdotal note. Teachers and other care providers often jot down information about children. For example, school personnel may be legally required to document serious behavior problems, using a behavior log, incident report, or some other schoolwide or districtwide format. This type of documentation can be useful for the functional behavioral assessment process if it includes information about antecedents and consequences. The example in Figure 6.2 illustrates useful anecdotal information. In this example, behavior in violation of school conduct was recorded when it occurred. Additional information was documented about the time and location of each incident, as well as how the incident was resolved. The information is not overly detailed, yet it provides important information about antecedents and consequences. This anecdotal information can then be examined to identify patterns associated with problem behavior (e.g., the time of day that such behavior most frequently occurs, activity associated with behavior occurrences). Anecdotal notes can yield extensive information about problem behavior; however, some find this format for documentation time-consuming and tedious. The time required makes it difficult to use for high-frequency behaviors. Also, unlike the example in Figure 6.2, many types of anecdotal notes are unstructured, and important information about antecedents and consequences may inadvertently be omitted.

Another format for collecting direct observation information is an *antecedent–behavior–consequence* (ABC) analysis. This is an arrangement where a data collection sheet is divided into three columns. The first column is for describing antecedents, the middle for indicating the particular behavior, and the last for indicating consequences following the behavior. Sometimes headings on ABC forms prompt the observer to include specific

Constitution High School
Behavioral Referral/Incident Log

Student: Dustin Lutz   Dates: 10/22/04–11/24/04

Grade: Ninth grade   Case manager: Mrs. Heckman

Date	Time/class period	Behavior	Resolution
10/22/04	Gym at 9:50 A.M.	Argument with peer during basketball game	Problem solving with teacher and returning to class
11/6/04	Reading at 10:35 A.M.	Leaving class and then school grounds without permission	In-school suspension for remainder of day; parent phone call
11/12/04	Computer class at 8:52 A.M.	Cursing at peer; leaving class without permission	Problem solving with teacher and returning to class
11/27/04	Study hall at 12:44 P.M.	Tearing up point sheet after receiving points for the period	Problem solving with peer and returning to class

FIGURE 6.2. Example of anecdotal information.

information, such as time of day, type of activity, or topography of behavior. Figure 6.3 shows an example of an ABC form. Like anecdotal notes, the ABC format can provide a great deal of information, but can also be time-consuming to complete. An advantage is that the format provides a prompt to include information about antecedents and consequences needed for support plan development.

Checklists can also be used to collect direct observation data. This format lists antecedents that are suspected of causing desirable or undesirable behaviors and common consequences. Observers simply check the relevant boxes each time they observe a target behavior. Checklists can be designed or modified so they are specific to a particular student, in terms of antecedents, behaviors, and consequences. Figure 6.4 depicts a trigger–behavior–response checklist for Claire. The checklist included events her support team believed to be triggers to undesirable and desirable behavior, all desirable and undesirable behaviors observed in the past, and consequences that staff members might provide. The checklist offers a very simple format for busy teachers or other observers; however, it may not provide detailed

Packer Middle School
ABC Observation Form

Student: Dan Perry   Observer: Mr. Shastry

Date	Antecedents What teachers/peers was the student interacting with? Class period? Specific activity?	Behavior Describe specific behavior in observable terms (what was said/done).	Consequences What did the teacher and/or students do? Any disciplinary actions taken?
2-04-04	Another student (Adam) touched Dan as he was leaving science class	Screaming, cursing, refusing to leave the room	Teacher verbally reprimanded Dan (and Adam); Adam laughed at Dan; teacher removed afternoon privileges for Dan and Adam
2-13-04	Dan and Adam were teasing each other before math class; Dan refused to take math quiz and watched as other students (including Adam) received free time when they finished their quizzes	Throwing book across the room and flipping desk	Teacher verbally reprimanded Dan and sent him to the office, where he received in-school suspension for remainder of day; Adam laughed at Dan
2-27-04	Dan was kicking Adam under the table before he went to blackboard to work on math problem	Kicking wall while working on math problem; refusing to sit down	Teacher verbally reprimanded Dan; Adam laughed
3-03-04	During transition from reading to math class, Dan reported being pushed by Adam	Walking around the classroom; making verbal insults toward classmates (but primarily Adam)	Teacher verbally reprimanded Dan; Adam made verbal insults back to Dan

FIGURE 6.3. Example of an ABC observation form.

Trigger–Behavior–Response Checklist

Child's name: _Claire_

Directions: For each instance, check all antecedents, behaviors, and consequences that apply.

Problem behavior

Location: _Classroom_	Date: _3/30/04_	Time: _10:00_
Trigger: **What happened before?**	**Behavior**	**Response:** **What happened after?**
☐ Asked to do something ☐ Bored—no materials or activities ☐ Could not get something he or she wanted ☐ Stopped from doing a liked activity ☐ Loud environment ☐ Another person provoked the child ☐ Child needed to move from one activity to another ☑ Attention being given to others ☐ Unclear ☐ Other (specify: _____)	☐ Fidgeting ☐ Noncompliance ☐ Going off task ☐ Physical aggression ☐ Verbal aggression ☐ Property destruction ☐ Provoking or teasing others ☐ Running away ☐ Screaming/crying ☑ Tantrum ☐ Other (specify: _____)	☐ Discussed problem behavior ☐ Nothing/ignored ☐ Interrupted/blocked ☑ Verbal redirection to activity ☐ Physical redirection to activity ☐ Physical restraint ☐ Removed from room/area ☐ Required to continue activity ☐ Time out (duration: _____) ☐ Other (specify: _____)

Desirable behavior

Location: _Playground_	Date: _3/30/04_	Time: _11:30_
Trigger: **What happened before?**	**Behavior**	**Response:** **What happened after?**
☐ Asked to do something ☑ Receiving attention (teachers/peers) ☐ Alone ☐ Preferred toys/activities available ☐ Another child initiated play ☐ Playing with another child ☐ Given transition warning (e.g., "In 5 minutes you will need to turn off the TV") ☐ Other (specify: _____)	☐ Following directions ☐ Sitting quietly ☐ Staying on task ☑ Waiting for turn ☐ Cleaning up ☐ Sharing ☐ Waiting ☐ Being kind to others ☐ Transitioning smoothly ☐ Playing nicely with other children ☐ Other (specify: _____)	☐ Given reinforcement ☑ Received attention from others ☐ Ignored ☐ Play continued ☐ Other (specify: _____)

FIGURE 6.4. Example of a checklist.

information. Also, each behavioral incident requires a separate checklist, making it impractical for high-frequency behavior.

The scatterplot is a direct observation strategy for data collection that can be structured to yield a visual depiction of times of the day when behavior is frequent and infrequent. Data are recorded according to both their occurrence and frequency. For example, Figure 6.5 was used to document Raoul's high frequency self-injury. A brief glance at these data across days reveals activities during which self-injury was both frequent and infre-

Scatterplot

Name: Raoul   Target behavior: Self-injury

Activity and time	11/1 Mon	11/2 Tues	11/3 Wed	11/4 Thurs	11/5 Fri	11/8 Mon	11/9 Tues	11/10 Wed	11/11 Thurs	11/12 Fri
8:00–8:30 Self-care			░							
8:30–9:00 Breakfast										
9:00–9:15 Cleanup										
9:15–10:00 Funct. academics		█	░		█		█		░	
10:00–12:00 Job exploration										
12:00–12:30 Lunch										
12:30–12:45 Cleanup										
12:45–1:30 Funct. academics	█		█		░		█	░		
1:30–2:15 P.E.										░
2:15–2:45 School jobs					░					█
2:45–3:00 Closing	░				█					█

☐ = 0 incidents   ░ = 1–5 incidents   █ = >5 incidents

FIGURE 6.5. Example of a scatterplot.

quent. Like a checklist, a scatterplot may not yield detailed information, such as individuals present, particular activities, specific types of instruction, and consequences. However, it is easy to complete and offers a starting point for determining when more detailed assessments should be conducted.

The Functional Assessment Observation (FAO; O'Neill et al., 1997) provides a format for collecting comprehensive observational data in everyday settings. The format prompts detailed data collection with regard to indicating a behavior that has occurred, the antecedents or predictors that preceded the behavior, the actual consequences provided to the person (e.g., redirection), and the perceived function of the behavior (i.e., *why* the observer thought the person engaged in the behavior, such as to get attention or to avoid or escape a task or activity demand). However, recording is done by checks or numbers, which makes for an easier data-recording process than the ABC approach. Research has demonstrated that the FAO can be a valid and reliable observational data collection procedure (Cunningham & O'Neill, 2000; Murdock, O'Neill, & Cunningham, in press).

Table 6.2 provides a summary of both direct and indirect assessment methodologies and recommendations for their use. Although direct methods can provide significant information in terms of detail and specificity, many of these methods require much time and attention from the observer. There are ways, however, to minimize the time requirements. One strategy consists of having the people who are naturally in the environment collect simplified direct observation data first, and then supplement the data with less frequent but more detailed direct observations by an outside person. Dividing data collection responsibilities across team members is another strategy. Table 6.3 highlights the advantages and disadvantages of direct and indirect methods.

CONSIDERATIONS FOR GATHERING FUNCTIONAL ASSESSMENT INFORMATION

There are many different methodologies and formats for gathering assessment information. Several considerations may help coordinate efforts and guide team decisions about how the process will be carried out. First, it is generally best to obtain information from multiple individuals. This is particularly important when working with individuals whose behavior problems are fairly intransigent, have occurred over a long period of time, or happen in multiple settings. Individuals who have come to know the student in different contexts or in different ways have unique information to offer. In addition, the perspectives held by various individuals will differ

TABLE 6.2. Strategies for Gathering Functional Assessment Information

Method	Level of effort	Considerations	Examples
Indirect methods			
Record review	High	Always recommended as a source of historical (and other) data	• SARS (Walker et al., 1991)
Adult interview	Moderate	Always recommended, but formality can vary	• FAI (O'Neill et al., 1997) • Dunlap et al., 1991 • Fad et al., 2000 • Nelson et al., 1998
Student interview	Moderate	Highly recommended for higher-functioning students	• Student Assisted Functional Assessment Interview (Kern, Dunlap, et al., 1994) • Student Completed Functional Assessment Interview (O'Neill et al., 1997)
Checklists	Low	Recommended in conjunction with other strategies	• MAS (Durand & Crimmins, 1988)
Meetings	High	Recommended in conjunction with other strategies	• Initial line of inquiry (Lohrmann-O'Rourke, Knoster, & Llewellyn, 1999)
Direct methods			
Direct observation	Level varies, depending on format	Always recommended	• Anecdotal notes • ABC forms • Checklists • FAO (O'Neill et al., 1997)

according to their belief systems and values, in addition to their history with the student. Varying perspectives offer a richer collection of information and yield a better understanding of the student. In the end, this will result in a support plan that reflects shared interests, is comprehensive, and is more likely to be durable and effective.

A second issue to consider is that it is generally advisable to use more than one assessment method, including at least one direct method. The value of using multiple methods is that converging information can be detected. For example, direct observation data that are consistent with information obtained from an interview offer stronger support for the factors associated with problem behavior. Some type of direct method is important to include, because the information it provides tends to be more reliable than information about events that happened at a previous time and has to be recalled.

TABLE 6.3. Advantages and Disadvantages of Indirect and Direct Assessment Methods

Advantages	Disadvantages	Recommendations
	Indirect methods	
• Access to broad information • Quickly gathers initial information that can direct further assessment • Gathers information across time, people, settings • Can obtain student's perspective	• Accuracy depends upon how well the sources know the target individual • May not be specific enough to guide intervention development • Commercially available instruments may not be relevant for all situations	• Use commercially available instruments as a starting point, then modify them to meet unique needs • Pair with direct methods
	Direct methods	
• Gathers information directly when it occurs • Conducted in the natural environment • Can provide rich detail about the environment, behavior, antecedents, and consequences	• More time-intensive • May be intrusive to daily routines to record information as the behavior occurs • May miss occurrences of behavior • Difficult to code high-frequency behaviors • Information gathered may be insufficient for low-frequency behaviors	• Use commercially available instruments as a starting point, then modify to meet each student's unique needs • Make as simple as possible for data collection during typical routines

A third pair of considerations are ease and preference. Observers who have multiple individuals to teach or care for simultaneously generally look for a format that is easy to complete, such as a checklist. However, preference is also important. Some people prefer to write detailed notes. More important than the particular method selected is that the format allows for the collection of critical information about antecedents and consequences surrounding inappropriate and appropriate behavior.

COORDINATING THE ASSESSMENT PROCESS

Prior to gathering functional assessment information, it is important to plan and coordinate among team members. A well-coordinated assessment process will yield highly useful information in an efficient manner. Decisions should be made about the assessment methods that will be used and the division of labor. Sometimes team members divide responsibilities equally, while at other times particular team members may be in a position to assume a larger role. Each team member's specific responsibility should also be determined; this planning can avoid redundancy and duplicative efforts. Finally, time lines should be established for completing assessments and reviewing information. A team whose members believe they already have a good understanding of an individual and his or her behaviors will want to meet early on to review information and determine whether it is adequate for progressing to Step 3 of the overall PBS process (hypothesis development). On the other hand, a team working with an individual with complex challenges or low-frequency behaviors may decide to collect extensive information across a long period of time prior to reconvening. Alternatively, the team might decide that a subgroup, such as the teacher and school psychologist, will convene frequently to review assessment information and then report back to the full team when patterns are evident. Planning and coordinating that establish a reasonable time frame and designate agreeable responsibilities are likely to make efforts smooth, productive, and efficient.

THE FINAL PRODUCT

The assessment process can be quite brief or very extensive. In some cases, it is relatively simple to determine environmental events associated with appropriate and inappropriate behavior. At other times, the process is extremely involved and time-consuming, and may appear along the way to be fairly ambiguous. When the process is successful, patterns will emerge from the assessment information that implicate specific antecedents and consequences frequently associated with undesirable and desirable behavior. If the information does not point to differences in behavior across environmental situations, collecting additional assessment information may be necessary. In the end, an adequate assessment will provide clear and converging information about the relationship between the environment and behavior.

SUMMARY

Developing a comprehensive PBS plan includes consideration of both broad and specific information. This information is gathered in a variety of ways and from a diversity of individuals. Assessment information allows the team to identify broad variables and quality-of-life issues that may have contributed in the past, or may currently be contributing, to the continuance of problem behavior. A well-conducted assessment also will identify the specific and more immediate variables related to desirable and undesirable behavior. Such information is crucial for developing a comprehensive, multicomponent support plan. When assessment is well planned and coordinated, the resulting information leads to a support plan that can have a meaningful and lifelong impact.

COMMONLY ASKED QUESTIONS

How long does the assessment process take? The amount of time it takes to complete the assessment process depends on a number of factors, including team members' expertise, the extent of their firsthand knowledge and experience with the student, and the frequency and severity of the student's challenging behaviors. Sometimes the process can be completed in a number of hours, particularly if behavior problems are just emerging and the team knows the student well. More often, it takes weeks or even months. This is because problem behaviors tend to be insufficiently addressed until they become severe. The assessment process becomes much more lengthy when problem behaviors are well established and occur across multiple environments, people, or activities.

Why should we spend time collecting assessment information when we can implement an intervention without it? Interventions implemented without the benefit of assessment are usually limited in several ways. First, without an understanding of antecedents, interventionists are left only with reactive intervention procedures. That is, they lack information that allows them to implement interventions that will prevent undesirable behavior. Reactive strategies require that others experience problem behavior prior to implementing an intervention. This can be unpleasant or even dangerous. In addition, reactive strategies tend to be punitive, rather than instructive or supportive.

Second, interventions are most effective if they teach an alternative response and build an individual's repertoire of skills. This requires information about an individual's weaknesses and limitations. Interventions that teach alternative skills usually result in long-lasting outcomes.

Third, a teacher will waste time implementing an intervention that will not work. This often happens when assessment information is not used to develop an intervention. Without assessment information, a trial-and-error approach to intervention is required, which can be a very time-consuming process.

What if the information we gathered doesn't tell us anything? It is sometimes the case that behavior patterns are not readily apparent in assessment information. In this case, it is best to collect additional information. Meanwhile, hypotheses and potential interventions can be tested on the basis of the limited information available (as described in Chapter 7).

What can we do if the behavior is serious, but occurs infrequently? Infrequent behaviors are difficult to assess, because they are not subject to regular and ongoing observation. It is very important that detailed information is collected when the behavior does occur, so that over time, patterns can be identified. Also, it is sometimes possible to obtain information about serious behaviors by collecting information about less serious behaviors. Less serious behaviors may be precursors to more serious behaviors and often occur more frequently. Support plans built around less serious behaviors are often successful at eliminating more serious behaviors.

What if the assessment process takes months? Does this mean we should do nothing at all to help the student in the meantime? No. It may take months to gather sufficient information to build a comprehensive support plan, but during the process useful information will be revealed a bit at a time. Team members may develop interventions around known information and then modify or expand the support plan as new information is revealed.

CASE EXAMPLES

Malik's Functional Assessment

Malik's team agreed that a functional assessment was critical to identify the variables associated with his challenging behavior. The team identified assessment activities to be conducted, the individual responsible for completing each activity, and a timeline for completing the activity. Because of his experience with PBS, Mr. Rodriguez (the behavior specialist) volunteered to coordinate the team's assessment activities, which included training the instructional assistant in data collection, being available for consultation, checking in with team members to make sure they were meeting deadlines, and scheduling the next team meeting as soon as all assessment activities were completed. Figure 6.6 describes the team's assessment plan.

The team members were timely in completing the assessment activities. A subgroup of team members, consisting of Mr. Rodriguez, Mrs. Nelson, and the instructional assistant, met to summarize the assessment data. The summary data were later presented to the core group for discussion and hypothesis development. Below are summaries of the key information obtained.

Functional Assessment Planning

Student: Malik   Date: November 2

Assessment activity	Person responsible	Target completion date
Record review	Mr. Rodriguez	November 9

Interviews:
  Special education teacher
  Instructional assistant
  Prior classroom teacher
	Mr. Rodriguez	November 16

Interviews:
  Grandparents
  Jenna
  Thomas
	Mrs. Nelson	November 16

Scatterplot (across day)	Mrs. Nelson Instructional assistant	November 3–10
Direct observation (times with high and low rates of behavior, based on scatterplot)	Mr. Rodriguez	November 10–17

FIGURE 6.6. Malik's team's assessment plan.

Summary of Record Review

- Several medications had been tried in the past; none seemed to have a significant impact on decreasing Malik's problem behaviors.
- Malik's individualized education program (IEP) goals and objectives for the past 3 years had remained the same. They focused on early academic skills, improving verbal language skills, and decreasing problem behaviors.
- Behavior intervention plans that focused on prompting Malik to work through difficult tasks were ineffective; in fact, the intensity and frequency of his problem behaviors seemed to be increasing over time.

Summary of Interviews

Interviews with grandparents, Jenna, and Thomas
- No problem behaviors occur at home.
- Malik loves to help around the house, especially cooking and cleaning.
- Malik was very independent and able to fulfill his own needs and wants (e.g., used the toilet independently, obtained food himself when hungry, engaged in indoor and outdoor leisure activities on his own).

- Malik likes to communicate with as few words as possible. Because his family members knows him well, they have learned to predict his needs and actions (e.g., they can tell when he isn't feeling well or doesn't like something).
- Malik follows a very structured schedule at home, with playtime, dinner, and established cleanup and bedtime routines at the same times each day.
- Malik is reluctant to go to school some mornings. Recently, his school refusals have been increasing. His grandmother motivates him to get up by offering to buy him breakfast at McDonald's before school.

Interviews with special education teacher, instructional assistant, and prior classroom teacher
- Malik loves to help in the cafeteria and do general classroom chores.
- Malik will often initiate communication with one or two spoken words, but will usually refuse to speak when prompted to elaborate (e.g., to speak in phrases or give more specific information). Mrs. Nelson introduced pictures. Malik seems receptive to using pictures as one mode of communication.
- Malik engages in problem behaviors throughout the day, but they are most frequent during instructional time.

Functional Assessment Summary

The interviews indicated that Malik's problem behaviors occurred only in school; therefore, the direct observations focused on the school setting. The members of Malik's teaching staff stated that problem behaviors occurred throughout the day, but were more frequent during instructional activities. To get a more precise idea of exactly when problem behaviors were most and least frequent, a scatterplot was completed (see Figure 6.7). The finished scatterplot showed that problem behaviors were most frequent during reading, outdoor activities, and math. Problem behaviors were completely absent during self-care, daily living, cafeteria assistance, and laundry activities. (During the month of November, Malik's class did laundry for the home economics room, washing dish towels. School jobs were shared and rotated across classrooms.)

Mr. Rodriguez decided to conduct more detailed direct observations during reading, outdoor activities, and math, to obtain more specific information about why these particular activities were associated with problem behaviors. In addition, he opted to observe during self-care and cafeteria assistance, to see how these activities differed from problematic activities. These direct observations revealed that problem behaviors were not constant throughout reading, math, and outdoor activities (see Figure 6.8). Isolated letter and number identification activities were most problematic, whereas letter and number matching were associated with fewer problem behaviors. In response to his problem behaviors during reading and math, staff members usually removed Malik from the classroom in order to avoid disturbing

Student: Malik

☐ = 0 problems   ▨ = 1–5 problems   ■ = >5 problems

Time of day and activity	Fri 11/3	Mon 11/6	Tue 11/7	Wed 11/8	Thu 11/9	Fri 11/10
8:00–8:15 Arrival					▨	
8:15–8:45 Breakfast			▨			
8:45–9:00 Self-care						
9:00–9:45 Reading	■	▨	■	■	▨	
9:45–10:00 Outdoors	▨		▨		▨	▨
10:00–10:45 Math		■	▨		▨	■
10:45–11:30 Daily living						
11:30–12:00 Cafeteria assistant						
12:00–12:30 Lunch						▨
12:30–1:00 Laundry						
1:00–1:30 Art	▨					
1:30–2:00 Group time				▨		
2:00–2:30 Leisure time		▨				
2:30–3:00 Closing				▨		

FIGURE 6.7. Results of scatterplot for Malik.

the other students (see Figure 6.9). Sometimes Malik was required to clean up the mess he made during a disruptive episode.

Combined, this information suggested that the work might be too difficult for Malik—an idea supported by the fact that over the past 3 years he had made little progress on academic objectives. Furthermore, Malik's very appropriate behavior during nonacademic activities suggested that he might prefer these activities. Direct observations conducted during outdoor activities revealed that Malik's behavior was very appropriate throughout such an activity until he was told that it was time to return to the classroom. Typically, staff members would reprimand Malik; however, to avoid escalation of problem behavior where many other children were present, the staff members were reluctant to require him to make an immediate transition. Thus he usually was able to play a little longer prior to returning to the class. The staff also noticed that transitions from other preferred activities were not nearly so problematic (art to group time, leisure to closing). This information suggested that transition from a preferred activity to a nonpreferred activity (math) was responsible for problem behavior. Direct observations also revealed that although problem behavior occurred infrequently in preferred activities, when it did, it seemed to be centered around Malik's communication. That is, when his teachers

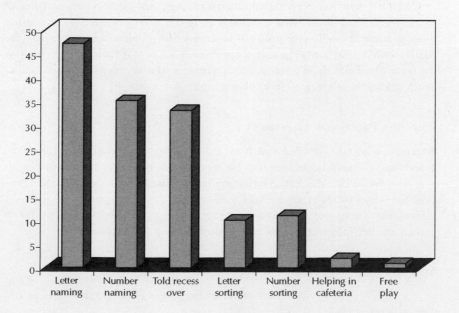

FIGURE 6.8. Results of direct observations: Observed antecedents to Malik's problem behavior (graphed by frequency).

Staff Responses to Problem Behavior				
Activity	Continued activity	Removed from activity or classroom	Made to clean up mess	Reprimand
Letter naming (48)	1	22	18	7
Number naming (36)	3	25	7	1
Told preferred activity ending (33)	23	8	0	13
Communication (prompted to use words) (10)	0	10	0	9

FIGURE 6.9. Results of direct observations: Summary of staff responses to Malik's problem behavior (graphed by frequency).

insisted that he use his words to communicate, Malik refused and sometimes attempted to hit or bite them. When this happened, teachers always backed off from their demands by terminating their requests.

Malik's functional assessment therefore suggested some clear patterns of when, where, and under what conditions problem behaviors were likely and not likely to occur, as well as the potential functions that problem behaviors served for Malik in these situations. The case description at the end of Chapter 7 shows how the team translated these patterns into hypothesis statements, which were used to develop Malik's behavior support plan.

Bethany's Functional Assessment

Bethany's team also decided that it would be valuable to conduct a functional assessment, to get a better idea of why her problem behaviors were occurring. It was determined that the special education teacher would lead the assessment process. She began by reviewing Bethany's records and conducting interviews with key individuals. These were followed by direct observations. The summaries below extract the key information that was used to develop her support plan.

Summary of Record Review

- Bethany's statewide testing indicates that she is close to grade level in academic areas.
- Bethany's grades have declined across her school years.
- Bethany's behavior problems have increased.

Summary of Interviews

Interview with Bethany's mother
- Bethany loves outdoor activities.
- Bethany likes to read, but refuses to complete homework.
- Bethany's mother sometimes has difficulty getting Bethany up and to school, particularly when she has been with her father for the weekend or out the night before.
- Bethany is often left alone in the afternoon, and she sometimes hangs out with older neighborhood kids.

Interview with Mrs. Lane, Bethany's neighbor
- Bethany frequently stops by their apartment in the afternoon to visit; Mrs. Lane believes she is lonely.
- Bethany loves to watch and play with Mrs. Lane's 3-year-old daughter.

Interview with Bethany's general education teacher
- Bethany has difficulty completing her classwork, although she sometimes partially completes her assignments, or will complete brief assignments.
- Because of Bethany's behavior, she frequently has missed recess and free-time activities; as a result, she has had little time to establish friendships with female classmates.
- Bethany often reports being tired.

Interview with Bethany
- Bethany reported she feels overwhelmed with school assignments and often avoids them altogether so she does not have to experience that feeling.
- Bethany stated that she hates classes in which she has to do a lot of writing.
- Bethany's favorite things to do are reading and playing sports.
- Bethany said that she likes to be with friends, but wishes she had more time to socialize.

Summary of Direct Observations

Direct observations of Bethany (see Figure 6.10) revealed that the following assignments were associated with appropriate behavior:

- Silent reading
- Hands-on group projects
- Explicit directions/requirements provided just prior to the beginning of a task

ABC Data Collection Form

Student: Bethany

Date/class	Antecedents	Behavior	Consequences
Feb. 8: Language Arts	Assigned chapter to read in book	Read chapter; no problems	No interaction
	Asked to predict and write ending of story	Wrote name on paper; did not begin assignment	Reminded to get working three times
Feb. 8: Science	Completed experiment with classmates	Engaged throughout	Nothing
	Asked to record findings in journal	Began wandering around classroom, disturbing others	Sent to office
Feb. 8: World Cultures	Class instructed to work on customs project	Pulled out reading book, rather than project	Ignored most of period; given detention at end of period
Feb. 9: Lunch	Seated with unfamiliar students in cafeteria (all boys)	Boys from another class were talking about girls they like	Bethany called boys "stupid idiots"

FIGURE 6.10. Results of direct observations for Bethany (partial).

162

The following assignments/activities were associated with inappropriate behavior:

- Written work
- Lengthy class assignments and extended "projects"
- Lunchtime—being seated with people she had nothing in common with

Functional Assessment Summary

Bethany's record review indicated that she scored near grade level on standardized testing; however, she was receiving poor grades. A close examination of the interviews and direct observation data revealed that extensive written work and lengthy assignments were associated with problem behaviors. In addition, projects requiring ongoing effort were rarely completed. Activities that were associated with engagement and appropriate behavior were reading, group projects that emphasized hands-on skills, and brief tasks that followed explicit and clear directions.

Social skills were also identified as a problem area. Although Bethany had friends at school and interacted appropriately with them, it was observed that when she was in unstructured situations with peers she did not know well, she sometimes interacted inappropriately, presumably to seek their attention.

Bethany's teacher indicated that fatigue was frequently a problem. Bethany reported being tired and sometimes fell asleep during class. Her teacher stated that in her recollection, this happened most frequently on Mondays.

With respect to Bethany's lifestyle, the assessment confirmed that she particularly enjoyed outdoor activities. In addition, Mrs. Lane, Bethany's neighbor, indicated that Bethany liked young children. But she also believed that Bethany was lonely and had little to do after school. Bethany confirmed that she would like to have more time with her friends.

REFERENCES

Cunningham, E., & O'Neill, R. E. (2000). A comparison of results of functional assessment and analysis procedures with young children with autism. *Education and Training in Mental Retardation and Developmental Disabilities, 35,* 406–414.

Dunlap, G., Kern, L., Clarke, S., & Robbins, F. R. (1991). Functional assessment, curricular revision, and severe behavior problems. *Journal of Applied Behavior Analysis, 24,* 387–397.

Durand, V. M., & Crimmins, D. B. (1988). Identifying the variables maintaining self-injurious behavior. *Journal of Autism and Developmental Disabilities, 18,* 99–117.

Fad, K. M., Patton, J. R., & Polloway, E. A. (2000). *Behavioral intervention planning: Completing a functional behavioral assessment and developing a behavioral intervention plan.* Austin, TX: PRO-ED.

Kern, L., Childs, K., Dunlap, G., Clarke, S., & Falk, G. (1994). Using assessment-based curricular intervention to improve the classroom behavior of a student with emotional and behavioral challenges. *Journal of Applied Behavior Analysis, 27,* 7–19.

Kern, L., Dunlap, G., Clarke, S., & Childs, K. E. (1994). Student-Assisted Functional Assessment Interview. *Diagnostique, 19,* 7–20.

Lohrmann-O'Rourke, S., Knoster, T., & Llewellyn, G. (1999). Screening for understanding: An initial line of inquiry for school-based settings. *Journal of Positive Behavior Interventions, 1,* 35–42.

Murdock, S. G., O'Neill, R. E., & Cunningham, E. (in press). A comparison of results and acceptability of functional behavioral assessment procedures with a group of middle school students with emotional/behavioral disorders (E/BD). *Journal of Behavioral Education.*

Nelson, J. R., Roberts, M. L., & Smith, D. J. (1998). *Conducting functional behavioral assessments: A practical guide.* Longmont, CO: Sopris West.

O'Neill, R. E., Horner, R. H., Albin, R. W., Sprague, J. R., Storey, K., & Newton, J. S. (1997). *Functional assessment and program development for problem behavior: A practical handbook* (2nd ed.). Pacific Grove, CA: Brooks/Cole.

Walker, H. M., Block-Pedego, A., Todis, B., & Severson, H. (1991). *School Archival Record Search (SARS).* Longmont, CO: Sopris West.

CHAPTER 7

♦♦♦

Developing Hypothesis Statements

♦

LEE KERN

It should be clear from Chapter 6 on functional assessment that information for developing an individualized support plan can be obtained from a variety of sources and in many different formats. As a result, the functional assessment conducted during Step 2 of the positive behavior support (PBS) process (conducting a functional assessment) often produces an abundance of information. The tricky next step is deciding how to use the information in ways that will inform the support plan. Unfortunately, all too often support plans bear little resemblance to the pertinent information collected during the assessment phase, and thereby fail to match the needs of the student. To avoid this disparity, Step 3 of the PBS process—developing hypothesis statements—is critical for creating a link between the information gathered and the final product, the support plan. The current chapter illustrates strategies to assist in developing hypotheses. In addition, procedures for evaluating the accuracy of hypotheses (i.e., *hypothesis testing*) are described.

THE IMPORTANCE OF A HYPOTHESIS STATEMENT

A hypothesis statement is the end product of the functional assessment or information-gathering process. Specifically, it provides a succinct summary of information gathered in the prior phase. A hypothesis statement serves the important purpose of assuring a link between the assessment information and the behavior support plan. It establishes this link by stating the relationship between environmental events and an individual's behavior. That is, it describes the antecedent and setting events that are most likely to cause the problem behavior, and it states the presumed function based on observed consequences as well as logical deductions. By offering a clear description of the events associated with problem behavior, it points to interventions that are likely to be effective. In other words, information about environmental events and behavioral function directly implicates classes of intervention approaches that will address the needs of the student and thereby reduce problem behavior. Correctly formulated, a hypothesis greatly facilitates the efforts of PBS team members to develop a behavior support plan. No longer is a trial-and-error approach to intervention necessary, which can be very time-consuming, in addition to creating delays in student progress. Instead, a support plan can be created with confidence, because it is based on data, comprehensive information, and familiarity with the student. The following sections detail strategies for completing this important step.

FORMAT OF HYPOTHESIS STATEMENTS

Specific hypothesis statements have been written in many different ways. Regardless of the specific format, what is important is that each one contains three pieces of information. First, it states events that occur prior to the target behavior, including setting events when relevant, as well as immediate antecedents. Second, it describes the target behavior. Third, it identifies the presumed function of the behavior. As described in Chapter 2, behavior can be viewed (albeit simplistically) as serving one of two functions. The first is to obtain something desirable. Attention, activities, tangible items, and self-stimulation are common things or events that individuals seek to obtain. The second function for behavior is to escape or avoid something unpleasant. Tasks or demands are a common requirement, particularly in school settings, that students attempt to escape or avoid by using problem behavior. Less frequently, a student may desire to avoid social interaction or even too much sensory stimulation. Based on assessment information gathered about antecedents, setting events, and consequences for behavior, a logical and parsimonious conclusion will be reached in a hypothesis statement about the function a particular behavior serves.

The most common format for a hypothesis statement is to list these three pieces of information sequentially, as illustrated in the following example: "When this happens [*setting event* and/or *antecedent*], [student's name] engages in [*problem behavior*], to [*presumed function*]. Figure 7.1 provides several examples to illustrate the structure of hypotheses.

When *given a difficult assignment,* Sally engages in *disruption,* to *escape the task.*
    (antecedent)   *(behavior)*   *(function)*

When *a classmate is playing with a toy Marty wants,* he engages in *aggression,* to *obtain the toy.*
    (antecedent)   *(behavior)*   *(function)*

When Ali *did not sleep well* and she *is left unattended,* she engages in *self-injury,* to *get attention.*
    (setting event)   *(antecedent)*   *(behavior)*   *(function)*

FIGURE 7.1. The structure of hypotheses: Sample statements.

GUIDELINES FOR HYPOTHESIS DEVELOPMENT

Several guidelines are important to consider when a team is developing hypotheses. First, hypotheses should implicate environmental events that can be modified in some way to formulate an intervention. It is sometimes tempting to attribute problem behavior to child characteristics. A common example pertains to diagnosis. Because many educational labels or psychiatric diagnoses (e.g., attention-deficit/hyperactivity disorder, or ADHD; anxiety disorder) are associated with particular constellations of behaviors, we often assume that a label or diagnosis is the single causal factor for a behavior. Such is the case in the hypothesis "Tommy engages in off-task behavior because he has ADHD." This is not a hypothesis that is useful for developing a support plan. It does not specify any environmental event associated with the problem behavior, nor does it suggest any changes that could be made to reduce the problem. A more appropriate hypothesis might be, "When given lengthy assignments (more than 15 minutes), Tommy engages in off-task behavior, to escape the continued work." The latter hypothesis specifies an environmental event associated with the target behavior that readily lends itself to an intervention.

A second guideline for developing hypotheses is that they should be grounded in data. Team members' experiences, personal philosophies, and values often shape and color their perceptions. Differing opinions are of great worth, which is exactly why a team process is the best approach for support plan development. However, it is also the case that an individual member's history or beliefs may cloud his or her ability to evaluate the information at hand objectively. Consequently, although each team member's opinion should be equally considered and carefully contemplated, in the end there should be consensus that a hypothesis is logical and rational in light of the available information. Take the case of Clayton's self-injurious behavior. Mr. Turner, Clayton's special education teacher, had had a student named Alexander in his classroom 4 years earlier who engaged in a high frequency of self-injury, just like Clayton. In fact, Mr.

Turner noted that the topography of Clayton's self-injury was identical to Alexander's: It consisted of slapping his cheeks and the back of his head and neck with an open palm. Mr. Turner recalled that Alexander's self-injury was determined to occur for biological reasons and was reduced with the administration of medication. Because of the similarities in topography, he was convinced that Clayton's self-injury also served a biological function. However, in Clayton's case, the assessment information indicated several distinctive antecedents that consistently preceded his self-injury; in addition, there were some activities during which self-injury rarely occurred. In light of these data, Mr. Turner agreed with the team that an alternative hypothesis was more accurate.

The third general guideline for hypothesis development is that hypotheses should reflect team consensus. All members should consider hypotheses to be *reasonable*. This does not mean that all hypotheses are equally valued by each team member, but rather that a hypothesis is viewed as logical based on the information available. If a team member does not consider a hypothesis reasonable, then further dialogue is warranted. Consensus by team members assures that all are actively contributing and working to achieve a common goal. Table 7.1 lists key questions that may guide the hypothesis development process.

MAKING SENSE OF ASSESSMENT INFORMATION

When a team is developing hypotheses, a critically important yet often complicated exercise is extracting meaning from the assessment information. Thus a key question is this: "How do team members organize assessment information to formulate hypothesis statements?" Ultimately, patterns of behavior should emerge, suggesting that a particular event or variable is associated with problem behavior. Identifying these events or variables requires that the support team carefully examine all the information gathered until the data reflect antecedents, setting events, and/or presumed functions that recur. This pattern of recurrence can emerge across days of observation or can be derived from different sources. The following

---

TABLE 7.1. Questions to Consider in Developing a Hypothesis

- Does the hypothesis specify an environmental event that can be altered to form an intervention?
- Is the hypothesis based on the data that have been gathered?
- Is there team consensus that the hypothesis is reasonable?

---

sections suggest strategies to go about organizing and analyzing assessment information.

Identifying Antecedents to Problem Behavior

The first question teams need to answer when sifting through assessment information is this: "Are there antecedent events that reliably precede the problem behavior?" A logical starting place for answering this question is to determine whether there are times of the day that are associated with particularly high (or particularly low) rates of problem behavior. After the problematic times are identified, the activities, people, and/or environmental features can be explored more thoroughly to specify just what it is about these particular times of day that are problematic. Table 7.2 provides an overview of suggested key questions and variables to look for when team members are parceling out antecedents associated with problem behavior. The following case examples illustrate how this process was followed to identify specific antecedents associated with problem behavior.

TABLE 7.2. Questions for Identifying Variables Associated with Problem Behavior

Key questions	Related questions
• What antecedent events reliably precede problem behavior?	• When does the behavior occur? • What activities are taking place? • What people are present? • How is the environment arranged?
• Are there antecedent events that are reliably associated with desirable behavior?	• When is problem behavior absent? • What activities are taking place? • What people are present? • How is the environment arranged?
• Are there setting events that reliably precede problem behavior?	• What earlier events seem to make the behavior more likely? • Is the student experiencing physiological symptoms? • Is the behavior cyclic? • Have there been changes at home? • Is the student having interpersonal conflicts?
• Do people respond to problem behavior in a way that is likely to encourage it?	• What happens following problem behavior? • Does the student escape or avoid a particular assignment or activity? • Does the student obtain a particular activity or item? • Does the student appear to receive sensory stimulation?

Tyler was a high school student described as having an emotional/behavioral disorder. He engaged in problem behavior at school, mainly in the form of inappropriate comments to others. A schedule analysis of Tyler's school day, shown in Figure 7.2, was completed across 5 school days. This analysis revealed that study hall was a time in which Tyler's problem behaviors were most frequent. Thus additional and more detailed antecedent–behavior–consequence (ABC) data were collected during study hall across the next 3 school days (Figure 7.3). The data from the ABC analysis suggested that a common variable during almost all of the incidents of problem behavior was the presence of another student, Mia. Further analyses indeed indicated that Mia was also in Tyler's homeroom and science class—the other two classes in which problems frequently occurred. She was not enrolled in any other classes with Tyler. In fact, Tyler's support team also noted that she was absent on December 5, a day when problem behaviors were absent. Additional information obtained from the Student-Assisted Functional Assessment Interview (Figure 7.4) supported the hypothesis that Tyler engaged in problem behavior to obtain attention, and that he might be attempting to gain attention from Mia. This pattern of information led to the hypothesis "When Mia is present, Tyler engages in problem behavior, to obtain her attention."

Yanna's data also revealed consistent patterns of problem behavior. Yanna was diagnosed with autism when she was 3 years old. Anxious to improve her social skills, her parents enrolled her in an inclusive preschool program. After a month of attendance, she began to engage in tantrums. The tantrums often lasted for long periods of time (up to 3 hours) and

Period/Class	Date: 12/2	Date: 12/3	Date: 12/4	Date: 12/5	Date: 12/6
Homeroom	//	///	//		//
Math	/				
Reading		/			
Gym					
Science	//	///	/		//
Lunch					
Social Studies					
Study Hall	///	//	///		//
Shop					

FIGURE 7.2. Tyler's schedule analysis.

ABC Data Collection Form

Antecedent (indicate date, time)	Behavior	Consequence
12/9 at 1:05 P.M.: Tyler was sitting at a table with three other students (Shane, Mia, and Damon). He was supposed to be doing his homework.	He whistled at a teaching assistant who entered the classroom.	Students laughed. I gave Tyler 1 day detention.
12/9 at 1:12 P.M.: Tyler asked me for help with his math.	As I was reading the assignment, he kept telling me to hurry. Then he said, "Can Mia help me?" I told him no, then he said, "You're stupid, you don't know how to do math."	I sent Tyler to study carrel at back of room.
12/9 at 1:20 P.M.: Tyler was working in study carrel. He asked to sharpen his pencil.	As he went toward the pencil sharpener, I saw him drop a note on Mia's desk. I intercepted the note. It said, "You're a babe."	Mia kept giggling. I gave Tyler a disciplinary referral and moved Mia's seat near my desk.
12/10 at 1:15 P.M.: Tyler was working on a group science activity (with Katie, Mia, Jake, and Scott).	Tyler fell out of his chair. He said Mia pushed him. She said he kept moving his chair too close to her.	Tyler and Mia were moved and told to work independently.
12/11 at 1:35 P.M.: Tyler was supposed to be doing homework independently.	He walked out of class without permission, then he kept banging on the classroom door.	I gave Tyler a disciplinary referral.

FIGURE 7.3. Tyler's ABC data.

Student-Assisted Functional Assessment Interview

Student: Tyler

Date October 28

Interviewer self-completed

Section I

When you do seatwork, do you do   (ALWAYS) SOMETIMES   NEVER
better when someone works with you?

Are there things in the classroom that   ALWAYS (SOMETIMES)   NEVER
distract you?

Section IV

What do you like about homeroom? My friends are in there.

What do you like about science? It's fun. We get to work in groups and I like
the people I work with.

What do you like about study hall? My girlfriend is in that class.

FIGURE 7.4. Selected information from Tyler's student interview.

included screaming at a volume that disrupted classroom activities. After
receiving numerous home–school notes about Yanna's behavior, her parents requested that a functional behavioral assessment be conducted. Interviews and direct observation data revealed that her tantrums invariably
occurred around noon. A further examination of the assessment data indicated that the tantrums occurred during the transition to the cafeteria for
lunchtime. One of Yanna's teachers noted that her tantrums had begun at
the exact time when new construction began on the north wing of the
building. Parent interview data confirmed Yanna's difficulties with transitions and change. Staff members noted that the route to the cafeteria had
changed as a function of the construction. From this combined information, Yanna's support team developed the hypothesis "When asked to
make a transition using an unfamiliar route, Yanna engages in tantrums, to
escape the unpredictability."

Judy's assessment data were a bit more complicated, because her self-
injury occurred throughout the day. The data alone, presented in Figure
7.5, were baffling to the team, partly because self-hitting seemed to occur
during activities that Judy enjoyed. Judy loved eating breakfast and lunch
in the cafeteria with her schoolmates. However, self-hitting occurred in this

ABC Assessment Form

Student: <u>Judy</u>

Antecedent (Indicate date and time, activity, and people in environment)	Behavior (Specify the form of the behavior)	Consequence (Describe all events that occurred in response to the behavior)
9/11 at 8:05: In the cafeteria, being supervised by volunteers; she was waiting for breakfast to be served	Punched herself in the head numerous times; episode lasted about 5 minutes	Was escorted out of cafeteria; breakfast was brought to her in the classroom
9/11 at 10:30: In the classroom; teaching assistant was preparing materials for lesson	Screamed and hit self five times in rapid succession	Teaching assistant ignored her and presented lesson
9/12 at 1:00: In line, getting ready to transition to the gym for P.E.	Hit her head twice	Was directed to seat; was given nonpreferred activity that she had to complete before gym
9/12 at 3:00: Unclear; class was getting jackets and backpacks in preparation to go home	Screamed and began hitting head	Teacher blocked head hitting; escorted Judy to bus when she calmed down
9/13 at 8:10: Dropped food tray in cafeteria; was told to go to the back of the line and get another tray	Screamed, yelled, dropped to the ground, and began hitting head on floor	Was taken to the classroom, where she ate breakfast
9/13 at 9:00: During fire drill, was waiting outside for signal to return to class	Screamed once and hit head	Teaching assistant took her for a walk around football field

FIGURE 7.5. ABC data for Judy.

setting. It was only after the ABC data were reviewed in conjunction with information from the interview conducted with Judy's mother (see Figure 7.6 for selected interview information) that the team was able to identify the common antecedent of waiting that was associated with Judy's self-injury.

In the cases of Tyler, Yanna, and Judy, particular events at school were identified that were commonly associated with problem behavior. Particular individuals may also be associated with problem behavior. This may happen for a variety of reasons. It may be that an individual interacts with a student in a way that is unpleasant. For example, data indicated that Alberta's screaming occurred most frequently when her teacher, Mr. Edwards, was scheduled to work with her. Further analysis indicated that screams happened each time Mr. Edwards provided a specific instruction. Observations of the instructions indicated that they were usually presented in a manner that was very harsh and demanding. Problem behavior may also occur in the presence of an individual who maintains closer physical proximity than the student can tolerate. Or, past teasing by a particular peer can cause a student to engage in behavior that will allow him or her to avoid situations where that peer is present. Conversely, inadequate interactions may likewise cause a student to engage in problem behavior in the presence of a particular teacher. For example, problem behavior may routinely occur to gain the attention of a teacher who sits at his or her desk and rarely interacts with the students.

Finally, particular environmental arrangements may serve as an antecedent that triggers problem behavior. Problems that occur during a partic-

---

Functional Assessment Interview

Student: Judy

Person being interviewed: Judy's mother

Person conducting interview: School psychologist

Date of Interview: November 20, 2003

Are there circumstances in which problem behaviors always occur?

Judy hits herself throughout the day, and I don't always know why. She can be very demanding. If she wants something and I cannot get it quickly enough, she will hit herself. Sometimes it appears that she wants something, but I don't know what it is.

FIGURE 7.6. Selected interview information regarding Judy.

ular time of day may be narrowed down to a classroom that is too crowded, too noisy, or illuminated with bothersome fluorescent lights.

Identifying Antecedents to Desirable Behavior

When a team is developing hypotheses, it is also helpful to consider this question: "Are there antecedent events that are reliably associated with *desirable* behavior?" The process of identifying when desirable behavior is most likely to occur will help not only to parcel out problematic events by way of contrast, but also to determine situations that are preferred by the student. The same process used to identify events associated with problem behavior can be used to determine events associated with desirable behavior. For example, assessment data indicated that Jesse's talking out and classroom disruptions occurred throughout the school day, with the exception of social studies period. In contrast to descriptions of highly disruptive behavior by all of Jesse's teachers, his social studies teacher never witnessed a single problem during class. Further observation indicated that social studies class was the only period in which small-group activities, such as cooperative learning, routinely occurred. All other academic classes employed primarily teacher lectures and/or independent work. This type of data analysis allowed his team to identify and place Jesse in the classes where teachers routinely used this type of small-group, cooperative format in which Jesse thrived.

Identifying Setting Events Associated with Problem Behavior

The emerging patterns of data may indicate that each occurrence of problem behavior is preceded by a particular event. However, sometimes when the particular event is present, problem behavior does not always occur. This data pattern may occur when behavior is indirectly influenced by a setting event. When antecedent events are inconsistently associated with problem behavior, a team may want to consider this question: "Are there setting events that reliably precede problem behavior?"

Identifying setting events requires team members to look beyond the immediately observable antecedents to determine whether other types of issues may be causing the student's difficulties. These may come in the form of physiological problems (e.g., illness, lack of sleep, allergies), cyclic events (e.g., menses), changes in the home environment (e.g., parent relationship problems, birth of a sibling, disruption caused by a move, recreational privileges removed), or interpersonal conflicts (e.g., fighting with a peer on the school bus, teasing by a sibling before school). The following example illustrates the process of identifying setting events.

Eve, a sixth-grade student, was identified as having a fairly significant learning disability. Her particular difficulty was in the area of reading. Intellectually, she was above average and was quite adept at learning and maintaining information when it was presented in an auditory mode. Because Eve was a very diligent and hard worker, she was able to remain in general education classes with accommodations, coupled with assistance on assignments one period a day from the learning support teacher. However, Eve's general education teacher noticed that she frequently failed to complete her class assignments. She also recalled that Eve frequently requested bathroom passes; was often out of her seat to sharpen her pencil, play on the computer, or attend to the activities of her classmates; and routinely fiddled with small trinkets that she kept in her desk. Having prior experience in support plan development, her teacher began to collect ABC data. After 3 weeks of careful data collection, no clear patterns were detectable. Although problems were noted only during academic activities, Eve seemed to have "good days and bad days." In particular, some days she attended to her work and completed almost all of her assignments. Other days, few assignments were completed, and associated behaviors (i.e., bathroom requests, out-of-seat behaviors, and fiddling with objects) were frequent. Puzzled, Eve's teacher called a team meeting. The team was unable to make sense of the data or to come up with any reasonable hypotheses. They agreed to continue data collection for an additional 2 weeks and then reconvene. During the intervening 2 weeks, Eve's mother noticed that Eve's bedroom light was sometimes on late at night, well after she was supposed to be sleeping. Eve explained to her mother that she had difficulties sleeping. Each morning when Eve awoke, her mother asked her how she had slept. She carefully documented Eve's response. When the team once again assembled, Eve's mother brought her notes on her daughter's sleep. Indeed, the teacher's data indicating off-task behavior and incomplete assignments corresponded exactly to the prior nights with sleep difficulty. Consequently, the team was able to develop the hypothesis "When Eve has not slept well and is given academic assignments, she engages in off-task behavior, to escape the work." Although developing this hypothesis was a lengthy process, Eve's teacher was now able to make additional accommodations on days when she had not slept well. More importantly, the process allowed Eve's mother to identify her daughter's sleep problem, which she sought a specialist to resolve.

Determining Consequences That Maintain Behavior

A final, yet equally important, consideration during hypothesis development is whether events that follow problem behavior may be reinforcing the behavior. To address this issue, team members must ask, "Do people respond to the student's behavior in a way that encourages the behavior?" As described in Chapter 6, assessment data should ascertain what occurs following the problem behavior. These data should be reviewed to determine whether there is a habitual response to the behavior. Problem behavior that continues, despite the imposition of a standard response following the behavior, suggests that the response may actually be contributing to the problem behavior. More specifically, the response may allow the student to escape or avoid a task or activity, obtain attention from others, acquire an item or activity, or gain sensory stimulation. Analyzing data to identify patterns of responding allows teams to determine whether events that follow behavior may be reinforcing the behavior, thereby suggesting the function of the behavior.

An analysis of Iris's assessment data focused on responses to problem behavior allowed her support team to clarify their hypotheses. A record review indicated that Iris's "noncompliance" almost always occurred around 10:40, during gym class. The activities during gym class that preceded noncompliance, however, differed and the exact antecedent could not be identified. Each time Iris refused to follow instructions, she was sent to the office, where she had to remain until the following class period. This routine response of an office referral led Iris's support team to hypothesize that sitting in the office might be preferable to being in class, and that noncompliance might function to help her escape from gym class. Iris's gym teacher changed the class procedures so that students could request two brief 5-minute breaks at any time during class. He noticed that Iris always used her breaks during endurance activities. Furthermore, her noncompliance disappeared. The team was able to determine that because Iris was not physically fit, she engaged in noncompliance during activities that required endurance, in order to escape these activities.

Tackling Troubling Data

Assessment information can sometimes be confusing. Occasionally patterns are not clear, or the patterns do not make sense on the surface. In this case, additional considerations and analyses may be necessary. Table 7.3 provides an overview of potentially problematic situations and strategies to help resolve the ambiguity. The following paragraphs provide illustrations of such situations.

In one type of situation that may result in unclear data, behavior occurs at relatively consistent rates regardless of differences in the environment, including the presence or absence of others who may respond to the behavior. In other words, no one event or response is reliably associated with the problem behavior. There are two possible explanations for this type of pattern. First, although epidemiological data suggest that such situ-

TABLE 7.3. Considerations When Data Are Unclear

Questions	Strategies
Does the behavior occur at relatively consistent rates across all settings, including when the individual is alone? Does the behavior appear to be physically reinforcing or pleasing to the individual? Is the behavior more frequent when the individual has little to do?	• Consider whether the behavior might serve a biological function. • Observe the individual to ascertain whether he or she appears to be receiving pleasurable sensory input. • Compare highly stimulating environments with low-stimulation environments to determine whether behavior might serve to provide stimulation.
Could idiosyncratic variables be influencing the behavior?	• Reexamine data to identify idiosyncratic variables. • Convene team to consider idiosyncratic variables.
Is the behavior low in frequency?	• Determine whether there are precursors to behavior that occur at a higher frequency. • Conduct record review for additional information about possible antecedents or reinforcers to low-frequency behavior.
Is the behavior difficult to observe?	• Obtain self-report data.

ations are infrequent (e.g., Iwata et al., 1994), sometimes behaviors can occur for biological reasons (Mace & Mauk, 1995). That is, a behavior results in some type of biological event, such as the release of endorphins, that is pleasurable to the individual. This explanation is more typical with behaviors directed toward oneself (e.g., self-injury) than with behaviors that are outwardly directed (e.g., aggression). It should be underscored that because biological explanations are infrequent, environmental explanations should be thoroughly explored first.

A second explanation is that behavior serves a self-stimulatory function. Rather than receiving reinforcement from the external environment, self-stimulatory behavior is self-reinforcing, which serves to maintain it. Typically, self-stimulation functions to provide access to internal stimulation, as in the case of Pat's eye poking, which provided enjoyable visual stimulation by distorting outside images. In addition to visual reinforcement, stimulation can come in the form of auditory, tactile, vestibular, or olfactory input. Self-stimulatory behavior also can function to avoid some sort of internal or external stimulation. For example, when Abe rocked back and forth with his eyes closed, it decreased sensory input when he was in noisy environments.

Engaging in self-stimulatory behaviors, such as hair twirling and leg swinging, is common among all individuals. However, when such a behavior interferes with learning or social interaction, or is socially inappropriate or stigmatizing, it becomes a problem needing intervention. Although self-stimulatory behavior may not be associated with predictable environmental events, it tends to occur more frequently in environments that provide low amounts of stimulation, such as when an individual is provided with little to do of interest. Thus, when behavior is suspected to be self-stimulatory, data should be examined to determine whether lower frequencies are· observed in highly stimulating environments.

In general, testing procedures to confirm whether behavior serves a biological or self-stimulatory function are difficult to implement, particularly in everyday settings. Typically, a self-stimulatory hypothesis is one of default, arrived at after all other potential environmental events have been ruled out. When a team is considering a sensory hypothesis, it should be kept in mind that sometimes behavior that appears to be self-stimulatory really is not. For example, although excessive self-talk appears self-stimulatory in form, it can serve to avoid social interactions with others (e.g., peers avoided Lea because they did not understand her nonsensical self-talking, which was odd to them) or to obtain attention (e.g., adults approached Suji when he began self-talk, in an attempt to stop it so he would not interrupt his classmates).

After determining that behavior serves a sensory function, it is important to attempt to figure out what type of sensory input the behavior provides, so that a related intervention can be developed. Again, this is not an easy endeavor. In a classic example, Rincover (1978) described a procedure to determine the sensory function of an individual's object spinning. When surfaces were carpeted, the spinning stopped, suggesting that it provided auditory input. Usually such testing is difficult, as in the case of eye poking. Careful observation and logic are needed.

A second type of situation that may result in unclear data is when a student's challenging behavior is influenced by highly idiosyncratic events. On these occasions, environmental events associated with the behavior may be difficult to determine. For example, Treat, a 16-year-old student with developmental disabilities, engaged in severe self-injury. Assessment information revealed that the self-injury regularly occurred with a specific teacher, Ms. Waters. However, Treat's team was unable to figure out the specific reasons why self-injury occurred with Ms. Waters. Even when Treat was involved in his most highly preferred activity, he still engaged in self-injury if Ms. Waters approached him. This was highly surprising to all of the school staff. Ms. Waters was considered one of the best teachers in her state, and she had received numerous teaching awards. Her classroom was a motivating environment full of interesting activities. She was well organized, and her students' daily programs were closely matched to their preferences and levels of functioning. Ms. Waters also had a very good rapport with her students. She was positive, encouraging, and warm. Her students clearly loved to be with her. She had excellent classroom control and rarely experienced problems with any student in her classroom. Perplexed, Ms. Waters called upon others for assistance. A team meeting was held, which was attended by Treat's new foster mother, Ms. Clausin. Immediately, Ms. Clausin noted the resemblance between Ms. Waters and Treat's natural mother, from whose custody he had been removed as a result of mistreatment. This clarified the cause of Treat's self-injury and allowed Ms. Waters to develop a plan for gradually building a trusting relationship with Treat, in order to reduce his self-injury while in her presence.

A third type of situation in which hypotheses may not be easily forthcoming is in the case of a low-frequency but high-intensity behavior. Because the behavior does not occur often, assessment data to identify antecedents and consequences are necessarily limited. One strategy given this situation is to determine whether there are precursors to the serious and low-frequency behavior that occur at a higher frequency. For example, fights at school are usually preceded by arguments or other inappropriate peer interactions, which may occur more often than the severe behavior of fighting. Interventions that decrease or eliminate such precursors should also decrease or eliminate the behaviors that follow. Thus the precursors should be the focus of assessment, hypothesis development, and intervention.

Another strategy for low-frequency behaviors is to rely largely on historical information when gathering assessment information. This was necessary in Pierce's case. The recess supervisor at Pierce's elementary school reported that she caught him fighting. She did not know how the fight started, she saw only the scuffle that ensued. Ms. Gonzales, Pierce's teacher, was very concerned, because this was Pierce's second fight this school year. In this case, because of the low frequency of the behavior, the support team could not afford to wait until the behavior occurred to collect direct observation data on the antecedents and potential function. Thus Pierce's teacher reviewed all of the accumulated disciplinary reports in his permanent file and found that he had been in fights three or four times each of the previous three school years. School staff members had observed many of those fights. In each case, the report indicated that Pierce began the fight in response to being teased or provoked by a peer. With this information, Ms. Gonzales was able to reduce Pierce's fighting by teaching him alternative ways to respond to teasing and provocation, and by promoting supportive and cooperative interactions among all of her students.

A final type of situation that causes difficulty is when a behavior occurs in a covert manner. Many behaviors, particularly those that are self-directed or "internalizing," may not be subject to observation. Examples of these behaviors include social withdrawal, cutting, drug use, and weapon possession. To date, the literature lacks examples where behaviors of this nature have been successfully reduced through the PBS process. However, we believe that the basic approach of identifying environmental events that appear to be associated with the behaviors, as well as enhancing lifestyle factors, should be central to the intervention process. The difficulty comes in identifying variables associated with the behaviors, given their concealed occurrence. It is likely that the assessment process will be focused on self-report. However, the accuracy of self-report is unknown at this time, and how it can be used to address internalizing behaviors is also unclear. Further research is needed to detail the process and outcomes.

Ambiguous Antecedents or Functions

Occasionally situations arise when the function for a problem behavior does not seem to conform to the categories that have been established in the literature (i.e., attention, escape, tangible, sensory). Similarly, antecedents to the behavior are not readily apparent. Such was the case with Jordan, a 12-year-old boy we recently encountered. Jordan had a history of encopresis, and data indicated that it occurred across all settings—at school, during his after-school program, and at home. Medical evaluations ruled out any physical explanation for his accidents. After many, many weeks of direct observation failed to yield any consistent antecedents to his accidents, we decided that our only remaining alternative to obtain information about his encopresis was to interview him. During the student interview, he told us that his peers or his parents sometimes teased him or made him mad, and that his accidents were a way to "get back" at them. In other words, in his eyes the purpose of his encopresis was revenge for what he saw as unfair treatment from others. The accidents usually occurred at a later time than the teasing or problematic interaction, making it difficult to identify the antecedent and suggesting that the behavior did not function to escape the interaction. In fact, at least with Jordan's father, the accidents resulted in additional reprimands.

This example illustrates the important point that occasionally the function of a behavior does not fall neatly into the commonly defined categories. As the PBS process is increasingly expanded to an array of challenges (e.g., psychiatric difficulties) and behavior problems, a wider scope of functions may need to be considered. When antecedents and/or functions are not entirely clear, teams may consider writing modified hypothesis statements—ones that are not complete, but identify at least some environmental variables that the team can address. In Jordan's case, we have developed the following hypothesis: "When Jordan is teased by his peers or parents, or when he is angry, he is likely to engage in encopresis." Although the behavior's function is not identified, this hypothesis has offered us a starting place for intervention. Our focus can be on giving Jordan alternatives for managing his anger and addressing peer and parent teasing. Once a behavior support plan is in place, we may learn more about other antecedents and gather enough information to formulate a hypothesis for the behavior's function. Then again, we may never completely understand its function, and we may not need to if our intervention efforts based on identified environmental factors are successful.

Considering Multiple Functions, Behaviors, and Environmental Events

For simplicity's sake, the prior examples for the most part have illustrated assessment information that points to a single hypothesis. However, it frequently happens that a student engages in problem behavior for more than one reason. For example, in some situations a student's disruption may allow him or her to escape from an undesired assignment, while in other situations that very same disruptive behavior may provide the student with attention from peers. This can be confusing because just when a team believes it has nailed down events related to problem behavior—say, lengthy assignments—disruption occurs when there are absolutely no academic demands. During the assessment process, it is important to review all possible types of reinforcement that follow behavior. Multiple functions for a behavior require the development of multiple hypotheses.

Likewise, an individual may engage in several different types of problem behaviors that serve a single function. For example, Dillon learned that he was able to get access to toys that his classmates were engaged with by verbally intimidating them, being aggressive toward them, or whining and crying. He had learned that particular peers responded differentially, depending on which of the three behaviors he exhibited. Although these three behaviors appeared outwardly to be very different, they all served the same function of obtaining a toy. This was reflected in his assessment data, which identified similar antecedents and responses, yet a variety of different behaviors. Thus all behaviors were the focus of a single intervention: learning to share.

Another point to keep in mind is that different behaviors may serve altogether different functions. In our work with Carla, we noted that her self-injury and aggression appeared to occur in very different situations (Kern, Carberry, & Haidera, 1997). Assessment information indeed indicated that Carla's self-injury, which consisted of punching her temples and cheeks with a closed fist, occurred in the cafeteria and functioned to obtain access to meals; aggression, in the form of clutching the clothing of staff members, functioned to help her escape from nonpreferred activities. In

Carla's case, this match between behavior topography and function made perfect sense when we considered that her clutching the clothing of others would actually hinder a staff member from being able to bring her lunch tray quickly. Instead, in order to avoid serious harm, the staff responded by quickly providing her with food as soon as self-injury began to occur. On the other hand, refusing to release staff members' clothing made it impossible for them to continue with a task. Thus, when a team is developing hypotheses, it is important to evaluate each different type or topography of problem behavior individually to ascertain whether they serve the same or different functions, as well as to consider that a single behavior may serve more than one function. When assessment data indicate that different antecedents and responses are associated with different behaviors, more than one hypothesis must be formulated.

A final note is that more than one type of antecedent event can contribute to problem behavior. For example, difficult work and lengthy (but not difficult) assignments may both result in unwanted behavior that serves an escape function. Thus hypotheses may identify multiple antecedent events, all of which are related to occurrences of problem behavior.

To summarize, sometimes assessment information yields behavior patterns that are very clear and consistent, and hypotheses are readily forthcoming. At other times, much more effort is required to determine the causes of behavior. Difficulties may arise because of the presence of setting events, different topographies of problem behavior, multiple functions, or more than one antecedent preceding behavior problems. It is important for a team to consider all of these possibilities when developing hypothesis statements, so that the impending support plan is sure to address all of the target individual's needs. Obtaining information from different individuals and using a variety of formats (e.g., interview, direct observation) are ways to increase the chance that all pertinent issues in the life of the student are considered. Furthermore, convergence of different data sources provides reassurance that problematic environmental variables have been detected.

WAYS TO SUMMARIZE ASSESSMENT INFORMATION

In order to interpret assessment information easily and generate hypotheses, it is often useful to summarize it, either in graphic or table format. A simple graph or table provides a visual depiction or simple summary that is less cumbersome than raw data and facilitates review by team members. When a graph or table is used to summarize assessment information, it is important to keep in mind that data should be displayed in such a way that the relevant findings are depicted. That is, a graphic display can depict the events, settings, time periods, individuals, or function linked to occurrences of the behavior of focus.

Figure 7.7 shows an example of Meredith's graphically displayed data. Meredith was a seventh-grade student who received numerous disciplinary referrals for disruptive classroom behavior. Each of her seven teachers agreed to collect data on the frequency and time of her disruptions across a full week of school. Figure 7.7 clearly depicts problematic and non-problematic class periods. During the observation week, Meredith engaged in disruptive behavior during reading, math, science, social studies, and writing classes. Few disruptions occurred during art or shop classes. Interviews with Meredith's teachers indicated that she usually started off well in her academic classes, but that her behavior worsened as each class period progressed. Based on this information, her support team reexamined the data collected, breaking it down according to 15-minute intervals during problematic class periods. This analysis, shown in Figure 7.8, confirms that disruptions were considerably higher at the end of class than at the beginning. These data led Meredith's support team to develop the hypothesis "When given a lengthy assignment that does not involve hands-on activities, Meredith engages in disruption to escape the assignment." Consequently, her support team was able to develop an intervention that involved increasing hands-on activities and allowing her to request one or two brief breaks during class.

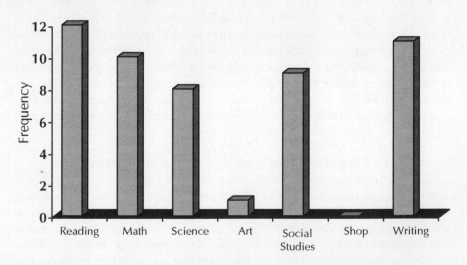

FIGURE 7.7. Graphic display of Meredith's class periods with disruptive behavior.

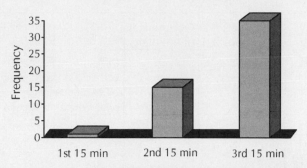

FIGURE 7.8. Graphic display of blocks of time when Meredith engaged in disruptive behavior.

Randy's assessment data are summarized in Figure 7.9. This more tabular format easily shows activities that were problematic and summarizes information from anecdotal notes and interviews suggesting the reasons why each activity may have resulted in self-injury. A quick review of this summary makes it clear that Randy's self-injury often occurred during difficult tasks or those that he was unable to complete easily and with success. It can also be seen that Randy liked activities involving water, and that he enjoyed being around people.

Figure 7.10 is a graphic display of Ivan's data. Depicted on the graph are events following his self-injury. As the first three bars indicate, the majority of the time staff members responded to Ivan's self-injury by blocking, reprimanding, or redirecting him. Each of these responses provided some type of attention, suggesting that the self-injury might serve to obtain attention. Of course, these data would need to be examined in combination with antecedents to provide further evidence of behavioral function.

TESTING HYPOTHESES

What Hypothesis Testing Is

Hypotheses are derived from assessment data. But because assessment information is collected during naturally occurring situations, it provides only correlational data about events associated with problem behavior. In other words, direct observations can suggest whether or not a particular event seems to co-occur with problem behavior. However, given that many events happen concurrently in classroom settings, it cannot clearly demonstrate that a particular event absolutely causes or maintains a problem

Daily activity observed	Number of times observed	Occurrences of self-injury	Notes
Brushing teeth	10	8	Difficulty removing toothpaste cap on three occasions; hands shaking on two occasions—couldn't get paste on toothbrush
Washing face	10	0	Randy seemed to enjoy activity
Dressing	5	3	All occurrences only during shoe tying
Hanging coat	4	1	Many people clustered around the coat rack, and Randy got impatient
Meal preparation	9	0	Seemed anxious to prepare meal so he could go to the cafeteria and eat with his classmates and staff
Washing dishes	9	0	Randy liked the warm water
Cleaning floors	3	3	Could not manipulate mop easily on one occasion; seemed upset when he could not get stains off the floor on two occasions
Washing clothing	5	0	Likes to watch water fill in washing machine
Money skills	6	4	Hard activity; consistently makes many errors
Community outing	4	0	Randy seemed very happy and greeted many people

FIGURE 7.9. Summary of Randy's assessment information.

behavior. Hypothesis testing can be used to confirm this relationship, and thereby to confirm or refute the accuracy of a hypothesis.

How to Test Hypotheses

A hypothesis can be tested by examining the frequency of behavior in the presence and absence of the variable identified during the assessment phase as potentially associated with problem behavior. The variable can be either an antecedent that precedes the problem behavior (e.g., presenting a math worksheet) or a response that follows the problem behavior (e.g., sending the student to time out). That is, occurrences of problem behavior during typical classroom conditions are compared with occurrences of problem

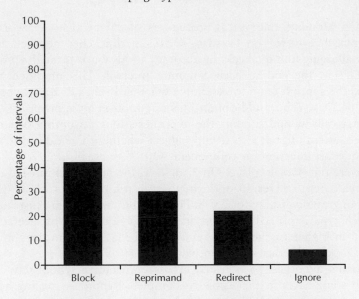

FIGURE 7.10. Summary of events following Ivan's self-injury.

behavior during modified conditions when the variable hypothesized to influence problem behavior is removed or modified in some way.

When a team is testing hypotheses, it is best to alternate a single variable at a time. For example, even though assessment information suggests that close teacher proximity, difficult work, and peer attention are all associated with problem behavior, each should be tested individually. This will provide a precise picture of the independent influence of each variable on problem behavior.

Typically, conditions are alternated across time for comparison purposes. From an experimental perspective, this process uses what is technically referred to as a *reversal* or *brief reversal* design. If the problem behavior systematically varies in response to changing environmental conditions (e.g., it decreases each time work difficulty is decreased), this provides evidence for the accuracy of the hypothesis.

To illustrate, Brian's support team hypothesized that his disruptive behavior occurred during independent seatwork and was designed to gain the attention of a particular peer, Eli; Brian reportedly wanted to befriend Eli, but lacked the social skills to do so. Brian's team developed the hypothesis, "When given independent seatwork, Brian engages in disruption, to obtain Eli's attention." Because math class was structured so that independent seatwork was required each day during the last 20 minutes, this class was selected for hypothesis testing. The hypothesis was tested across 4 days. On Monday, the typical procedures of independent seatwork were left in place. However, on Tuesday, Brian's math teacher modified the routine by allowing him to check the accuracy of his work through comparing it to Eli's at the end of each 5-minute interval. This modified routine allowed the support team to determine whether Brian's disruptive behavior would decrease if he could obtain Eli's attention in an appropriate way. If so, it not only would support the hypothesis that disruption occurred to gain peer attention, but also would suggest whether the modification could be used as an intervention component. On Wednesday, the typical procedures were put back in place. On Thursday, the peer check procedure was again evaluated. The results of the hypothesis testing across school days are shown in graphic display format in Figure 7.11. As the data illustrate, days in which typical procedures were in place, denoted by "no peer check," resulted in higher frequencies of disruptive behaviors than days in which "peer check" procedures were in place.

Brian's hypothesis was tested across consecutive school days. However, in some cases it is possible to complete hypothesis testing across a shorter period of time. In the case of Courtney, hypothesis testing was completed in a single morning. Her support team hypothesized that she engaged in refusal behavior (screaming and stomping her feet) when an instruction to complete a task was issued in a stern and demanding manner. This hypothesis was based on the observation that there was no consistency across tasks that were refused and those that were completed; however, the behaviors occurred most frequently with a particular staff member. This

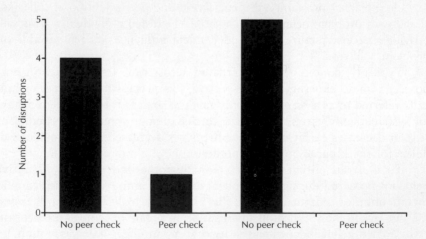

FIGURE 7.11. Results of Brian's hypothesis testing: Number of disruptions during independent seatwork.

particular staff member had a very demanding style of interaction when she assisted Courtney with task completion. To test the hypothesis "When a request is issued in a demanding way, Courtney engages in refusal behavior, to escape the request," six tasks were selected that she routinely completed. The request to complete the first task was issued in the usual demanding way by the staff member. She stated, "Courtney, put your coat away," in a brisk, loud manner. The next task request was modified so that it was presented in a calm, quiet, and less demanding way. The staff member approached Courtney, greeted her, and then calmly suggested that she complete the next task by stating, "Courtney, it's nice to see you today. Why don't you give Ms. Diehl your lunch money?" These two styles of instructional requests were alternated across the six selected tasks. As Figure 7.12 shows, stern requests were associated with refusal behavior and failure to complete the task, while calm requests were associated with the absence of refusal behavior and task completion.

Name: _Courtney_　　　　　　　　Person testing hypothesis: _Amy_

Date: _January 15_

Hypothesis tested: _When a request is issued in a demanding way, Courtney_
engages in refusal behavior, to escape the request.

Task	Condition	Task Completed? (Yes or No)	Incidents of Problem Behavior	Comments
Hang coat	Harsh	No	1	Screamed for 3 minutes until I hung coat for her
Pay for lunch	Calm	Yes	0	Very compliant and pleasant
Go to seat	Harsh	No	3	Never went to seat; I had to physically escort her
Complete daily schedule	Calm	Yes	0	Good behavior
Set table	Harsh	Yes	2	Screamed and stomped for several minutes, then set table
Clear table	Calm	Yes	0	Complied right away

FIGURE 7.12. Results of hypothesis testing for Courtney.

When to Test Hypotheses

Testing hypotheses can either confirm or refute their accuracy. There are certain situations when hypothesis testing is prudent and desirable, and others in which it is not recommended. Hypothesis testing may be advantageous in situations where a support team is not certain of the accuracy of a hypothesis. In cases where behavior appears to be relatively complex or intransigent, it may be practical in the long run to test hypotheses prior to developing a support plan. However, prior to making a decision to test hypotheses, the potential danger of the behavior must first be considered. It is never advisable to create a situation in which an individual may cause harm to him- or herself or another. If this is likely, it is usually better to develop and introduce a support plan based on available information, which can be modified if it is not adequate. In all cases, the potential benefit of hypothesis testing must be weighed against the possible damage that could result. A team may determine it is worth enduring some problem behavior to be sure that a hypothesis is correct and will lead to an effective support plan. This is a decision that must be made by team members, taking into consideration the severity of the problem behavior, the ease and feasibility of testing a hypothesis, and the long-term benefit of data-driven support for the hypothesis and ultimately the support plan.

Another consideration when a team is determining whether to test a hypothesis is whether the behavior can easily be reversed. Hypothesis testing requires behavior to change in response to varying environmental conditions. When the hypothesis involves teaching a new skill, such as providing a strategy to facilitate completion of difficult math word problems, it may not be possible to test whether the intervention is effective; once the strategy is learned, it cannot be withdrawn. Likewise, a behavior problem, such as making inappropriate noises or faces, may occur to obtain attention from peers. One component of an intervention might involve teaching peers to ignore the behavior and continue their work. After teaching peers to ignore it, it may not be possible or reasonable to ask them to respond once again to the behavior.

Analogue Functional Analysis

An alternative to the procedure described above for evaluating the function of problem behavior was developed by Iwata, Dorsey, Slifer, Bauman, and Richman (1982) and has been demonstrated and replicated numerous times in the literature. Known as *analogue functional analysis*, this procedure tests potential reinforcers for problem behavior in an analogue or contrived setting, such as an empty classroom or therapy room. Typically, four different types of conditions are tested during sessions that last 5–15 minutes.

During an attention condition, the staff member diverts his or her attention from the focus individual. When problem behavior occurs, the individual is provided with a brief period of attention (e.g., 30 seconds). Theoretically, high rates of problem behavior during this condition suggest that the behavior occurs to obtain attention, and that it continues or is maintained by the provision of attention. Similarly, during an escape condition, work demands are placed on the individual. If problem behavior occurs, the demands are briefly removed. Elevated rates of problem behavior during this condition indicate that problem behavior serves an escape function. In a tangible condition, a preferred item or activity is removed from the individual. When problem behavior occurs, temporary access to the item or activity is given. Observed problems under these circumstances imply that it functions to obtain tangible items or activities. These three conditions are compared with a play or control condition, in which the individual is provided with preferred activities and attention and the session is free from demands. Problem behavior that occurs for environmental reasons should be absent during play sessions.

When a team is conducting an analogue functional analysis, sessions are repeated in random order, using what is referred to as a *multielement experimental design*, until patterns emerge within and between conditions. For instance, high and consistent rates of self-injury during only the escape condition, when demands are removed following occurrences of self-injury, would indicate that the behavior is maintained by escape from demands.

Analogue functional analysis has several advantages. It usually can be completed in a relatively short period of time. Sessions are typically 10–15 minutes in duration; this means that the analysis can be completed in a few hours, including brief breaks between sessions. This may appear to be attractive when compared with the prospect of collecting data across several days or even weeks. In addition to being relatively brief, the procedures are standardized and unambiguous. This contrasts greatly with the multitude of formats, methodologies, and procedures that have been used to conduct functional assessments in school settings, which can be confusing and overwhelming. Finally, in many cases the analysis yields a readily apparent function without a great deal of data analysis and interpretation. Definitive answers are gratifying when a team is addressing problem behavior.

In spite of its strengths, this methodology also has limitations. Perhaps the most worrisome is that with any procedure conducted in an atypical setting, one can never be sure that the variables present in the testing environment are the same as those in the natural environment. A simple example is that analogue functional analysis is conducted on a one-to-one basis, which excludes the possibility of peers as a source of reinforcement for problem behavior. It is well known that peers can exert a great deal of influence on the behavior of their classmates, and thus they constitute a variable that should not be neglected. Among the many other variables that may differ between the testing environment and the natural environment are room size, décor, lighting, noise, staff, materials, and tasks. Because it is virtually impossible to replicate variables in the natural setting within a testing environment, it may be difficult to identify the precise antecedents of problem behavior—particularly when they involve combinations of variables, such as a lengthy and difficult assignment in the context of a noisy, distracting environment. It may be extremely frustrating to a team to develop an intervention based on the results of an analogue functional analysis, only to find that it is not effective in the setting where an individual typically spends time.

A second concern with analogue functional analysis is that it requires providing reinforcement for problem behavior. Theoretically, problem behavior continues because it has been reinforced in the past, and analogue functional analysis simply tests this assumption in a rapid way by providing a dense schedule of reinforcement (i.e., every time problem behavior occurs) across a brief period of time. However, providing reinforcement for problem behavior makes it possible for an individual to learn, during the analysis, that engaging in the problem behavior will result in access to a preferred situation or escape from a nonpreferred situation. That is, problem behavior emerges during the testing situation, but is not indicative of why an individual typically engages in problem behavior in the natural setting. This becomes a particularly salient concern with individuals who fall into the higher range of cognitive functioning and can readily recognize that by simply engaging in a particular problem behavior, they can avoid any demand placed upon them. Furthermore, many teachers and practitioners are reluctant to reinforce problem behavior under any circumstances, even if only during a testing situation. For example, a teacher may find it objectionable to purposefully remove a student's assignment and say that the student can take a break after the teacher has just been hit. An equally important consideration when a team is considering reinforcing problem behavior is whether the behavior will cause serious injury or damage. If such an outcome is likely, team members may decide to avoid this procedure. Ultimately, the team must weigh the potential value of the information the analysis will provide against the risk involved.

Analogue functional analysis is also limited in that it focuses exclusively on immediate contextual variables. The analysis is conducted in a way that attempts to isolate antecedents occurring immediately prior to the problem behavior and reinforcers occurring immediately after. However, as we discuss throughout this book, setting events as well as lifestyle issues play a significant role in the occurrence of problem behaviors and must be considered when teams are developing support plans that are comprehensive and will address the lifelong needs, rights, and well-being of individuals with disabilities.

A fourth limitation of this methodology is that it requires resources that may not be available in school settings. Because it is conducted away from the classroom setting in a one-to-one situation, it requires a vacant room, a staff member to implement the procedures, and another staff member to collect data. Most schools are hard pressed to find these resources, even if only for a few hours of the school day.

A final limitation of analogue functional analysis is that although it may identify the general circumstance (e.g., demands issued) and function (e.g., escape) of a problem behavior, it is less helpful at pinpointing specific antecedents (e.g., lengthy tasks) or potentially effective interventions. Such an analysis focuses only on problem behavior; therefore, it does not include the opportunity to develop an understanding of contexts in which problem behavior is absent, or of situations that are enjoyable and productive for an individual. Nor does it specify particulars regarding the environmental events associated with problem behavior, such as the reason why a particular task is associated with problem behavior. This important information, gathered during a more comprehensive functional assessment, is usually critical for developing a comprehensive support plan.

Several recent surveys indicate that analogue functional analyses are seldom used in school settings (e.g., Derochers, Hile, & Willams-Mosley, 1997; Ellingson, Miltenberger, & Long, 1999; Scott, Meers, & Nelson, 2000). In addition, we believe that testing hypotheses in the natural context, as described earlier, is a more comprehensive and feasible approach. For this reason, we do not delineate the procedures for analogue analyses in detail in this book. However, it is a methodology with a great deal of empirical support that may be very valuable in certain circumstances. We encourage readers who believe the methodology will be useful to consult the original article (Iwata et al., 1982) for a procedural description.

CONSIDERING BROAD INFORMATION

When a team is developing hypotheses regarding the role of antecedents, setting events, and consequences that influence problem behavior, it is equally important to consider lifestyle issues. Variables that have a broad but unfavorable impact on an individual's life, such as an absence of close friends, limited opportunities to engage in preferred leisure activities, or health problems can significantly influence an individual's tolerance of or response to more immediate problematic events. Thus it is critical to concurrently summarize broad information and hypothesize about the possible influence of lifestyle issues on behavior. Chapter 11 provides detailed information about the link between broad information and lifestyle issues, as well as their place in support plan development. It is important to note that the process of hypothesis development described in the current chapter can be applied in much the same way to identify lifestyle issues that are having an objectionable effect on an individual's well-being. Readers are referred to Chapter 11 for additional direction.

SUMMARY

Developing hypothesis statements is a critical step in the process of support plan development. Such a statement serves to summarize assessment information and to assure a link between the assessment information that was gathered and the support plan. A hypothesis statement recognizes the immediate environmental events that are associated with problem behavior, while broad information tends to pertain to the development of problem behavior and lifestyle issues. In certain circumstances, a team may decide that it is important to test the accuracy of a specific hypothesis. This can be accomplished by manipulating the variables that are hypothesized to be associated with problem behavior. Hypotheses that are correctly formulated directly suggest interventions that will result in behavior improvement and greatly facilitate the development of a support plan.

COMMONLY ASKED QUESTIONS

How many hypotheses will we need to develop for any particular student? Eliminating problem behavior requires in some way addressing all of the variables that are associated with problem behavior. Each cause and function of problem behavior should result in its own hypothesis. This means that it is often necessary to develop numerous hypotheses for a given student. The specific number will be very individualized. Although this can become a time-consuming process, it is essential for comprehensive and long-lasting improvements.

What should we do if we cannot develop hypotheses based on the assessment information? Assessment information should yield consistent and detectable patterns of behavior that lead directly to hypotheses. If hypotheses cannot be easily developed from the information gathered, it is advisable to continue to collect additional information until patterns are evident.

What if some of our assessment information supports a specific hypothesis, but not all of it is consistent with that hypothesis? When an individual engages in problem behavior for a variety of reasons, sometimes some of the assessment information results in clear patterns, while other information does not. When this happens, it is usually prudent to develop hypotheses as patterns emerge. This way, intervention components can be developed that will reduce problem behavior in some contexts. Meanwhile, further information can be gathered to clarify additional variables associated with problem behavior.

Once hypotheses have been developed and confirmed, will they ever change? As individuals mature, or events in their lives change (such as attending a new classroom or school), the causes for problem behavior may also change. Thus a hypothesis developed by a team that led to an effective intervention may no longer be valid. It is important for teams to consider new and different hypotheses when problem behavior reemerges, particularly when team members are sure that the existing support plan is being implemented as designed.

CASE EXAMPLES

Malik's Hypotheses

Hypothesis Development

Malik's core team met to discuss the summary information from the functional assessment. The team's purpose was to come to a consensus on hypothesis statements that would offer data-based explanations for Malik's problem behaviors. Malik's team came up with three hypotheses that would guide their support activities. Although each hypothesis identified escape as a function of problem behavior, they differed with regard to antecedents.

- *Hypothesis 1: When prompted through difficult work (e.g., letter and number naming, verbal communication), Malik is likely to refuse/aggress, to escape the activity.* Although Malik encountered many difficult tasks in school, currently the most difficult tasks (as revealed by the functional assessment data) were (a) letter and number recognition and (b) communication, particularly when Malik was prompted to use words rather than gestures or to speak in two- or three-word strings rather than one word. Interestingly, all these activities required recall, which the team speculated might be difficult for him.
- *Hypothesis 2: When asked to complete nonfunctional activities, Malik is*

likely to refuse/aggress, to escape the activity. This hypothesis was based on several bits of information. First, although problem behaviors were less frequent with letter- and number-sorting activities, they sometimes still occurred during these and other academic activities (although the team never observed that Malik refused to participate in academic games, such as Math Bingo). Second, problem behavior was nonexistent during outdoor recess, classroom chores, or any "assistant-type" activities (e.g., serving as a cafeteria assistant or teacher assistant). The team speculated that Malik enjoyed chores and assisting with activities because they were similar to things he did at home. His grandmother explained that Malik enjoyed being active, liked feeling "special" by helping out, and felt proud of his accomplishments when activities (e.g., helping around the house) were completed. In contrast, the team wondered whether Malik found value in or saw the purpose of some of his academic activities, particularly when they were presented in isolation, stripped from any meaningful activity. When the team thought about it, it made sense that he would enjoy Math Bingo, because the game had a purpose . . . to win! But what about other activities, such as letter sorting? Did Malik find the meaning in that? Did he understand its purpose? The team defined *nonfunctional activities* as those did not have a clear, meaningful outcome or value for Malik.

- *Hypothesis 3: When required to make a transition from a highly preferred activity to a nonpreferred activity, Malik refuses/aggresses, to maintain the preferred activity and avoid the nonpreferred one.* This hypothesis was based on the evidence that problem behaviors occurred around transitions, particularly when Malik was asked to leave an activity that he enjoyed.

Taken together, all three of these hypotheses would help the team select effective interventions for each component of Malik's support plan. Strategies for antecedent interventions, alternative skill training, responses for problem behavior, and long-term supports designed specifically for Malik are described at the ends of Chapters 8, 9, 10, and 11 respectively.

Bethany's Hypotheses

Hypothesis Development

Bethany's special education teacher summarized the assessment data collected, and a conference call was scheduled to discuss the outcomes with the other members of Bethany's core support team. Four hypotheses were developed during the conference call.

- *Hypothesis 1: When Bethany is given written assignments, she engages in off-task behavior, to escape.* There was consensus among the team members that written work was difficult for Bethany. During her interview, Bethany directly stated that she did not like writing. Ms. DeLope observed that most of Bethany's homework assignments were written, which might account for her homework completion problems. Direct observation supported written work as a problem. Higher rates of problem behavior occurred during written assignments than during nonwritten assignments. Finally, her records revealed difficulty with fine motor skills, which might partly explain the problem.

- *Hypothesis 2: When Bethany is given lengthy assignments, she engages in off-task behavior, to escape.* Direct observation data showed that Bethany often began her work, but failed to complete it. In addition, Bethany revealed during her interview that she often felt overwhelmed with her schoolwork.

- *Hypothesis 3: When Bethany has visited her father over the weekend, she engages in off-task behavior, to escape work (because of fatigue).* Bethany's teacher indicated that Bethany often complained about being tired. She seemed to recollect that this happened more often on Mondays. The team thought that Bethany might be fatigued on Mondays after arriving home late from visits with her father.

- *Hypothesis 4: When Bethany is in unstructured situations (e.g., lunch, free time) with unfamiliar peers, she engages in inappropriate interactions, to obtain their attention.* Observations indicated that Bethany sometimes had problems with peers. Bethany's mother suggested that this might be because it took her a while to get used to new situations and new people. The school staff agreed that problems generally occurred around peers who were not Bethany's friends.

Hypothesis Testing

Bethany's team decided to test the hypotheses before developing a support plan. In spite of the fact that several of the hypotheses were supported by multiple types of assessment information, this decision was made because Bethany's behavior problems had been ongoing for a long period of time; the hypotheses appeared relatively easy to test; and the team members wanted to make sure that they were accurate so an effective intervention could be developed that would allow Bethany to stay in the general education program.

Hypothesis testing took place during naturally occurring situations in Bethany's class, and was planned and implemented jointly by the general education and special education teachers. It was determined that testing would continue as briefly as possible and only until behavior patterns were evident.

Testing of Hypothesis 1 was conducted to confirm whether written work was associated with more problem behaviors than nonwritten work. This hypothesis was tested during daily 15-minute journal writing—an activity associated with problem behavior during direct observations. This hypothesis was tested across 4 school days by alternating written and nonwritten assignments. During written assignments, Bethany was required to complete her journal writing in her journal, using a pencil or pen. During nonwritten assignments, Bethany completed her journal activity by recording into an audiotape. Figure 7.13 shows the results of this hypothesis testing.

Hypothesis 2 was tested by comparing Bethany's engagement during short and long assignments. This hypothesis was tested in Bethany's spelling class. The typical routine during spelling was to assign a single activity each day of the week. Daily assignments were to write the spelling words 10 times each, write sentences using the spelling words, complete word searches and word games with the spelling words, and unscramble the spelling words on a computer program. In the testing of Hypothesis 2, rather than have Bethany complete a single activity each day, the teacher divided the activities across the days. Thus, instead of spending Monday writing all of the spelling words, Bethany wrote only a quarter of the words. Completing only one spelling game, writing sentences with a quarter of the words, and unscrambling a quarter of the word list followed. So, rather than spending roughly 40 minutes on a single activity, Bethany completed four activities, each lasting about 10 minutes. Figure 7.14 displays the results of Hypothesis 2 testing.

Hypothesis 3 pertained to Bethany's fatigue and lack of engagement following visits with her father. The team did not deliberately schedule visits versus no visits with her father, but instead gathered data as visits naturally occurred. Ms. DeLope sent a note to the teacher each Monday indicating whether Bethany had visited her father the prior weekend. Data were collected each Monday morning across 5 weeks to compare engagement on the Mondays following a visit and on the Mondays following no visit. Figure 7.15 shows the results of these naturally occurring events.

The final hypothesis that was tested concerned Bethany's interactions when she was with familiar or unfamiliar peers. Bethany's teachers noted that she often

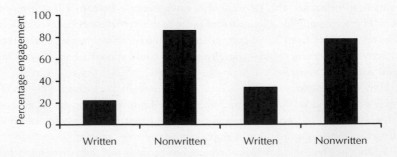

FIGURE 7.13. Hypothesis 1: Bethany's engagement during written versus nonwritten work.

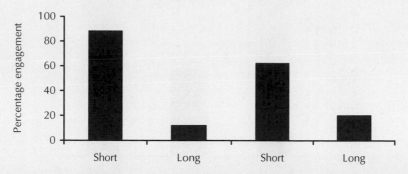

FIGURE 7.14. Hypothesis 2: Bethany's engagement during short versus long assignments.

was delayed in getting to lunch because she was completing her classwork. Because students were seated in the order in which they entered the cafeteria, the delay often caused Bethany to be seated with classes other than her own. The school psychologist agreed to collect data on Bethany's interactions in the cafeteria on days when she was seated with her classmates and when she was not. Figure 7.16 reflects these observations across 3 school days.

To summarize, the hypothesis testing confirmed each of the hypotheses. Bethany's team now had direct data to verify that they had identified variables associated with her problem behavior. The team members also felt reassured that they could develop interventions that would result in behavioral improvements. In addition, the hypothesis testing gave the team ideas about how they could make classroom changes, such as providing a number of short academic assignments rather than a single long assignment.

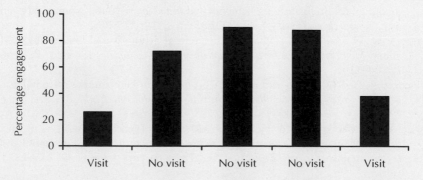

FIGURE 7.15. Hypothesis 3: Bethany's engagement on Mondays following a visit with her father versus Mondays following no visit.

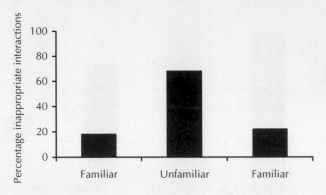

FIGURE 7.16. Hypothesis 4: Bethany's inappropriate interactions with familiar peers versus unfamiliar peers.

REFERENCES

Derochers, M. N., Hile, M. G., & Williams-Mosley, T. L. (1997). Survey of functional assessment procedures used with individuals who display mental retardation and severe problem behaviors. *American Journal on Mental Retardation, 101,* 535–546.

Ellingson, S. A., Miltenberger, R. G., & Long, E. S. (1999). A survey of the use of functional assessment procedures in agencies serving individuals with developmental disabilities. *Behavioral Interventions, 14,* 187–198.

Iwata, B. A., Dorsey, M. F., Slifer, K. J., Bauman, K. E., & Richman, G. S. (1982). Toward a functional analysis of self-injury. *Journal of Applied Behavior Analysis, 27,* 197–209.

Iwata, B. A., Pace, G. M., Dorsey, M. F., Zarcone, J. R., Vollmer, T. R., Smith, R. G., et al. (1994). The functions of self-injurious behavior: An experimental–epidemiological analysis. *Journal of Applied Behavior Analysis, 27,* 215–240.

Kern, L., Carberry, N., & Haidera, C. (1997). Analysis and intervention with two topographies of challenging behavior exhibited by a young woman with autism. *Research in Developmental Disabilities, 18,* 275–287.

Mace, F. C., & Mauk, J. E. (1995). Bio-behavioral diagnosis and treatment of self-injury. *Mental Retardation and Developmental Disabilities Research Reviews, 1,* 104–110.

Rincover, A. (1978). Sensory extinction: A procedure for eliminating self-stimulatory behavior in psychotic children. *Journal of Abnormal Child Psychology, 6,* 299–310.

Scott, T. M., Meers, D. T., & Nelson, C. M. (2000). Toward a consensus of functional behavioral assessment for students with mild disabilities in school contexts: A national survey. *Education and Treatment of Children, 23,* 265–285.

CHAPTER 8

♦ ♦ ♦

Antecedent and Setting
Event Interventions

♦

LEE KERN
SHELLEY CLARKE

This chapter addresses the first component of a positive behavior support (PBS) plan: *antecedent and setting event interventions*. As discussed throughout this book, interventions for problem behavior have long focused on reactive strategies alone, usually in the form of punishment, that are implemented after problem behaviors occur. Only recently have the value and importance of antecedent and setting event interventions been fully appreciated. The strength of these approaches lies in their ability to prevent problem behaviors from occurring. Such an outcome is beneficial not only to the student (whose behavior may cause self-harm, isolation, stigmatization, and the like), but also to others (who may experience environmental disturbance, intrusion, or injury resulting from disruptive and aggressive acts). Furthermore, reducing problem behavior through prevention provides opportunities to teach new and alternative skills—a task that is virtually impossible amidst problem behaviors. In this chapter, we first provide a definition and overview of antecedent and setting event interventions. We then give descriptions of numerous types of antecedent interventions that have been documented in the research literature to effectively reduce challenging behavior. Embedded are strategies for selecting antecedent interventions that match the needs of a particular individual. Setting event interventions are then briefly described. Finally, we suggest circumstances when antecedent or setting event interventions should be faded, and offer strategies for successful fading.

OVERVIEW OF ANTECEDENT AND SETTING EVENT INTERVENTIONS

Description

Chapter 2 has presented the concept of the *four-term contingency*. That is, a setting event influences the likelihood that an antecedent, or immediate environmental event, will trigger a problem behavior; the problem behavior is then responded to in some way, causing the behavior either to continue or increase or to decrease. Antecedent and setting event interventions focus on the first two terms of the four-term contingency. This intervention approach clearly differs from reactive approaches, which focus on the last term of the contingency by imposing some type of consequence following a problem behavior, with the hope that the consequence will reduce the problem behavior. Rather than attempting to reduce problem behavior by implementing a consequence after it occurs, antecedent and setting event interventions instead are designed to restructure the environment to prevent problem behaviors from occurring in the first place.

Preventing problem behaviors requires either eliminating or in some way modifying setting events or antecedent events that precede the problem behavior. That is, either they are removed altogether, or they are changed so that they are either no longer recognized as triggers for problem behavior by the student or they are no longer contain the same array of aversive properties that set off problems.

In addition to eliminating or modifying specific events identified as precursors to problem behavior, antecedent/setting event interventions may also involve modifying, increasing, or introducing events identified to. be associated with desirable behavior. That is, preferred, rewarding, or meaningful events can be incorporated into nonpreferred activities so that they become more preferred and/or less aversive. This strategy reduces problem behavior in the same way as modifying a problematic setting event or antecedent does. Either the specific trigger for problem behavior is masked, or, when blended with pleasing events, it becomes less objectionable.

Advantages of Antecedent and Setting Event Interventions

Antecedent and setting event interventions hold many advantages that are not seen in other interventions (see Table 8.1). The primary advantage of

TABLE 8.1. Advantages of Antecedent and Setting Event Interventions

Purpose	Importance
• Prevent problem behavior	• Reduce likelihood of harm/injury
• Quick-acting	• Assure appropriate curriculum
• Correct faulty environment	• Create pleasant atmosphere
• Enhance instructional environment	• Increase student motivation

these interventions is that they are *preventive*. That is, they serve the specific purpose of preventing problem behaviors from occurring by eliminating or changing the triggers that precede them. Prevention of problem behaviors creates a safe environment for both the student and those in his or her environment. This end is particularly important in circumstances where severe problem behavior places an individual at risk of harming him- or herself or others, or where the behavior puts an individual's educational placement at jeopardy.

In addition to preventing problem behavior, antecedent and setting event interventions tend to be very quick-acting. Problem behaviors generally are rapidly reduced when antecedents or setting events are removed or modified. As is the case in prevention, a hasty reduction of problem behavior is particularly appealing in circumstances of dangerous or extremely disruptive behavior.

Another advantage of antecedent and setting event interventions is that they can correct environmental problems. Many problem behaviors result from external features of the environment that do not fit an individual's needs or are simply unreasonable. For example, a mismatch between the difficulty level of assigned work and a student's skills is a common cause of problem behavior. Similarly, a very lengthy bus ride may function as a setting event for problem behavior. In many cases, antecedent or setting event interventions can resolve these types of inadequacies, creating an appropriate curriculum and reasonable expectations for the student.

Finally, antecedent and setting event interventions are advantageous because they can work to create an improved environment for students. Increasing antecedents and setting events associated with desirable behavior, in conjunction with decreasing those associated with undesirable behavior, can make the resulting environment much more pleasant and motivating for the student. Creating a pleasant and motivating environment throughout the day enhances the individual's general well-being and happiness, thereby reducing the overall likelihood of problem behavior. In addition, learning occurs much more readily in a motivating environment. This is particularly important, because alternative and general skills must be taught to replace problem behavior (described in Chapter 9). Thus the various components of the support plan, such as antecedent/setting event interventions *and* instruction of alternative skills, can work synergistically to achieve desired outcomes rapidly.

Because there has been much more research on antecedent interventions than on setting event interventions, and because it is often more difficult to identify or modify setting events than antecedents, most of the remainder of this chapter focuses on antecedent interventions. We do discuss setting event interventions briefly in a later section.

DEVELOPING ANTECEDENT INTERVENTIONS

Before we describe the specific varieties of antecedent interventions, a bit of general explanation is warranted. Because the types of antecedent events that can trigger problem behavior are numerous, so are the types of antecedent interventions to address the behavior (for a review, see Kern, Choutka, & Sokol, 2002). In essence, almost any type of antecedent event that is identified to be associated with problem behavior can be changed in some way to create an intervention. Likewise, there are many different ways in which any particular antecedent event can be modified to create an intervention. By way of a simple example, the problematic instruction "Recess is over; line up" can be modified by preceding it with a warning (e.g., "In 5 minutes, recess will be over"); by using behavioral momentum, or issuing the instruction following a series of unproblematic instructions ("Point to your line location. What's your line number? Tell me who you are behind. Get in line"); by pairing peers to encourage one another to line up quickly when instructed; or by scheduling a highly preferred activity to follow the difficult transition from recess to class time. Exactly what is changed and how it is changed depend on many factors, such as the predicted effectiveness of the modification, the contextual fit or preference of the team, the resources needed, the long-term goals for the individual, and the ease with which the intervention can be faded. Parameters to consider when a team is selecting an intervention are described in more detail in Chapters 3 and 4. The remainder of this section describes general strategies for narrowing down the intervention options that are likely to be effective. The specific intervention that is ultimately selected remains a decision of the support team, which has an intimate understanding of the many factors that will influence its implementation and effectiveness.

Antecedent interventions rely on hypotheses about antecedents related to problem behavior. Chapter 7 has described the importance of linking intervention to assessment information—a process facilitated through hypothesis development. Readers should now be versed in how to evaluate assessment information to identify patterns that will lead to hypotheses regarding problem behavior. With hypotheses in hand, antecedent interventions can be developed to prevent the occurrence or frequency of undesirable behavior and increase desirable behavior.

When a team is selecting or developing an antecedent intervention to address a specific hypothesis, a parsimonious first step is to consider the function that the behavior serves. This will narrow the class of intervention options that the team will consider. When behavior serves an attention function, the antecedent intervention will be addressed toward assuring that adequate attention is available and/or that situations leading to attention-seeking behavior are modified. Problem behavior serving an escape function means that intervention will be directed toward eliminating or modifying some aspect of instruction, demand, or expectation placed on the student. The class of antecedent interventions that addresses behavior functioning to obtain a tangible item or activity will focus on preparing the student for removal/loss of the item or for activity change, and/or on arranging the environment to make the loss or change less aversive. Finally, interventions to address behavior serving a biological or self-stimulatory function will arrange a more stimulating environment or provide sensory stimulation to match the sensory input obtained through the problem behavior.

Although it is helpful first to identify a behavior's function, this information usually is not sufficient to develop an antecedent intervention. Consider the case of behavior that serves an escape function. Knowing that behavior is escape-motivated is helpful information, but knowing only the function is not sufficient to determine *why* the individual is behaving to escape. At this point, intervention options are limited to strategies such as ignoring the behavior, punishing the behavior, providing periodic breaks, or perhaps teaching the individual to request a break. These interventions may have limited success, but they do not allow the support team to correct problems that are triggering challenging behaviors and create a motivating environment for the student; nor do they enable the team to include approaches that will prevent problem behavior. Take the case of Laura, who regularly screamed when her teacher placed demands on her. Determining that screaming served an escape function was useful information; however, it was not sufficient for developing a comprehensive intervention. Further analysis revealed that Laura's teacher routinely provided multiple-step directions that she was unable to comprehend and follow. Without this specificity of information about the precise event that triggered the screaming, it would not have been possible to develop an antecedent intervention that corrected the problem of Laura's difficulty following multiple-step directions. Thus, after the function of a behavior has been determined, the specific antecedent events that trigger the behavior also must be identified.

After identifying the behavioral function and specific antecedents triggering problem behavior, the team should have adequate information to select an antecedent intervention. The antecedents identified in the hypothesis statement will serve as the conduit for this selection process. Selecting an antecedent intervention involves evaluating the match between information about both antecedents and function on the one hand, and potential interventions on the other. Sometimes the process is relatively easy, as in the case of providing easier work when too difficult work is the trigger. However, at other times the process is more extensive, when the hypotheses encompass a broad class of events that cut across activities, and any number of interventions appear suitable. For example, Jay was a 14-year-old student who exhibited aggressive and disruptive behaviors, in conjunction with noncompliance, which also served an escape function. Unlike the data for Laura, Jay's assessment information indicated that his assigned work was appropriate in content and well matched to his skill level. The assessment revealed that Jay had been in a classroom throughout his elementary school years where teachers seldom placed any demands on him. Jay's problem behavior appeared to be unrelated to any particular demand per se, but rather to the fact that he suddenly was expected to complete many tasks throughout the day in his current classroom. Considering the broad assessment information in conjunction with the hypothesis "When ongoing demands are placed on Jay throughout the school day, he engages in aggression and disruption, to escape the demands," the team identified a number of antecedent interventions that they believed were matched to Jay's needs. One proposed intervention was to decrease the overall number and frequency of demands during the day. Once fewer demands were completed without problem behavior, the frequency could be gradually increased. The team also believed that choice making might be effective. Staff members working directly with Jay referred to his actions as "rebellious," noting that problem behaviors occurred even when simple requests were made of him. They hypothesized that the problem behaviors were his attempt to exert control over his new environment with changed expectations. The team agreed that choice of the task he could complete would give Jay a greater sense of control over his environment. Finally, the team determined that Jay's general motivation could be increased and his problem behaviors reduced by fashioning a curriculum rich in highly preferred and interesting activities. In the end, his team included all of these antecedent intervention strategies in his support plan, and used all of them whenever possible. This example illustrates the complexity that sometimes may accompany intervention development. It also underscores the importance of broad information when a team is developing antecedent interventions.

TYPES OF ANTECEDENT INTERVENTIONS

In this section, we provide detailed descriptions of common antecedent interventions that are supported by research evidence. Many of the illustrations include some information about the assessment and hypotheses pertaining to problem behaviors as a way of further illustrating the importance of linking together each step in the PBS process. The intervention examples are organized first by function to facilitate narrowing down the intervention options, as suggested above. They are subdivided by categories of antecedent interventions whenever possible. Table 8.2 provides an overview of intervention strategies and examples in relationship to behavioral function.

When reviewing the intervention examples, readers should keep in mind that antecedent interventions represent only one component of a behavior support plan. In very few cases are antecedent interventions in isolation adequate, such as when work is too difficult. Alternative behaviors must simultaneously be taught, as described in Chapter 9. For example, it is likely that difficult demands will be made of a student at some time in the future. Thus the student also must be taught how to obtain assistance appropriately. As we have stressed throughout this book, comprehensive support involves multicomponent plans. However, for purposes of clarity, the examples below describe only selected information about the individual that pertains to his or her antecedent intervention. In almost every example, the support plan of the individual described involved many more components.

Interventions Matched to an Attention Function

Problem behavior that serves an attention function is generally exhibited under circumstances where a student (1) has been required to experience a period of time without any attention; (2) desires attention from a particular individual, who is unavailable; or (3) sees that others are getting attention or interaction when he or she is not. It should be kept in mind that school-age children often seek to obtain attention from their peers, not just adults. The following antecedent interventions address problem behavior exhibited to gain attention.

Scheduled Attention

One antecedent intervention that can change conditions associated with attention-motivated problem behavior is to ensure that adult or peer attention is made available on some type of schedule. This is referred to as *scheduled attention*. The effectiveness of this intervention relies on the fact

TABLE 8.2. Overview of Antecedent Interventions

Function	Intervention strategy	Example
Attention	Schedule adult attention	• Have adult work with student • Have adult provide periodic attention
	Schedule peer attention	• Pair student with peer • Use peer tutoring
	Increase proximity to student	• Move seating arrangement • Periodically move about classroom
	Provide preferred activity	• When adult is occupied, assign more preferred work
Escape	Adjust demand difficulty	• Provide easier work

	Offer choices	• Allow student to choose:
		  • Task to complete
		  • Sequence of tasks to be completed
		  • Materials to use
		  • Where to complete task
		  • When to complete task
		  • With whom to complete task

	Increase student preference/interest in activity	• Incorporate student hobbies/interests into activities
	Assure that activities have functional or meaningful outcomes	• Provide activities with a valued outcome
	Alter task length	• Shorten activity • Provide frequent breaks
	Modify mode of task completion	• Change medium/materials • Replace pencil and paper with computer, etc.
	Use behavioral momentum/task interspersal	• Present easy requests prior to difficult request
	Increase predictability	• Provide cues for upcoming or change in activities (instructional, visual, auditory)
	Modify instructional delivery	• Use pleasant tone of voice
Tangible	Provide a warning	• Indicate that activity is about to end
	Schedule a transitional activity	• Schedule a moderately preferred activity between highly preferred and highly nonpreferred activities
	Increase accessibility	• Put highly preferred items within student's reach
Sensory	Provide alternative sensory reinforcement	• Offer radio to student seeking auditory reinforcement, or visual stimuli to student seeking visual reinforcement
	Enrich environment	• Fill environment with interesting and stimulating activities

that attention is provided before problem behavior occurs; this should eliminate the need to seek attention via problem behaviors.

Developing this type of intervention requires careful planning. Sometimes interventions are put in place hastily because of the urgency of reducing problem behavior, resulting in the overuse or unnecessary use of valuable time and resources. For example, too frequent attention burdens staff
members, and students may become accustomed to ongoing and readily
available attention; this may make it difficult for them to adjust to more
typical conditions, where attention must be shared among a classroom of
students. This type of attention, on an unnecessarily dense schedule, can be
detrimental to a student over the long term. A better approach is to carefully determine the conditions under which a student solicits attention
(appropriately or inappropriately) and the length of time he or she is able
to carry on without attention. Based on this information, a schedule can be
developed that supersedes problem behavior. For example, Mr. Winters's
assessment data indicted that Jonathan regularly engaged in self-injury in
the cafeteria. Unlike Jonathan's classroom, with a staff-to-student ratio of
1:5, all of the middle grades convened for lunch in the cafeteria, where each
lunchtime monitor was expected to supervise approximately 30 students.
The data also indicated that Jonathan's behavior was appropriate for a
good 10 minutes before the self-injury began. Therefore, a schedule was
put into place whereby lunchtime monitors began to provide Jonathan with
attention at just under 10 minutes, and did so at intervals throughout the
rest of the lunch period. Through these brief interactions with Jonathan,
self-injury was eliminated.

Peer attention can also be scheduled to reduce inappropriate attention-
seeking behavior. When planned well, scheduled peer attention has the benefits of improving peer-to-peer social interactions, as well as reducing the
demands on classroom staff. Zachary's case offers an example of a scheduled peer attention intervention. Assessment information indicated that
Zachary's talking out and inappropriate noises occurred primarily during
teacher lecture, regardless of the content. After a close examination of the
assessment data, it was concluded that Zachary's disruptive behaviors were
attempts to gain the attention of two particular classmates. When these two
classmates were not present in the classroom, Zachary's disruptive behavior decreased dramatically. Zachary's team developed the hypothesis "In
the presence of Miles and Stephen, Zachary talks out and makes noises, to
obtain their attention." Zachary's teacher developed an antecedent intervention that allowed him periodically (every 15 minutes) to check his lecture notes against those of one of the two peers whose attention he desired.
This provided him with adequate attention in an appropriate manner,
while also having the benefit of increasing his work productivity. As this
example illustrates, the antecedent intervention was linked to an attention

function, and was specifically matched to the particular type of attention Zachary sought to obtain through his problem behavior.

There are many examples of ways to schedule peer attention that capitalize on routine or classwide peer-to-peer activities. Examples of these include cooperative learning and peer tutoring. Support teams may use these strategies creatively, so that all students experience a rich variety of social interactions.

A caveat to scheduled attention interventions is that the schedule, although data-driven, is not created by the student. Regardless of the frequency of attention provided, it still may not coincide with the specific timing of a student's desire for attention. Thus it is critical to simultaneously teach appropriate methods for soliciting attention, as described in Chapter 9.

Change Staff Proximity

Staff proximity also has been found to influence student behavior. Attention-seeking behaviors can be reduced by placing students in close proximity to staff. This can signal that attention is more likely; alternatively, it may be effective simply because some individuals prefer having someone nearby. For example, Duane, an 11-year-old, displayed challenging behavior during his daily reading activity, which required independent completion at his desk (located at the back of the classroom). During assigned reading activities, Duane was often off task, crying, whining, or displaying self-injurious behaviors. Because Duane enjoyed being close to others, his team believed that his challenging behavior would be reduced if a staff member remained physically proximal to him. Thus his desk was moved to the front of the class, near his teacher's desk. Once this move was made, Duane's engagement during reading worksheet activities increased, and there was a substantial reduction in his disruptive behavior.

Provide Preferred Activities

Sometimes a highly preferred activity will compete with an individual's demands for attention. This should not replace an intervention that focuses on creating an interesting curriculum. However, some students find it very difficult to engage independently. Careful scheduling of highly preferred activities may allow a teacher to complete necessary classroom activities while avoiding problem behavior. For example, Foster demanded very high levels of staff attention, making it almost impossible to provide high-quality instruction to his classmates. However, he would engage for relatively long periods of time without problems when he was given computerized games and activities to operate. Therefore, his day was scheduled so that work periods with frequent adult attention were alternated with computerized activities, during which time instruction for Foster's classmates was scheduled.

Interventions Matched to an Escape Function

Because educational settings focus on skill building, a student's school day necessarily comprises a collection of instructional demands. The high frequency of demands to learn material that is new or difficult can be very taxing for students. In addition, students with disabilities often have histories of failure with tasks or assignments, making demands to follow requests or complete assignments all the more aversive. Furthermore, for many students, learning requires frequent prompting or direction from adults in circumstances where demands are practically constant. These situations increase the likelihood that problem behavior in school settings will serve the function of escaping, avoiding, or delaying a task. A variety of antecedent interventions matched to an escape function may be considered.

Adjust Task Difficulty

When a team is considering intervention for escape-maintained behavior, it is first important to be sure that the level of difficulty of the task or activity is appropriate. A number of research studies (Gunter & Denny, 1996), have implicated too-difficult work as the cause of problem behavior. This has been shown for students with developmental disabilities, learning disabilities, and emotional and behavioral disorders.

A high rate of student success is important, not only because success is both self-satisfying and likely to produce reinforcement from others, but also because errors may actually interfere with learning. Independent work should be completed with a high percentage of accuracy, whereas a slightly lower accuracy percentage is acceptable during instruction. However, it may be important to consider a student's history of failure to determine his or her tolerance for mistakes. When team members are modifying instruction to decrease the difficulty, the level of accuracy should be individually determined.

Provide Opportunities for Choice

Creating opportunities for choice making is a common antecedent intervention for changing conditions associated with escape. Offering choices is important for several reasons. First, research has documented that choice making can reduce problem behaviors (see Kern et al., 1998, for a review). Second, and equally important, choice making is a right that should be afforded to all individuals—with or without disabilities. Historically, however, choice-making opportunities for individuals with disabilities have routinely been overlooked or denied. Some individuals, particularly those with severe disabilities, were viewed as being incapable of making appropriate choices. In addition, the highly structured nature of many special education programs and practices preempts opportunities for choice about even the simplest decisions. The opportunity to make choices is critically important, however, because it allows people to arrange an environment that reflects their personal preferences. In other words, choice making allows individuals to be with people they enjoy, engage in activities they like, and take pleasure in a variety of other environmental arrangements. Finally, a growing body of research indicates that the act of choice making itself may be reinforcing, regardless of what is selected. Thus providing opportunities for choice addresses escape behavior by (1) allowing an individual to select more enjoyable activities, and/or (2) providing a sense of control through the act of choosing.

There are countless ways that choices can be provided during typical and ongoing activities to reduce problem behavior associated with escape. Dunlap et al. (1994) described an example of choice of academic task. Wendall, a fourth grader diagnosed as having an emotional/behavioral disordered, engaged in noncompliant behavior by refusing to complete or destroying his assigned work. Wendall's support team noted he was able to complete the assigned work without difficulty, but appeared to have problems accepting instructions. When instructed to complete his work, he often made statements such as "Don't tell me what to do," or "I'll do what I want." Wendall's support team developed the hypothesis "When instructed to complete an assignment, Wendall engages in noncompliant or destructive behavior, to escape being told what to do." Because of his difficulty accepting instructions, his team determined that choice making had a good probability of being effective. Thus, at the start of each academic period, he was given a choice of the specific academic task within the respective academic area. For example, during spelling, Wendall was usually required to complete independent seatwork that consisted of writing 20 assigned spelling words three times each, writing words in alphabetical order, and writing definitions for each of the 20 words. The assignments were teacher-selected, and changing tasks was not permitted. At intervention, these usual procedures were modified to incorporate choice making by providing him with a menu of five different spelling tasks (equivalent to those during typical spelling assignments) from which he could choose which task he would complete each day. In addition, he was provided the option of changing tasks at any time during the spelling activity. This small change resulted in a decrease in problem behavior, while still maintaining the integrity of the assigned work.

Offering a choice of the sequence of tasks also has been shown to reduce escape-related problem behaviors. Use of choice in this manner is advised when there are activities or assignments that students must complete. One study (Kern, Mantegna, Vorndran, Bailin, & Hilt, 2001) demonstrated the effectiveness of this approach for students with a range of diagnoses, including a student with developmental disabilities and another with attention-deficit/hyperactivity disorder (ADHD). Three tasks were selected for each student, and completion of all three was required. The tasks ranged from activities of daily living for the student with developmental disabilities to academic activities for the student with ADHD. The sequence in which the students completed the three tasks was either student-selected or teacher-selected. When the students selected the task sequence, problem behavior was lower, and engagement was higher.

Offering student a choice of the type of materials to be used during an activity is another variation of choice procedures that can make unpleasant work more desirable. Ronnie, a 6-year-old boy diagnosed with reactive attachment disorder, was fully included in a first-grade classroom. He was performing slightly behind his grade level in academic subjects; therefore, his team determined that additional review in the evening was necessary for him to keep up with his classmates. Each night Ronnie would work with his aunt at the kitchen table and was required to complete two homework pages consisting of beginning reading skills, such as matching sounds to objects. When his aunt asked him to complete his homework, Ronnie would refuse to sit down, hold onto his aunt, or stare off into space. If his aunt tried to redirect him back to the homework assignment, he would begin crying, which eventually led to a tantrum. To make his assigned work more enjoyable, his team developed an intervention that included a choice component presented at the start of the homework task. Instead of completing his practice sheets with a pencil, Ronnie was given the opportunity to choose fat colored markers or crayons, and he could select any color he wanted. Ronnie was also allowed to change markers or crayons at any time during his homework task. This choice intervention made the activity more preferred, and Ronnie readily began and completed the work upon his aunt's requests.

Opportunities for choice can be provided in many different ways. For example, variations of choice include providing the option of a peer to work with, allowing a student to select where to complete a task, and providing the opportunity to choose the mode of task completion. Additional suggestions are provided in Table 8.2.

Increase Student Preference/Interest

Revising the curriculum content to reflect student preference or interest is another antecedent intervention that has been shown to effectively reduce escape-maintained problem behavior. Additional desirable outcomes of this particular intervention often include an increase in appropriate behaviors, including engagement and work productivity. This approach is similar to choice-making interventions in that the outcome for the student is work that is preferred. However, it differs in that the student's opportunity to make a choice is removed. Thus, providing preferred or high-interest activities is likely to be effective for students who find a task or assignment unpleasant or irrelevant. Conversely, if a student finds the act of choice making itself to be reinforcing, then a choice intervention is a better option. Another caveat is that constructing a curriculum with preferred or high-interest activities requires knowledge of the student's interests and preferences. This information can sometimes be obtained through the functional assessment and/or preference assessments. If clear information about preferences cannot be ascertained, a choice intervention may be a better option. A final note is that students' preferences change over time. Ongoing assessments will detect changing preferences and assure that the intervention remains effective over time.

High-interest/preference interventions can be relatively easy to develop and are highly effective. But the key is individualizing the modification to assure that it reflects a student's specific preferences or interests. In one study (Dunlap et al., 1993), a goal for Ann, a 6-year-old student with developmental disabilities and behavioral challenges, was learning to count. Her typical assignment consisted of counting objects on a worksheet and then coloring the objects. She frequently exhibited off-task behavior, including leaving her desk, talking out, or yelling in order to escape the activities. Ann's team developed the hypothesis "Because of a history of failure with academic-type tasks, when presented with worksheet activities Ann engages in problem behaviors, to avoid the types of activities she perceives she cannot complete successfully." Ann's team developed her intervention after observing that she enjoyed playing with Legos. To introduce preference within the math assignment, Legos were used for counting instead of objects on a worksheet. Ann was required to count Lego blocks by color as she constructed objects. Following this modification, Ann because highly engaged in the counting activity and did not display problem behavior. The simple intervention allowed Ann's teacher to maintain her academic goals and daily task requirements, which, for a change, Ann began to complete regularly. In fact, Ann seemed to look forward to her math activity following the curriculum revision.

A high-preference/interest intervention was developed for Ahmad, a 5-year-old diagnosed with a severe emotional disturbance. During seatwork activities he was often observed to engage in off-task and disruptive behaviors, including aggression, noncompliance, property destruction, and leaving his work area without permission. These behaviors occurred during daily activities focusing on language arts. During his typical language arts assignment, Ahmad was instructed to complete a two-page matching assignment, which consisted of tracing and copying letters of the alphabet. He was then required to color the accompanying picture on the worksheets. His assessment indicated that Ahmad was highly interested in cars and motorcycles, and this interest was subsequently incorporated into his daily language arts tasks. In the revised assignment, Ahmad was instructed to complete two modified sheets of tracing and copying upper- and lowercase letters of the alphabet and coloring the pictures. In the modified assignment, the worksheets consisted of cars and motorcycles that corresponded to the assigned letters. When the sheets were completed, Ahmad was instructed to place them into a folder covered with pictures of cars and motorcycles. The requirements of the assignment remained the same, but the revised activity was associated with higher rates of engagement and lowered disruptive behavior.

The examples above illustrate the infusion of student interests into math and language art assignments. Student preferences and interests can be incorporated throughout the curriculum, for students of all ages. For example, Clarke et al. (1995) demonstrated a successful intervention by replacing handwriting book exercises with copying instructions from preferred video games' bonus point booklets. Problem behavior exhibited by a 12-year-old with severe disabilities during transitions was reduced by adding a preferred activity (listening to a tape player with preferred music) when the student was required to walk across her school campus (Clarke, Worcester, Dunlap, Murray, & Bradley-Klug, 2002).

Assure That Activities Have a Functional or Meaningful Outcome

In addition to considering student interest when developing antecedent interventions, the task itself may be modified to produce a functional or meaningful outcome. This means that completion of the task is associated with an event or product that in some way has value to the student or others. Working toward a valued outcome can reduce a student's desire to escape from a task that is aversive or without apparent meaning. For example, one study (Dunlap, Kern-Dunlap, Clarke, & Robbins, 1991) described Jill, a 13-year-old student with multiple disabilities and serious behavior problems. Jill experienced difficulty completing most academic activities, particularly written assignments. During assignments she displayed off-task and disruptive behaviors, including bizarre speech, inappropriate social interactions, screaming, aggression, noncompliance, and running around or leaving the classroom without permission. Jill's writing was barely legible, and an instructional objective was for her to demonstrate correct letter formation and word spacing in manuscript handwriting. To accomplish this goal, Jill was required to copy words (approximately 35 at a time) from a handwriting book onto a blank sheet of lined paper.

Jill's support team hypothesized that she was simply bored with this task because it had no meaningful outcome. Thus the handwriting activity was modified to result in a functional outcome, while maintaining the integrity of the instructional goal. Each day during handwriting practice, Jill developed and wrote captions onto a blank sheet of lined paper to accompany photographs that she had taken earlier in the week. After completing all of the captions, Jill affixed them to a photo album she was creating. The outcome resulted in a completed photo album, which Jill could share with others. Because Jill was creating a permanent product that would be shared with others, she was particularly motivated to generate her very best handwriting. Consequently, not only did she meet her handwriting requirements without problem behaviors; her handwriting also improved greatly, and the frequency of her appropriate social interactions increased as she proudly shared and discussed her photo album with her classmates.

Similar interventions were implemented across the curriculum with Jill. For example, math was also targeted to reflect a functional, concrete outcome. During typical math assignments, Jill was required to complete 20 word problems that involved fractions from a third-grade textbook, with the answers to be written on a separate blank sheet of paper. This assignment was associated with high rates of problem behavior. The intervention maintained problems that reflected math concepts in the original curriculum, but involved a functional activity with a concrete outcome— such as baking a cake (e.g., fractions for measuring, using measuring cups, dividing a stick of butter into fourths), or reading a bus schedule to determine the increments within an hour-long bus ride and then taking a bus ride. These interventions—addressing the same skills as the typical tasks, but with a meaningful outcome—were effective in reducing disruptive behavior and increasing her engagement during math activities.

A comparable approach to modifying an activity to include a functional outcome was described in another study (Dunlap, Foster-Johnson, Clarke, Kern, & Childs, 1995). Jary was a 13-year-old boy diagnosed with autism and mental retardation. His teacher noted that he was off task frequently and displayed a number of inappropriate and disruptive vocalizations while working on a daily assembly task. His instructional objective of multistep assembly was to be accomplished by putting together component parts of ballpoint pens for a nearby factory. Jary's team noted several facets of this task that might be problematic for Jary. First, he had worked on this task throughout the school year, and team members did not believe that the work resulted in an outcome that was meaningful for Jary. Furthermore, Jary was a very social person, but the activity did not allow for socialization. The members of his support team suggested that when Jary was given tasks without a functional outcome or tasks that required independent completion, he engaged in problem behaviors, to escape the tasks. They believed he might become more involved in an alternative assembly task that included a functional outcome and allowed for socialization. Thus the pen assembly task was replaced with the assembly of peanut butter and jelly sandwiches. Parts of the task were laid out sequentially, just as with the pen assembly task, and Jary was required to complete the steps of sandwich assembly. However, rather than packaging the assembled items for factory delivery as he had the pens, Jary instead distributed the completed snacks to his classmates. This modified task produced a functional outcome that Jary could share with peers, and it also provided him with the opportunity to socialize. As a result, disruptive behavior was nearly eliminated.

These examples illustrate how activities with functional or meaningful outcomes can be incorporated in many different ways across the curriculum, and with students at a variety of skill levels. This intervention does not require forgoing or attenuating instructional objectives. In addition to reducing problem behaviors, desirable collateral effects may emerge, such as performance improvements (as illustrated with Jill's handwriting).

Alter Task Length

Many students are capable of completing an assigned task, but presentation of one that appears unbearably lengthy may be overwhelming, resulting in problem behavior as a means to escape the assignment or avoid it altogether. In these situations, modifying the task duration or dividing the task into smaller increments is a quite simple antecedent intervention that can reduce problem behavior. This strategy was used with Duane, a high school student with ADHD, who engaged in problem behaviors in the form of cursing and threatening others. When independent seatwork was given, he refused to begin, his face reddened, and he appeared tense. He would eventually begin cursing, mostly about the work, and also threatened others ("If you don't quit staring, I'll punch you in the nose"). Duane's teacher observed these behaviors primarily when he was asked to begin ongoing assignments, such as projects or activities that would last several days. This observation generated the hypothesis "When given lengthy assignments, Duane engages in inappropriate language and interactions, to avoid and escape the work." Intervention consisted of dividing lengthy assignments or projects into smaller portions that were manageable for Duane. Each new portion was assigned only after the prior portion was completed and handed in. For example, in World Cultures class, students were each assigned a country for which they were to research the language, economy, governmental structure, and customs, using at least three sources. They were to compile a 10-page written paper, followed by a class presentation. This extended assignment was divided into manageable portions for Duane by having him identify only one source at a time, select a single topic (e.g., language), and note factual information in bulleted form. This work was then turned in, and a second, similar step was assigned. After completion of all steps, the information gathered was complied into a finished document that was identical to those of his classmates. Similar accommodations were made in all of Duane's classes, which greatly reduced problem behaviors.

This type of intervention can be similarly accomplished in a number of different ways. For example, the length of an assignment can be reduced by decreasing the number of problems on a page (e.g., Dunlap et al., 1991). A 30-minute reading period for a student with difficulty in sustaining attention can be divided into two 15-minute periods, distributed in the morning and afternoon. The daily schedule can be rearranged to include short work periods interspersed with brief breaks, rather than long work periods followed by a long recess.

Modify Mode of Task Completion

Modifications can be made that change the medium or materials used to complete a task. For example, pencil-and-paper tasks require fine motor skills and can be laborious after a time. This typical medium can be replaced in many instances with the use of a computer or tape recorder to encode responses (e.g., Ervin et al., 2000). Similarly, a pencil can be replaced with colored pens or crayons (e.g., Moes, 1998). Interventions of this nature can address escape-related problem behavior that occurs for a variety of reasons. Skill deficits such as fine motor difficulties can be circumvented, or task attention problems can be reduced, by increasing interest in a task.

We (Kern, Childs, Dunlap, Clarke, & Falk, 1994) used this procedure with Eddie, an 11-year-old student functioning above average, who had difficulty attending to his work (as described previously in Chapter 6). The intervention was implemented during his composition class. Typically, the first 15 minutes of class were devoted to completing a daily writing assignment in his composition book. Eddie often had difficulty getting started, and when he failed to complete the task in the allotted time, he would often cry, have tantrums, and sometimes engage in self-injury. Based on a review of Eddie's records, fine motor skills were identified as a particular problem. This led to the hypothesis "When Eddie is given tasks that require fine motor skills, he engages in problem behaviors, to escape the task." Writing tasks were modified to permit Eddie to complete his assignment in ways that avoided the need for fine motor skills. Instead, Eddie was provided with a tape recorder in which he could dictate his stories, or a laptop computer to type his stories. This modification to the mode of task completion enabled Eddie to complete his assignment, in addition to reducing his problematic behaviors. As with many other antecedent interventions, this strategy does not require adjusting instructional objectives.

Introduce Behavioral Momentum or Task Interspersal

Behavioral momentum and *task interspersal* are similar strategies, in that the goal is to create a "momentum" of compliance or willingness to complete a nonpreferred or difficult task. In the case of behavioral momentum, this is accomplished by presenting a series of brief and simple tasks that the student has a history of readily completing, just prior to issuing a request to complete a task that the student has difficulty completing. Task interspersal involves arranging an instructional sequence so that it offers variation. Typically, easy tasks are interspersed among more difficult tasks; however, sometimes variation alone, regardless of the relative difficulty of interspersed tasks, may reduce the redundancy inherent in some tasks. Both strategies increase the likelihood that the student will complete the nonpreferred or difficult task. Thus they are ideally matched to problem behavior that serves an escape function. When considering this intervention, team members should keep in mind that it should be used only if the requested tasks are already a part of the student's repertoire. Tasks that a student has not yet learned to complete require an instructional intervention.

Horner, Day, Sprague, O'Brien, and Heathfield (1991) combined behavioral momentum and task interspersal during nonacademic tasks for individuals identified as having cognitive impairments. Three adolescents with severe mental retardation displayed high frequencies of self-injurious behavior when presented with what appeared to be difficult tasks. An interspersal intervention involved introducing "easy" tasks, defined as those that the students could complete independently with high accuracy, among difficult tasks. Examples of easy tasks included pouring water from a pitcher into another container, putting on a T-shirt, and following a simple request to do something (e.g., "Put the glass on the table"). Examples of difficult tasks were sorting silverware, putting on underwear, or following a two-step instruction. The activity began with three to five easy tasks. During instruction, a similar series of easy tasks was interspersed following three difficult tasks or upon any sign of resistance from the students, such as whining or grunting. The behavioral momentum and interspersal modifications implemented during the target activity resulted in reductions in self-injurious behavior, as well as increased attempts at completing tasks.

A study by Logan and Skinner (1998) illustrated the use of task interspersal for sixth-grade students with low achievement in the area of mathematics. The students had a low completion rate on assignments consisting of 25 four-digit × one-digit multiplication problems. An interspersal procedure was introduced whereby a one-digit + one-digit addition problem was interspersed following every third multiplication problem. When the interspersal procedure was used, the students completed significantly more problems. Furthermore, the students rated the assignments with interspersed problems as requiring less effort overall. When given the option, significantly more students chose to complete the assignment with interspersed problems.

Increase Predictability

Some students engage in problem behaviors to escape unpredictable routines, activities, or events. More specifically, problem behaviors may occur when students cannot anticipate when an activity will begin or end, when they do not know what activity is scheduled next, or when predictable routines are changed or disrupted in some way. Interventions can be implemented to increase predictability on an ongoing basis or when a student's regular schedule must be adjusted.

An intervention increasing predictability was successful for Mindy, a 12-year-old girl with an autistic-spectrum disorder and other disabilities, including a visual impairment and motor skill deficits (Clarke et al., 2002). Mindy was required to make transitions to different settings and routines throughout the school day, and this was extremely difficult for her. Most of the time, when instructed to move to the next routine, she engaged in challenging behavior, including falling to the ground and hitting herself. Her team hypothesized that when a request to make a transition was issued, Mindy engaged in problem behaviors, to escape from the unpredictability associated with the transition. An intervention was developed that modified teacher instruction presented to Mindy immediately prior to transitions. Typically, when it was time to make a transition, Mindy's teacher merely directed her to do so (e.g., "Let's go to P.E."). The instructional procedure was modified in the following ways. Distractions in the classroom were minimized 5 minutes prior to transition (e.g., audio and visual aids, the computer, and the television were turned off). A warning was provided several minutes prior to the transition (e.g., "We are going to P.E. in 5 minutes"). When it was time to make the transition, the teacher provided clear instructions of each step needed for a successful transition (e.g., "You will stand up, walk to the door and wait for your classmates, then walk the to locker room"). These steps were accompanied by a picture schedule with sequentially ordered photographs that illustrated a specific object related to each transition step, as well as the next activity. An additional modification addressed Mindy's motor skill deficits and visual impairment. Mindy was provided additional time to complete the transition at her own pace, without being rushed or physically guided. These instructional modifications provided increased predictability for Mindy, as well as addressing her skill level and pacing issues; they thereby allowed Mindy to be successful and independent during transition activities.

Flannery and Horner (1994) illustrated how specific predictability signals or features were associated with low and high levels of problem behavior for adolescents with developmental disabilities and autism. Intervention consisted of providing information about the content, duration, timing, and/or consequences of future events. Increasing predictability in this way improved the students' behavior throughout the school day.

Modify Instructional Delivery

At times, problem behavior may result not from a request or instruction per se, but rather from the manner in which it is issued. Requests that are delivered with a demanding or harsh tone can be a cause of challenging behavior. Many students are more likely to find requests stated in a pleasant way less objectionable.

Interventions Matched to a Tangible Function

In some instances, removing a highly preferred object or asking a student to discontinue a very enjoyable activity can lead to problem behavior. In this case, problem behavior is intended to send the message that the student wants to return to the item or activity. When problem behavior follows removal or denial of an item or activity, the behavior is said to serve a tangible function. In these instances, the antecedent interventions described below may diminish undesirable behavior.

Provide a Warning

Preparing a student for the upcoming termination of an activity or confiscation of an item can help to avoid problem behavior. It may also be the case that multiple warnings are more effective than a single warning (Mace, Shapiro, & Mace, 1998). For example, a warning can be provided indicating that computer time will end in 5 minutes, then 2 minutes, then 1 minute prior to a request to return to seatwork. This warning can be given either verbally alone or with an additional visual or auditory cue, such as a countdown clock or an egg timer.

Schedule a Transitional Activity

Transitions from highly preferred activities to nonpreferred activities can be particularly difficult. Scheduling a moderately preferred transitional activity can reduce problem behavior by helping to ease the transition. For example, Mr. Bean noticed that Holly frequently refused to leave gym class to return to her classroom for reading. She would flop to the floor and scream when instructed to go to reading. To ease the transition from gym, which she loved, to reading, which she found difficult, Mr. Bean scheduled a game each day at the beginning of reading. Holly did not mind ending gym to play a short game of Reading Bingo or Reading Concentration. Following the game, she readily began nonpreferred reading activities.

Increase Accessibility of Items

At times, individuals without communication will engage in problem behaviors to obtain items that are not accessible. For instance, a child's Legos may be stored on a high shelf, out of the child's reach. Rearranging the environment so that preferred items are accessible can eliminate problem behaviors.

Interventions Matched to a Sensory Function

Offer Alternative Sources of Stimulation

Challenging behaviors exhibited in the form of self-stimulation or self-injury are sometimes related to a need for sensory reinforcement. Examples of such behaviors include finger sucking, object mouthing, head banging, and hand flapping. Such behavior may be difficult to decrease as it is motivated by a self-produced intrinsic variable. As explained in Chapter 7, when sensory stimulation is the driving force for behavior, antecedent interventions can be arranged to provide specific alternative reinforcement that is matched to the type of sensory stimulation the child obtains through the undesirable behavior. For example, if a student's eye poking is assessed to provide visual stimulation, the classroom environment may be rearranged to include activities that provide rich alternative sources of visual stimulation, such as highly visual computer games or toys such as Lite-Brite. Some students may engage in self-stimulatory behavior to satisfy a sensory need for full body movement, such as swaying back and forth or arm waving. An early study (Kern, Koegel, Dyer, Blew, & Fenton, 1982) demonstrated that the inclusion of vigorous exercise (jogging) in the daily schedule of children with autism reduced the self-stimulatory behaviors of hand flapping and body rocking. Luiselli (1994) provided a chewable stick made of soft rubber to a 10-year-old-girl who frequently displayed object grabbing and object mouthing, as an alternative means of obtaining oral sensory reinforcement.

Enrich the Environment

It is also well established that self-stimulatory behaviors more frequently occur in environments that are relatively barren or devoid of preferred activities, objects, or individuals. Self-stimulatory behavior in these contexts is probably a way to reduce boredom. Creating an environment that is rich in stimulating and preferred activities and persons will decrease undesirable behavior, enhance engagement and learning, and improve such an individual's overall quality of life.

COMBINING MULTIPLE ANTECEDENT INTERVENTIONS

For illustrative purposes, many of the examples above describe application of a single antecedent intervention. Often support plans include multiple antecedent interventions. There are three reasons why a support team may want to consider more than one antecedent intervention. First, in some cases, multiple interventions may increase the likelihood that a support plan will be effective. For example, shortening task length *and* offering a choice of tasks may both reduce unwanted behavior.

A second reason multiple interventions may be considered is that multiple events often influence the occurrence of problem behaviors. Dharma offers an illustration of multiple variables associated with problem behavior. Dharma was a high school student with developmental disabilities. Her school routine included assisting with breakfast and lunch preparation in the cafeteria. Dharma's support team considered this to be an ideal opportunity to teach her skills she would need in the future to live independently. However, incidents of self-injury during cafeteria work time began to escalate, putting her at risk of losing this school job. Assessment data indicated that self-injury was limited to the cafeteria and occurred when instructions were provided, supporting an escape function. Further analysis of Dharma's assessment data helped to isolate particular activities that were problematic, and allowed her team to develop reasonable explanations clarifying why they were problematic. Three specific activities were identified as immediate antecedents to self-injury. These were opening cans prior to food preparation, serving prepared foods onto individual trays, and refilling napkin holders. Anecdotal notes that accompanied direct observations, as well as interviews with cafeteria workers and others, suggested that Dharma's self-injury associated with opening cans and filling napkin holders resulted from her poor fine motor skills, which made these tasks extremely difficult. It was also noted that self-injury increased when serving food required reaching down into deep pots to obtain the food. It was hypothesized that Dharma's short stature might contribute to difficulty with this task. Her expanded support team, including the cafeteria workers, developed a support plan that included multiple antecedent interventions. First, the team determined that filling napkin holders was not a skill Dharma would need in the future. The cafeteria workers had no problem assigning this job to other students. Thus it was eliminated from her assigned work duties. To address Dharma's difficulties with can opening, the school purchased an electric can opener. Finally, Dharma borrowed a stepping stool from shop class during breakfast and lunch; she used this to reach various items and objects, such as food in deep pots, more easily. This example shows how information related to both the function and the specific antecedents of behavior allowed problematic tasks to be eliminated or modified in a way that averted problematic features of the task.

A third reason for considering multiple antecedent interventions is to offer an array of interventions when the support plan will be implemented in different settings. In our work with Eddie (Kern et al., 1994), his support team consisted of three teachers, each of whom taught a different subject. During the intervention-planning process, his support team generated a list of intervention strategies. To assure a good contextual fit, each teacher selected interventions to use in his or her classroom. The teachers' choices differed, reflecting individual preference, feasibility, and anticipated effectiveness depending on the class structure.

SETTING EVENT INTERVENTIONS

The sections above have described interventions to alter antecedents, or variables that precede problem behavior in relatively close proximity. As discussed in earlier chapters, more distal events, referred to as *setting events*, may also influence problem behavior. In general, it is considerably more difficult to isolate setting events and determine exactly how they influence problem behavior. It is often equally difficult to develop effective interventions to decrease or eliminate setting events. For example, physiological events, such as sleep difficulties, may be difficult to change. Furthermore, events that occur outside the school day generally are beyond the influence of school personnel, and other people must be relied upon to carry out an intervention consistently. Nonetheless, a comprehensive support plan must address all variables that contribute to problem behavior and influence an individual's well-being. Effective interventions for setting events require a carefully assembled support team, including members within all domains in which an individual lives and learns, working collaboratively to identify influential variables and assure that the interventions are consistently implemented.

When a setting event is identified, clearly the preferred course of action is to eliminate it. Sometimes this can be accomplished, as in the case of shortening a lengthy bus route (Kennedy & Itkonen, 1993). However, more often, setting events are unfortunately difficult to change. For example, a cold may have to run its course (e.g., Lohrmann-O'Rourke &

Yurman, 2001), or menstrual cramps may have to self-resolve (Carr, Smith, Giacin, Whelan, & Pancari, 2003). When a setting event cannot be eliminated, an alternative accommodation can help to nullify the effect of the setting event. As noted in Chapter 2, setting events work in conjunction with immediate antecedents. For instance, a lack of sleep may make the presentation of an otherwise innocuous assignment particularly aversive. Thus intervention can target the immediate antecedent, as in providing a shorter or less difficult assignment when the student is fatigued from inadequate sleep. Another option is to intervene in a way that ameliorates the setting event. Menstrual cramps may be reduced with a heating pad or aspirin. A student who is upset because his or her parents fought most of the night may be calmed by the opportunity to talk with a teacher or counselor. Figure 8.1 offers a schema depicting courses of intervention when setting events are identified.

The following example illustrates the strategy outlined above for developing a setting event intervention. Dora was a 9-year-old girl described as having oppositional defiant disorder. At age 6, social services removed her from a home that could be described as very chaotic. Dora's father worked two jobs and was seldom home. Her mother experienced significant mental health difficulties that left her incapable of asserting order and discipline. In fact, two of Dora's older siblings had previously been removed from the home and placed in residential settings. Dora was

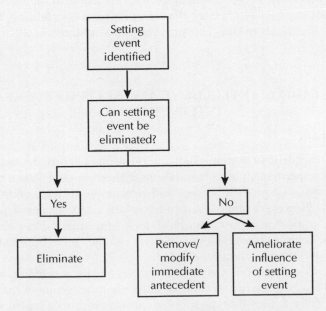

FIGURE 8.1. Intervention approaches for setting events.

placed in the home of an aunt and uncle, which provided substantial stability. However, Dora's aunt and uncle had an arrangement with Dora's mother whereby they occasionally babysat on weekends for Dora's younger sister, who remained in her mother's home.

Meanwhile, Dora's school staff noted that her behavior was extremely variable. Usually she had only minor difficulties throughout the school day, but occasionally she engaged in severe tantrums that could last up to 2 hours. Dora's teacher kept diligent records, which revealed that lengthy tantrums almost always occurred during circle time on Monday mornings, when the class members shared their weekend activities. Her team convened to attempt to sort out this boggling concern. Dora's aunt described troubling weekend circumstances in which Dora's mother dropped off her younger sibling without stopping to say hello. The aunt explained that this upset Dora tremendously and that she would periodically cry throughout the weekend. The team determined that Dora's unpleasant experience with her mother functioned as a setting event, and that the antecedent of asking students to share their weekend experiences resulted in tantrums. The team first questioned whether the setting event could be eliminated. Dora's aunt did not believe that she could eliminate the setting event by changing Dora's mother's behavior; she had tried unsuccessfully to do so in the past. Instead, the team chose to remove the immediate antecedent. A home–school communication log was initiated, and Dora's aunt informed the teacher when Dora's mother had failed to greet Dora on the weekends. On those Monday mornings, rather than participate in circle time, Dora was given school errands to run. This intervention eliminated Monday morning tantrums.

FADING ANTECEDENT AND SETTING EVENT INTERVENTIONS

Why to Fade

Not all antecedent or setting event interventions need to be faded. Some may become permanent accommodations if they are determined to be necessary to maintain student success and reasonable to implement over the long term. However, other such interventions are considered temporary solutions for decreasing problem behaviors. Once the student has learned alternative skills and behaviors or lifestyle changes have been made, these interventions can and should be faded.

Several key questions are pertinent when a team is deciding whether it is in a child's best interest to fade an antecedent or setting event intervention (see Figure 8.2). A first question to consider is this: "Has the modification eliminated a skill or behavior that the individual ultimately will need

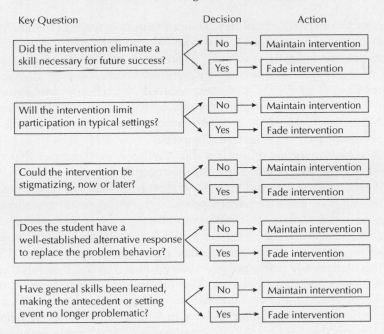

Key Question	Decision	Action

FIGURE 8.2. Key questions before fading antecedent or setting event interventions.

to succeed in the future?" For example, Mr. Gleason's data showed that Bernard engaged in frequent behavior problems when completing pencil-and-paper tasks. Bernard's records revealed difficulty with fine motor skills, and he often reported fatigue and aggravation with lengthy writing assignments. Mr. Gleason decided it was important to eliminate written assignments from Bernard's curriculum to reduce problem behavior and assure that Bernard continued to progress academically. Instead of completing assignments via pencil and paper, Bernard used a computer, a tape recorder, or an adult or peer for dictation purposes. Although this resulted in the behavior improvements that Mr. Gleason wanted, he determined that Bernard might need to be able to complete handwritten work in his future. Thus he developed a strategy for gradually increasing the amount of handwritten work, while simultaneously working in a systematic way, with help from an occupational therapist, to improve Bernard's fine motor skills.

Dakota, a student with severe cognitive disabilities, provides an example of someone for whom fading was deemed to be unnecessary. Dakota's functional behavioral assessment indicated that she had difficulty and exhibited self-injury when her routine changed and her daily schedule was unpredictable. This happened when school assemblies took place, holiday or birthday parties occurred in her class, or teacher inservice sessions mandated an abbreviated school day. Dakota's support team determined that events resulting in schedule changes could almost always be foreseen. They found that periodically informing Dakota of each upcoming schedule change, in addition to providing her picture schedule the previous evening for her parents to review with her, reduced her self-injurious behavior. Given that Dakota had no other way of accessing information about schedule changes, the antecedent intervention was a reasonable accommodation that was built into her long-term supports.

A second important question is this: "Will the intervention exclude the individual from participation in typical settings?" Fading is essential if the modification in any way will limit the student from fully functioning in typical or inclusive settings. Jeremy provides an example of a student for whom an antecedent intervention was likely to result in exclusion. Although he was near grade level academically, Jeremy had difficulty maintaining his attention to assigned tasks longer than a few minutes. Therefore, his special education teacher allowed him to take 1-minute breaks following every 5 minutes of work. This intervention helped Jeremy attend to the task at hand and was not difficult to implement in a classroom of eight students whose assignments were individualized. However, Jeremy's teacher knew that breaks of this frequency would be disruptive in a general education classroom and would result in his missing important material. Therefore, a plan was developed for gradually increasing the duration of time Jeremy worked prior to taking a break.

A third question to consider when choosing whether to fade an intervention is this: "To what degree is the intervention stigmatizing to the target individual?" In the example below, Josh's support team considered his intervention to be stigmatizing; therefore, it was implemented only temporarily, with a plan to fade it. Josh's intervention was designed to increase predictability pertaining to his daily schedule. Because Josh was not yet proficient with a picture schedule, objects were used to indicate the upcoming activity. A chart was developed that contained objects ordered to correspond to daily activities, such as a toothbrush to indicate morning care routine, a sponge to designate cleaning, and a toy van to correspond to community outings. The bulkiness and size of the chart made it difficult to transport and was stigmatizing when Josh carried it about. Thus a plan was developed to fade the chart once Josh became accustomed to the routine. Josh's support team also began teaching him to recognize more portable photographs to replace the objects, in case Josh preferred having a schedule.

When to Fade

When to fade an intervention is a very important decision. If an intervention is faded too soon, problem behaviors are likely to reemerge. Prior to fading an intervention, a few questions should be considered (Figure 8.2). One question is this: "Does the individual have a well-established alternative response to replace problem behavior in the presence of problematic antecedents or setting events?" The importance of appropriate replacement behaviors that serve the same function as problem behaviors is discussed in detail in Chapter 9. If replacement behaviors are well established, intervention fading is highly likely to be successful.

Interventions that focus on teaching general skills may render an antecedent or setting event intervention unnecessary. For example, as a student becomes proficient at math facts, a once difficult assignment may no longer be so. Thus, if the question "Have general skills been learned so that the antecedent or setting event is no longer problematic?" can be answered affirmatively, then fading should be considered.

How to Fade

Fading antecedent or setting event interventions in a way that avoids the recurrence of problem behavior is best accomplished gradually and systematically. Gradual fading requires slow rather than abrupt change. Systematic fading is accomplished by establishing criteria to guide the fading process. For example, an intervention was implemented with Kirsten, an 18-year-old girl identified as having a developmental disability, during her daily living skill activity of washing a load of clothes at her home. Prior to implementation, she frequently exhibited self-injurious behavior (wrist biting), as a means to escape the activity. A visual photo schedule that depicted and broke down each step of the activity (separating clothes, loading washer, adding soap, etc.) was introduced; in addition, the requirements for completing activity were modified to ensure student success. Kirsten's transition teacher initially instructed Kirsten to complete the first step of the activity each day. A criterion of 3 days of completing Step 1 without self-injurious behavior was utilized as a requirement to increase task demands. Following 3 days without self-injurious behavior, Kirsten was instructed to complete an additional step of the routine. She was now instructed to complete two of the six steps of the routine. The 3-day criterion for adding each new activity step continued until Kirsten was completing all six steps of the laundry task. Following 3 days of task completion (all six steps) without challenging behavior, the number of instructions and the visual schedule were both faded. The number of instructions that the teacher issued to Kirsten for each step was reduced until only one instruction was given for Kirsten to wash a load of laundry. Fading of the detailed visual schedule continued until only one picture of the washing machine was necessary to represent the entire six-step activity.

SUMMARY

Antecedent and setting event interventions constitute an effective and quick-acting approach for reducing challenging behavior. These interventions are vital to a behavior support plan because they prevent problem behavior. In doing so, they create an environment where alternative behaviors can be learned readily. Antecedent and setting event intervention strategies have also been demonstrated to have a positive impact on desirable behaviors, including increasing task performance, productivity, engagement, and student happiness. Many different types of antecedent interventions have been described in the literature and are accompanied by a strong empirical research base. This critical and powerful component of behavior support has not only reduced problem behavior, but also diminished the need for reactive procedures. The examples provided demonstrate that antecedent and setting event interventions can be effective with students who exhibit various problem behaviors and/or represent diverse characteristics, including cognitive, emotional, behavioral and/or intellectual differences.

COMMONLY ASKED QUESTIONS

Will antecedent interventions lead to a watered-down curriculum? Many antecedent interventions allow instructional goals to be maintained. However, sometimes interventions decrease the number or difficulty of tasks presented. The important thing to remember is that the objective is to reduce problem behavior, which often interferes with learning. After problem behavior has been reduced, a plan for fading should be considered.

Is it fair to other students in the class to change the expectations for a student with problem behaviors? Students who exhibit severe behavioral challenges require individualized intervention strategies. Universal approaches, such as schoolwide behavior systems, are unlikely to offer adequate support. Furthermore, individualized intervention is supported and required by the Individuals with Disabilities Education Act (IDEA).

Once an effective antecedent intervention is identified, will it work in all settings? The fact that an intervention is effective in one setting does not necessarily mean it will be effective in others. Environments can differ greatly, in terms of expectations, people, activities, and so forth. If an intervention works in one setting but not in another, it may be necessary to collect additional assessment information to determine whether different variables are influencing behavior in different settings.

What should we do if problem behaviors reemerge when an antecedent or setting event intervention is faded? The reemergence of problem behaviors during fading probably means that the fading was initiated too soon or occurred too quickly. The intervention as initially designed should be reimplemented, or fading should resume at a slower pace.

CASE EXAMPLES

Antecedent Interventions for Malik

When developing a behavior support plan for Malik, his team focused on antecedent interventions first, because their quick-acting nature could bring immediate relief for both Malik and the team. The team's ultimate goal was to eliminate the situations that were problematic for Malik, while at the same time building in preferred activities so that he would once again enjoy participating in school. The team's selection of antecedent interventions was summarized in Malik's behavior support plan (see Figure 8.3). Behavior support plans may be presented in many different formats; the format used in Figure 8.3 is just one example if a template for summarizing each of the four support plan components. The same figure format is used in Figure 8.4 for Bethany, and in subsequent chapters to show how each component builds on the others.

When coming up with antecedent interventions for Malik, the team members kept several questions in mind:

- How can we eliminate or change the triggers to problem behavior?
- What strategies will bring about the quickest results? Can the strategy be easily implemented in the classroom?
- Are we addressing Malik's interests and preferences, as well as his needs?

As shown in Figure 8.3, the team came up with six antecedent strategies. The first three interventions addressed difficult and nonfunctional activities that provoked problem behaviors. After giving consideration to Malik's overall curriculum, the team decided to eliminate letter- and number-naming activities entirely. These activities had appeared on Malik's individualized education program (IEP) for the past 3 years. They were not only difficult for him, but also seemed repetitive and boring. After many years of traditional academic instruction and little progress, Malik's team also concluded that in the very near future they would need to consider an alternative curriculum that emphasized functional academics, where pre-

Malik's Behavior Support Plan

Hypotheses:
1. When prompted through difficult work, Malik is likely to refuse/aggress, to escape the activity.
2. When asked to complete nonfunctional activities, Malik is likely to refuse/aggress, to escape the activity.
3. When required to make a transition from a highly preferred activity to a nonpreferred activity, Malik refuses/aggresses, to maintain the preferred activity and avoid the nonpreferred one.

Antecedent/setting event interventions	Alternative skills	Responses to problem behavior	Long-term supports
Eliminate letter- and number-naming activities from curriculum; avoid recall in academic activities.			
Embed academics in functional activities; ensure meaningful outcomes.			
Prompt Malik to use alternative forms of communication (pictures, gestures) when he has difficulty with verbal expression.			
Use a daily picture schedule to mark classroom activities.			
Provide a transitional warning prior to ending a preferred activity.			
When it is necessary to make a transition from a preferred to a nonpreferred activity, begin activity with a brief preferred activity (e.g., math game).			

FIGURE 8.3. Malik's antecedent interventions.

requisite skills such as letter naming could be bypassed entirely. For example, rather than learning letter names, Malik could be taught to recognize words that frequently occurred in his daily living, school, and community activities. Malik's team also agreed that his academic instruction should take place in the context of meaningful activities where the outcomes would have some functional value to Malik. Letter sorting, for example, could be taught by having Malik sort and place mail in the teachers' mailboxes in the school office. Number identification (pointing to numbers) could be taught during cooking activities or dialing a telephone.

Similarly, with regard to communication, the team decided to stop prompting Malik to use words as his only form of communication. Rather, when Malik's communication was unclear, he would be encouraged to use alternative forms such as gestures and pictures to express himself.

The last three antecedent interventions addressed transitions. Although most transition difficulties occurred when Malik was leaving preferred activities, the team decided to introduce a daily picture schedule that could be viewed each morning and between activities, to increase the predictability of what would happen next. At home, Malik's routines were highly preferred and followed a predictable schedule. However, at school, schedule changes due to special events and snow days made activities more difficult to predict. With regard to Malik's difficulties in making transitions to less preferred activities, the team reasoned that the first three antecedent changes would eliminate most of the problems. However, just to be sure that transitions would be successful, they added two further strategies: (1) a transitional warning about 3 minutes before an activity would end (e.g., "Malik, in a few minutes, it will be time to go to math. We have a fun game planned"), and (2) a fun activity to initiate a less preferred activity (e.g., "Let's start by playing this game").

Antecedent/Setting Event Interventions for Bethany

Bethany's team developed five preventive intervention strategies (see Figure 8.4). First, to accommodate the fine motor difficulties that made written work problematic for Bethany, the team decided to minimize the amount of written work she was required to complete and to provide an alternative strategy for work completion (e.g., a tape recorder) whenever possible. In addition, Bethany requested that she be given shorter assignments, so the team agreed that academic activities would be presented in small increments rather than in lengthy assignments. Finally, Bethany's teachers would make sure that instructions for assignment completion were clear and explicit.

To address inappropriate interactions in the cafeteria, Bethany requested that she be able to sit next to classmates during lunch. The team agreed with this suggestion and believed it would encourage her to develop friends. The team also recognized her need to develop appropriate ways of gaining the attention of people with whom she was not familiar. Thus they decided to introduce new students gradually to Bethany's seating area, while prompting her to initiate appropriate interactions.

Bethany's Behavior Support Plan

Hypotheses:

1. When Bethany is given written assignments, she engages in off-task behavior, to escape.
2. When Bethany is given lengthy assignments, she engages in off-task behavior, to escape.
3. When Bethany has visited her father over the weekend, she engages in off-task behavior, to escape work (because of fatigue).
4. When Bethany is in unstructured situations with unfamiliar peers, she engages in inappropriate interactions, to obtain their attention.

Antecedent/setting event interventions	Alternative skills	Responses to problem behavior	Long-term supports
Minimize amount of written work; provide alternative strategy for work completion (e.g., tape recorder).			
Break work into small increments.			
Make sure instructions are clear and explicit.			
Seat Bethany near classmates in cafeteria; gradually introduce new people while prompting appropriate interactions.			
Have Bethany return home earlier on Sundays after visiting her father.			

FIGURE 8.4. Bethany's antecedent/setting event interventions.

234

Finally, a setting event intervention was implemented: Bethany's father agreed to bring her home earlier on Sundays so she could follow her usual bedtime routine and be in bed by 9:00. This required his parents (with whom the father lived) to move their family dinner 2 hours earlier, which they were glad to do.

REFERENCES

Carr, E. G., Smith, C. E., Giacin, T. A., Whelan, B. M., & Pancari, J. (2003). Menstrual discomfort as a biological setting event for severe problem behavior: Assessment and intervention. *American Journal on Mental Retardation, 108,* 117–133.

Clarke, S., Dunlap, G., Foster-Johnson, L., Childs, K., Wilson, D., White, R., et al. (1995). Improving the conduct of students with behavioral disorders by incorporating student interests into curricular activities. *Behavioral Disorders, 20,* 221–227.

Clarke, S., Worcester, W., Dunlap, G., Murray, M., & Bradley-Klug, K. (2002). Using multiple measures to evaluate positive behavioral support: A case example. *Journal of Positive Behavior Interventions, 3,* 131–145.

Dunlap, G., dePerczel, M., Clarke, S., Wilson, D., Wright, S., White, R., et al. (1994). Choice making to promote adaptive behavior for students with emotional and behavioral challenges. *Journal of Applied Behavior Analysis, 27,* 505–518.

Dunlap, G., Foster-Johnson, L., Clarke, S., Kern, L., & Childs, K. E. (1995). Modifying activities to produce functional outcomes: Effects of the problem behaviors of students with severe disabilities. *Journal of The Association for Persons with Severe Handicaps, 20,* 248–258.

Dunlap, G., Kern, L., dePerczel, M., Clarke, S., Wilson, D., Childs, K., et al. (1993). Functional analysis of classroom variables for students with emotional and behavioral disorders. *Behavioral Disorders, 18,* 275–291.

Dunlap, G., Kern-Dunlap, L., Clarke, S., & Robbins, F. R. (1991). Functional assessment, curricular revision, and severe behavior problems. *Journal of Applied Behavior Analysis, 24,* 387–397.

Ervin, R. A., Kern, L., Clarke, S., DuPaul, G. J., Dunlap, G., & Friman, P. C. (2000). Evaluating assessment-based intervention strategies for students with ADHD and comorbid disorders within the natural classroom context. *Behavioral Disorders, 25,* 344–358.

Flannery, K. B., & Horner, R. H. (1994). The relationship between predictability and problem behavior for students with severe disabilities. *Journal of Behavioral Education, 4,* 157–176.

Gunter, P. L., & Denny, R. K. (1996). Research issues and needs regarding teacher use of classroom management strategies. *Behavioral Disorders, 22,* 15–20.

Horner, R. H., Day, H. M., Sprague, J. R., O'Brien, M., & Heathfield, L. T. (1991). Interspersed requests: A nonaversive procedure for reducing aggression and self-injury during instruction. *Journal of Applied Behavior Analysis, 24,* 265–278.

Kennedy, C. H., & Itkonen, T. (1993). Effects of setting events on the problem behavior of students with severe disabilities. *Journal of Applied Behavior Analysis, 26,* 321–327.

Kern, L., Childs, K., Dunlap, G., Clarke, S., & Falk, G. (1994). Using an assessment-based curricular intervention to improve the classroom behavior of a student with emotional and behavioral challenges. *Journal of Applied Behavior Analysis, 27,* 7–19.

Kern, L., Choutka, C. M., & Sokol, N. G. (2002). Assessment-based antecedent interventions used in natural settings to reduce challenging behavior: A review of the literature. *Education and Treatment of Children, 25,* 113–130.

Kern, L., Koegel, R. L., Dyer, K., Blew, P. A., & Fenton, L. R. (1982). The effects of physical exercise on self-stimulation and appropriate responding in autistic children. *Journal of Autism and Developmental Disorders, 12,* 399–419.

Kern, L., Mantegna, M. E., Vorndran, C. M., Bailin, D., & Hilt, A. (2001). Choice of task sequence to increase engagement and reduce problem behaviors. *Journal of Positive Behavior Interventions, 3,* 3–10.

Kern, L., Vorndran, C., Hilt, A., Ringdahl, J., Adleman, B., & Dunlap, G. (1998). Choice as an intervention to improve behavior: A review of the literature. *Journal of Behavioral Education, 8,* 151–169.

Logan, P., & Skinner, C. (1998). Improving students' perceptions of a mathematics assignment by increasing problem completion rates: Is problem completion a reinforcing event? *School Psychology Quarterly, 13,* 322–331.

Lohrmann-O'Rourke, S., & Yurman, B. (2001). Naturalistic assessment of and intervention for mouthing behaviors influenced by establishing operations. *Journal of Positive Behavior Interventions, 3,* 19–27.

Luiselli, J. K. (1994). Effects of noncontingent sensory reinforcement on stereotypic behaviors in a child with post-traumatic neurological impairment. *Journal of Behavior Therapy and Experimental Psychiatry, 25,* 325–330.

Mace, A. B., Shapiro, E. S., & Mace, F. C. (1998). Effects of warning stimuli for reinforcer withdrawal and task onset on self-injury. *Journal of Applied Behavior Analysis, 31,* 679–682.

Moes, D. R. (1998). Integrating choice-making opportunities within teacher-assigned academic tasks to facilitate the performance of children with autism. *Journal of The Association for Persons with Severe Handicaps, 23,* 319–328.

CHAPTER 9

◆ ◆ ◆

Teaching Alternative Skills

◆

JAMES HALLE
LINDA M. BAMBARA
JOE REICHLE

This chapter addresses the second component of a positive behavior support (PBS) plan: *teaching alternative skills*. As discussed in earlier chapters, students typically engage in challenging behavior because they do not have the requisite social skills to influence people in their environment in intended ways, or because they have learned that challenging behaviors are more effective than other means to achieve this influence. An important goal of PBS is to identify the intended outcomes of challenging behavior with functional assessment, and to assist students to achieve these outcomes by teaching alternative skills that are more effective, efficient, and socially acceptable. Teaching alternative skills can help students get their needs met, change situations that trigger problem behaviors, and cope with difficult situations as they arise. Having acquired these skills, students become more independent and resilient (or adaptive) in their everyday encounters and less dependent on others' efforts to help them address difficult situations. The beauty of teaching alternative skills is that the skills targeted for instruction (e.g., communication, social skills, independence, problem solving, and coping/tolerance) are the same skills we hope to teach to all students; taken together, they define a high-quality education.

CONCEPTUAL FRAMEWORK FOR TEACHING
ALTERNATIVE SKILLS

There are three types of alternative skills, each with a different purpose: (1) *replacement skills*, (2) *coping and tolerance skills*, and (3) *general adaptive skills* (Bambara & Knoster, 1998). Replacement skills are those alternatives that serve exactly the same functions as problem behaviors. In teaching a replacement skills, the goal is to identify a socially acceptable behavior that will allow the student to achieve the same outcome as the problem behavior. For example, if DeShawna shouts to obtain assistance during independent math work because she cannot solve two-digit multiplication problems, her teacher can teach DeShawna to ask for help to directly replace shouting for assistance. If in another situation DeShawna grabs a toy held by a peer, a polite request to share can serve as a replacement to gain access to the toy. Before a replacement skill is taught, however, a decision needs to be made about whether the replacement can or cannot be reliably honored.

Coping and tolerance skills, the second type of alternative skills, enable students to cope with difficult situations and remain in them without engaging in problem behavior. Situations that cannot or should not be addressed by teaching replacement skills are ideal candidates for teaching coping and tolerance. For example, we would not want to teach a replacement behavior for escaping a doctor's office. Honoring a replacement in such a situation would mean that a student might fail to receive needed medical services. Also, situations in which replacement skills may not be immediately honored are ideal occasions for teaching coping or tolerance skills. If DeShawna's polite request does not consistently produce the desired outcome (e.g., the peer says, "I just got the toy; you can have it later"), her team will need to consider what other skills need to be taught to compete with the problem behavior. In this case, she may need to be taught how to ask and wait for a turn with the toy.

General adaptive skills are the third type of alternative skills. Once acquired, these skills eliminate the need for problem behaviors by teaching students how to change situations or conditions associated with the problem behaviors. For example, DeShawna's teacher can teach her how to solve two-digit multiplication problems, removing the need for engaging in problem behavior to obtain assistance. Teaching general adaptive skills includes identifying and remediating factors or skill deficits that contribute to problem behaviors. Targets may include enhancing general communication and academic competence, teaching organizational or time management strategies to enhance work efficiency and completion of assignments, and expanding social skills to facilitate rewarding social relationships with peers and adults.

When designing PBS plans, teams may wish to consider all three types of alternative skills. As summarized in Table 9.1, each skill type has a distinct purpose and associated limitations; the limitations can be offset by combining two or more types of alternative skills in a single behavior support plan. Table 9.1 also provides guiding questions that teams can use when considering what types of alternative skills to teach.

In the remainder of this chapter, we provide specific recommendations and examples for teaching each of these three types of alternative skills. Replacement skills are organized by the functions of (1) escape, (2) accessing or obtaining something, and (3) sensory or self-stimulation. Recommendations for teaching coping and tolerance cut across functions and include several different self-management strategies. We then provide an overview and rationale for teaching general adaptive skills. Finally, we use two case scenarios to compare and contrast how each of the three alternative skill types can be combined in one behavior support plan.

TEACHING REPLACEMENT SKILLS

Teaching Considerations

If the function of a problem behavior can be reliably honored, then a functionally equivalent replacement skill can be taught. For example, letter recognition was an objective in Juan's IEP (individualized education program). However, a functional assessment revealed that this task was not preferred by Juan due to its difficulty, and that it often triggered problem behavior (i.e., screaming and pounding his desk with his fists), resulting in his teacher's immediately providing assistance to Juan. His teacher taught Juan to raise his hand (a replacement skill) to obtain assistance. When he used this new skill, his teacher immediately provided him with the assistance he requested.

Before teaching a replacement skill, team members should ask themselves several pertinent questions in their planning. First, "What skill or behavior will be taught as a replacement?" Second, "How should the replacement skill be taught?" Third, "How can we be sure that the replacement skill will compete successfully with the problem behavior?" And fourth, "Once the replacement skill has been acquired, how can we ensure that the student continues to use it over time?"

What Skill Will Be Taught?

The replacement skill must have the same (communicative) function as the problem behavior. The behavior's function, identified in the hypothesis

TABLE 9.1. Three Types of Alternative Skills

Alternative skill type	Guiding questions	Purpose and limitations
Replacement skills	What skill will serve exactly the same function as the problem behavior?	*Purpose:* • To provide student with an effective way of achieving the same outcome as the problem behavior. *Limitations:* • The function of problem behavior cannot always be honored. • A single replacement skill rarely addresses the skills needed to prevent or change problem situations (e.g., work is too difficult).
Coping and tolerance skills	What skills will help the student cope or deal with difficult or unpleasant situations?	*Purpose:* • To teach socially acceptable ways of coping with situations that should not or cannot be changed. *Limitations:* • Usually not effective alone. Works better when students have alternative ways of achieving desired outcomes or can modify problem situations by themselves (e.g., have the skills to address difficult work situations). • Caution: Expecting a student to tolerate unpleasant situations without teaching replacement skills, teaching general adaptive skills, and/or making antecedent/setting event changes may be unethical.
General adaptive skills	What related skills will prevent the need for problem behavior? What skills will result in meaningful lifestyle improvements for the student?	*Purpose:* • To expand social, communicative, and academic competence, in order to prevent problem situations and help the student pursue preferences and interests. *Limitations:* • Instruction is more labor-intensive than teaching replacement skills. • A student may need to learn replacement skills first to address immediate needs.

statement, will suggest what the new skill needs to accomplish. When identifying a replacement skill, team members should consider the student's current repertoire of skills to determine whether the student already possesses a response that can be adopted or adapted as a replacement for the problem behavior. It is much easier to encourage a student to use an existing skill than it is to teach an entirely new one.

Let us digress momentarily to describe a crucial concept that may assist teams in making decisions about what skills to teach. When a group of responses produces the same outcome (i.e., has the same function), the group is called a *response class*, and each response is a member of the class and is said to be *functionally equivalent*. Thus, when a person says "Hi" or "How are ya?", waves, or smiles, each of these four responses functions as a greeting and, in the presence of another person, produces the same functional outcome (see Figure 9.1 for a visual display of a greeting response

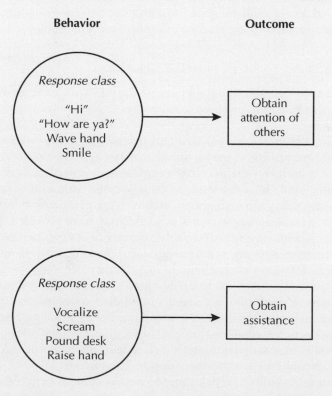

FIGURE 9.1. Examples of response classes: Greeting others and requesting help. Note that in each class, topographically different behaviors produce the same effect on the environment (i.e., have the same outcome).

class). Figure 9.1 includes a second example of a response class. Remember Juan, who requested help by screaming and pounding his desk? His teacher taught him the replacement behaviors of making a sound and raising his hand for help. This figure reveals that Juan already vocalized to request help, and that the teacher needed only to pair this response with hand raising—a response that was in his repertoire, but had not been used previously for requesting help. After the teacher modeled this new help-requesting method ("Make a sound and raise your hand"), and reinforced it repeatedly by providing assistance, hand raising became a member of Juan's response class for requesting help.

When team members are answering the question about what skill to teach, it is imperative to assess the behaviors in the student's repertoire and identify existing behaviors that are already members of the relevant response class (i.e., share the same function). If no existing behavior is a "good fit" to replace problem behavior, then teaching a new skill is necessary. A "good fit" means that the skill can serve exactly the same purpose, can be used across multiple situations, and can be readily understood by a wide range of social partners (both familiar and unfamiliar).

How Should the Replacement Skill Be Taught?

Although there are an infinite number of considerations for teaching, only a few of the most relevant are discussed here.

- *Teach in the same situations that provoke problem behavior.* This is important, because all of the factors that may cause the problem are present, and it is in these situations that a replacement is needed. The triggering antecedents (and, in some cases, setting events) will inform when and where to teach. In Juan's situation, teaching took place during independent work periods when letter recognition worksheets were provided. However, sometimes it helps to teach in rehearsal or practice settings before introducing the training into the actual triggering situation. This is appropriate when the new behavior takes time to acquire or when the actual situation provides little flexibility for teaching. Juan's teacher, for example, might have chosen to teach him to raise his hand during one-to-one instruction where she had more time to work with him, before teaching him to use it during independent activities.
- *Teach in conjunction with antecedent interventions.* Alternative skills can be enhanced with other support components in place, especially antecedent interventions, which can make instruction more pleasant for the student and give the teacher greater control over the teaching opportunities. As an antecedent strategy, Juan's teacher limited his exposure to difficult letter recognition tasks when he worked alone. She did this by inter-

spersing only a few letter recognition tasks (matching letters to word pictures) with other reading tasks he could do successfully (putting picture sequences in the correct order). This antecedent intervention reduced Juan's frustration and decreased the number of occasions that Juan needed to request assistance. Juan's teacher could not possibly have responded to all of Juan's requests for help if he raised his hand every minute.

• *Teach or prompt the alternative skill before problem behavior occurs.* During situations when problem behavior is likely, it is best to prompt the replacement skill before the student has the opportunity to engage in problem behavior, rather than after the problem behavior occurs. During independent seatwork, Juan's teacher carefully observed Juan's response to triggering antecedents (letter recognition tasks). Before he had a chance to scream, she prompted him by saying, "Remember, Juan, if you need help, raise your hand." When Juan raised his hand, she offered immediate assistance. This was a far better strategy than waiting for Juan to scream and then prompting him to raise his hand, which could have inadvertently led to Juan learning a chain: "First I scream [engage in problem behavior], and then I raise my hand to get my teacher's help."

How Can We Be Sure That the Replacement Skill Will Compete Successfully with the Problem Behavior?

Given that problem behaviors and replacement skills are members of the same response class, it is important to ensure that the student will choose to use the alternative skill and not the problem behavior to achieve desired outcomes. In the last 15 years, groundbreaking research (e.g., Horner & Day, 1991; Neef, Mace, & Shade, 1993) has revealed answers to this question. Researchers have identified at least five criteria that influence this competition. These criteria, taken together, determine the *efficiency* of a response and must be considered when replacement skills are being taught.

The first criterion, *effort,* is defined by the physical movements (calories of energy expended, according to Horner & Day, 1991) or the cognitive challenge required to produce a response. With all other factors being equal, students will choose to engage in the most efficient response—in this case, the one involving the least effort. The rule for instruction is to select a replacement skill that takes less effort than the problem behavior. For example, Sal's flinging his textbook to the floor requires less effort than making a sound to obtain his teacher's attention and then pointing to two pages in his communication book—first the "help" page and then the "math" page. If Sal's teacher wants him to ask for help without flinging his text, then she will have to consider teaching another replacement skill that requires less effort than the problem behavior.

The second efficiency criterion, *quality* or *magnitude* of the outcome, refers to the level of preference or the reinforcing value of the events or objects delivered as consequences. The rule for instruction is to be sure that the outcome or reinforcer for the replacement skill is the same quality as, or better quality than, the outcome produced by the problem behavior; otherwise, the student will not use the alternative skill. Chad, who has not acquired spoken words, likes interacting with other students and has multiple ways of obtaining their attention, including making loud noises, spitting, clapping his hands, and touching them on the arm. Noises, spitting, and clapping cause others to look up momentarily and see what Chad is doing. However, tapping them on the arm often produces either a question like "Do you need something?" or some other type of social response that is of a longer duration and is more interactive than a momentary glance. Both the quality and magnitude of peers' responsiveness are greater when Chad taps them, thus we would predict that this member of the response class for *obtaining peer attention* would be the most probable.

The third efficiency criterion, *immediacy* of the outcome, is also an influential factor in determining efficiency of responses. Logically, if a particular response produces the desired outcome more quickly than others, we would anticipate that the student would use this response option. The rule for instruction then is to ensure that responsiveness to the replacement skill is as immediate as, or more immediate than, responsiveness to the problem behavior. For example, Alonzo contributes to class discussions in either of two ways: (1) he raises his hand and waits to be recognized, or (2) he speaks out without being recognized. Both behaviors produce the same outcome of giving his perspective. However, often when he raises his hand, he has to wait to be recognized by his teacher; whereas no waiting is required when he talks out. Thus we would expect him to speak out more often, because it permits more immediate access to giving his perspective. If Alonzo's teacher wants him to raise his hand, then she will need to consider how she can respond immediately to his hand raising and/or change the outcomes for talking out (e.g., interrupt his response, ignore his response, or remove him from the class discussion).

The fourth efficiency criterion, the *consistency* of the outcome, refers to the number of student responses required before the consequence is delivered. The rule for instruction is to respond each time the student uses a replacement skill—the first time, every time. This is especially important during the initial stages of instruction, when the goal is to establish that the replacement skill is more efficient in helping the student to achieve the desired outcome. If the replacement skill is responded to inconsistently, then the student may choose to use the problem behavior to achieve what he or she wants. Unfortunately, examples abound of inconsistent and inadvertent ignoring of socially appropriate behavior and consistent attention to problem behavior. One of us (James Halle) can recall numerous occasions when his young children would ask in a nice way, "Daddy, will you play with me?", and he would sometimes stop what he was doing and engage with them; more often, however, he would say, "I'm busy, but I can play later." In effect, his children learned that perhaps once for every four or five times they would ask nicely, he would play. In contrast to this ideal picture, his young children also learned that almost every time they screamed and cried with great intensity, he would abruptly stop what he was doing and interact with them. Once again, the two options constituted a response class in which both asking nicely and "asking" coercively were functionally equivalent, producing the same outcome (i.e., Dad's interacting). We would anticipate that if the children wanted to interact with their father, they would scream and cry because the consistency or rate of reinforcement was greater.

The final criterion, *probability of punishment*, refers to the likelihood that a response will be followed by a consequence that is aversive or unpleasant. It is a well-known principle of learning that responses followed consistently by unpleasant events will diminish in frequency. Thus the rule for instruction is to ensure that replacement behaviors are *not* followed by unpleasant events. A corollary to this rule might be to ensure either that the problem behavior for which a replacement has been identified is followed by an unpleasant event, or that nothing changes as a result of engagement in the problem behavior (i.e., extinction, as described in Chapter 10). Probability of punishment has not often been discussed in the context of response efficiency, for at least two reasons: (1) It has rarely been identified as a factor; and (2) some researchers believe that it influences responding, but do not consider it part of efficiency. We include it as a criterion for two reasons. First, we believe it has a pervasive influence on the response options students select; therefore, we want to emphasize the importance of ensuring that punishing consequences are *not* associated with the teaching of the replacement skill. Second, the probability of punishment may explain what otherwise would be inexplicable outcomes. For example, Lucy is socially sensitive and cares greatly about "fitting in" and being accepted by her peers. When participating in classroom group activities, Lucy prefers to work with her friend Cynthia. She has learned that she can ask the teacher to be in Cynthia's group; she can ask the group leaders for the activity to choose Cynthia and her; or she can engage in a tantrum. Each of these three responses is sometimes effective at producing the desired outcome: Lucy's being on the same team with Cynthia. Tantrums require more effort, but they produce the outcome more immediately and more often than making a verbal request. Even though it would appear that tantrums are more efficient, Lucy *asks* to be grouped with Cynthia much more often than she has tantrums, because occasionally when she has tantrums the teacher will isolate Lucy, directing her to sit in a corner of the classroom while the rest of the class participates in the group activity. Lucy finds such isolation embarrassing, and it functions as a punisher (Alberto & Troutman, 2003). Thus, although tantrums may be more efficient in reference to reinforcement (immediacy and rate) criteria, because the response is occasionally punished, it becomes less probable and less efficient relative to asking.

In summary, these five criteria that define efficiency depend primarily on the consequences delivered by others in the environment with the student (e.g., teachers, peers, staff, parents); therefore, they require an interplay or reciprocity between teaching students replacement responses and ensuring that the social environment is more responsive to the replacement skills and less responsive to their functionally equivalent problem alternatives. This is a critical concept, and is highly relevant for the fourth and final question we have posed earlier—the one about ensuring the maintenance of replacement skills relative to problem behavior. Maintenance of the use of replacement skills relative to problem behavior is determined in large part by the responses provided by peers and adults. Are social partners responding immediately? Consistently? To the extent that social partners ensure that the replacement skills are more efficient than problem behavior in producing desired outcomes, their maintenance will be assured. Figure 9.2 provides a checklist for ensuring efficiency.

Replacement Skill Interventions

Numerous strategies exist for teaching replacement skills. In this section, we highlight common intervention approaches grouped according to behavior function. Most of the replacement interventions are predicated on a

---

☐ Does the replacement skill require *less effort* than the problem behavior? From the student's perspective, is it easy to use?

☐ Does the replacement skill produce *outcomes of the same quality or magnitude* as the problem behavior?

☐ Do others *respond immediately* when the student uses the replacement skill, especially during initial instruction?

☐ Do others *respond consistently* when the student uses the replacement skill?

☐ Are procedures in place to ensure that replacement skills are encouraged and *not inadvertently punished?*

FIGURE 9.2. Checklist for ensuring response efficiency.

procedure referred to as *functional communication training* or FCT (Carr et al., 1994; Carr & Durand, 1985; Durand, 1990; Wacker et al., 1990). Chapter 2 has explained how problem behavior can often be considered a form of communication, because it enables people to influence others in their environment in intended ways—which is the definition of *communication*. FCT involves three general steps. First, a team must conduct a functional assessment to determine the function of the problem behavior (i.e., what the student is trying to communicate). Once the function has been identified, the second step is to select a socially acceptable communicative replacement that serves exactly the same purpose. Finally, this communicative replacement must be taught, and the team must ensure that the newly acquired behavior is more efficient than the problem behavior. FCT, as well as other replacement interventions, must be designed to accommodate the varying environmental situations or contexts that make problem behavior likely. In this section, we identify the most common of these contexts and describe replacement skills that are crafted individually to address each specific context.

Interventions Associated with Escape from Activities or Social Interactions

Escape-associated problem behavior occurs when students encounter unpleasant or difficult situations. They have learned that they can avoid, postpone, or escape these situations by engaging in problem behavior. In addition to modifying the situations to make them more pleasant through antecedent or setting event interventions, instructors can teach alternative, socially acceptable ways of avoiding or escaping from these unpleasant situations. There is a range of distinctly different replacement skills, each matching a set of environmental contexts that can be taught in an effort to replace challenging behavior with functionally equivalent communicative alternatives. Selecting the most appropriate alternative will be determined by the specific events identified in the hypothesis for each problem behavior.

Escape by rejecting is a viable option for students when the rejected activity, object, or attention is not necessary for the achievement of important educational and social goals. The selected replacement behavior might be the words "No, thank you," a back-and-forth head movement, the sign for "no," or whatever form minimizes response effort and maximizes the probability of the intended outcome for the student. The latter can be facilitated by ensuring that the replacement is understood by a wide range of social partners. Lola hated singing solos in music class and often swore at the teacher when she was told to sing a song by herself. When she swore, she was removed from class (and did not have to sing the solo). Mr.

Capella, Lola's teacher, used an antecedent cue to prompt a replacement when he asked her to sing a solo: "If you'd rather not sing, please say, 'No, thank you, Mr. Capella!' " Lola complied by saying these words and was not required to sing. After the antecedent cue was faded, Mr. Capella's intervention was effective and satisfactory for both him and Lola, because he did not really care if she sang solos and she could successfully avoid singing.

In other situations, an activity or an interaction may become unpleasant when it continues beyond a length of time or a number of repetitions that the student finds acceptable. In this instance, *escape by requesting a break* from the activity or from the interaction may be appropriate. We (Halle, Ostrosky, & Silliman, 1995) worked with a young boy named Asher who would tolerate counting tasks for brief periods of time, but would begin to scream and pinch his teacher after a small number of practice trials. Asher had no words and few ways to communicate that he wanted a break, so we introduced a symbol of a red circle with an "x" in the center. Using physical prompts, we taught Asher to touch the symbol when he wanted to leave the task, and then immediately removed the task materials and assisted him to leave his chair and move to a play area of the classroom. With time, Asher touched the symbol independently and waited for our permission to leave. Returning readily to a task is not something one can expect, but at least two features of this approach can enhance the likelihood of it. First, as students learn that they can leave the task when they want (they are in control), they find it easier to return to it; second, team members can ensure that upon their return something they enjoy is present (e.g., counting locomotives for a math task).

In a third context, the difficulty of the task may cause it to be unpleasant for students, resulting in problem escape behavior. For example, when a worksheet contains difficult problems, the task quickly becomes unpleasant. On such occasions, teaching the replacement *escape by requesting assistance or asking for help* may be warranted. Ms. Brenner, Jerry's preschool teacher, taught him to replace whining and crying with a simple phrase ("Help, please") when he could not find the proper places for puzzle pieces. Both crying and "Help, please" led to Ms. Brenner's providing the needed assistance; however, she was careful to ensure that she provided her help immediately and consistently in response to "Help, please," but not to crying.

A fourth escape context is encountered when students wish to communicate that they are finished with an activity or do not want to engage with the current task/activity any longer. Escape-motivated problem behavior often occurs in such situations—especially when students lack the communicative means of saying, "I've had enough," or when they perceive that the only way to terminate an activity is by engaging in problem behavior (the latter situation often occurs when ambiguous requests to stop are ignored). These are ideal occasions for teaching students to *escape by terminating an activity* through socially appropriate ways. If students use words, they can be taught to say, "I've had enough," or "No more, thank you." Students who do not communicate verbally may be taught to sign "Stop" or "Done," or to gently push away materials to signal "done."

A fifth and final context discussed here is more subtle than the previous ones. In this situation, a student may be engaged in an activity that is perfectly acceptable; however, a competing activity that is far more enjoyable becomes available, creating a reason to terminate or escape from the less preferred activity. Engaging in problem behavior may be a means to end the less preferred activity and gain access to the more preferred activity. For example, let's assume that students in a fifth-grade class are writing their autobiographies—an activity that Leonardo finds somewhat enjoyable, but is lagging behind the rest of the class in completing. Let's assume further that the entire group, except for Leonardo, is then excused for recess, and recess is far and away Leonardo's favorite time of the school day. Leonardo is likely to engage in challenging behavior because it provides escape from an activity that was tolerable for a while, but has become unpleasant now that a more enjoyable activity is available. Teaching Leonardo to negotiate with his teacher a time when he will finish his autobiography (e.g., at home tonight and handed in first thing in the morning) so he can go to recess is an example of a replacement skill that will allow Leonardo to temporarily terminate a less preferred activity to engage in a more preferred one.

Interventions Associated with Obtaining or Accessing Materials or Activities

Problem behavior associated with obtaining or accessing occurs when students want something that they cannot access themselves without the help or permission of another. As in cases of escape-motivated problem behavior, many different socially acceptable replacement skills, each matching a distinct environmental context, can be taught to help students access the materials or events that they desire. Selecting the most appropriate replacement skill for each context or situation is a decision that must be informed by a careful functional assessment.

Teaching replacement skills to gain access to materials or activities can be conceptualized in three general ways. First, students may be taught to *request desired materials or activities*. This strategy simply involves prompting students to use a communicative replacement skill (i.e., providing them with FCT) in those situations where they currently use problem behavior to obtain desired items or events. For example, at the completion of a meal, Tommy came to expect that he would be given a dessert. If dessert did not arrive immediately, he began crying, which rapidly escalated to a tantrum. To establish a communicative replacement, Tommy's parents used a physical prompt: They physically guided Tommy's hand to touch a symbol, representing dessert, prior to Tommy's initiation of a tantrum. Immediately after this response was prompted, a dessert was delivered. Across successive teaching opportunities, his parents gradually and systematically reduced the magnitude of the physical prompt from full physical guidance to lightly tapping Tommy's hand. When the only prompt required was tapping Tommy's hand, they began delaying the prompt by waiting 3 seconds to see whether Tommy would initiate the response independently. The second time they delayed the prompt, Tommy initiated a request. Tommy soon learned that touching the symbol enabled him to access dessert after every meal; touching the symbol was more efficient than having a tantrum.

Similarly, in the second strategy, students may be taught to *request assistance from others to obtain desired materials or activities*. Earlier, during our discussion of escape, we had identified requesting assistance as a means of reducing the difficulty of a task or an activity. Requesting assistance can also be a useful intervention strategy with students who engage in challenging behavior to obtain access to goods and services that require the help of others. Some examples of services requiring assistance include unwrapping a candy bar, zipping a coat before going outside, or inserting a videotape or DVD to watch a favorite movie.

Interestingly, research suggests that teaching requests for assistance in the context of one function of behavior (e.g., escape) will not necessarily guarantee that the same form of requesting assistance (e.g., "Help, please") will be used to replace challenging behavior associated with other social functions (e.g., obtaining/accessing) (Reichle, Drager, & Davis, 2002). Thus teams should be prepared to teach students how to request assistance across varying purposes (functions) and in the situations that require its use.

A third general strategy to replace problem behaviors associated with obtaining access to materials or events is to *teach the student to obtain desired activities/materials directly, without seeking permission or asking for assistance*. Students with disabilities sometimes engage in problem behavior if they perceive that their access to a desired event or material is blocked. Rather than being taught to request help, the students can be taught to obtain the material or engage in the activity independently without the assistance or permission of others. Walter, a 17-year-old with autism, paced frantically in the school locker room when he noticed the other boys in his gym class showering. Until Walter's pacing escalated to the point of disruption, it never dawned on his gym teacher that Walter might enjoy showering with the other boys. From Walter's perspective, showering was not seen as an option after gym class, because it was never offered to him. Walter's gym teacher considered teaching him to request showering; however, teaching Walter that he could shower without permission was more age-appropriate and consistent with what his peers did. His gym teacher simply prompted Walter to engage in the replacement behavior as soon as gym class ended (e.g., "Walter, you may shower if you want. Go ahead"). After several prompts, Walter realized that he could take a shower without the permission of his teacher.

Interventions Associated with Recruiting Attention and Social Interaction

Daily opportunities for students to seek and maintain the attention of others are too numerous to count. For most of us, the attention of another (e.g., talking, playing, sharing an idea) is an enjoyable and highly desirable event. The strategies we use to obtain attention or initiate social interaction with others are critical for establishing ongoing positive interpersonal relationships. Often students with disabilities who have not yet acquired more sophisticated strategies will recruit peer and adult attention through inappropriate means. Making silly noises or faces in class, teasing others, bragging, or engaging in rough play may be viewed as clumsy attempts to engage others.

Selecting and teaching alternative replacement skills for attention-seeking problem behaviors can be a complex endeavor, perhaps more complex than teaching replacement skills for other functions. As in implementing other replacement skill interventions, team members must pinpoint the exact situation or context that triggers the student's attention-seeking in order to identify appropriate teaching opportunities, and they must select a suitable replacement skill that will work in that situation. Moreover, team members must make reasonable guesses about the type of attention or social interaction that the student is seeking. Just knowing that the student is seeking attention is not enough. It is important to understand the type of social attention sought in order to select the most appropriate replacement skill. For example, is the student seeking attention to receive praise or approval from others (e.g., "Look what I did," "Watch what I'm doing")? Is the student seeking to initiate play or conversation (e.g., "Do you wanna play Uno?" "Hey, wassup?")? Is the student seeking comfort or sympathy (e.g., "I don't feel well")? Is the student seeking to share ideas, feelings, or experiences (e.g., "You'll never guess what happened to me over the weekend")? Is the student seeking attention to have fun (e.g., joking, "I lost your homework—sorry!")? These examples illustrate that not all attention-seeking behaviors are the same. Thus team members must be very careful about the specific purpose of attention seeking. The replacement skill targeted for instruction must match the specific type of attention that the student is seeking to be a functionally equivalent replacement, and therefore to be effective (Carr & Durand, 1985; Carr et al., 1994). The only way to pinpoint the type of attention the student is seeking is with careful assessments, such as thorough interviews and focused observations.

A few examples illuminate the continuum of complexity required in the assessment to identify socially adaptive replacement skills for attention seeking. When Charlie wants the attention of another, he screams or stands in close proximity with the peer or adult whose attention he's seeking and places his hand on the other person's chin, forcefully turning the person's head until he or she is facing him. Both of these responses are considered problematic by peers and adults. Charlie can be taught to use either of two replacement responses: (1) to lower the decibel level of the scream to a vocalization that can be heard by his social partner, and (2) to tap the partner on the arm or shoulder, instead of forcefully moving his head. If the new responses are to replace the problem behaviors, however, they need to meet the efficiency criteria described earlier. Although Charlie may no longer engage in these problem behaviors, his social partners may still encounter difficulties understanding exactly what Charlie wants. Thus, even though he has obtained their attention, they now need to determine his precise purpose; this often leads to a process similar to a game of Twenty Questions.

To be responsive to this new challenge, replacement interventions that are located midway on the continuum of complexity are warranted. These replacements involve teaching Charlie a two-part request: first, to gain attention (as described above), and then to specify the type of attention he wants. This requires chaining together two responses. Let's assume that Charlie has requested the attention of his teacher, Ms. Chan, and he wants her to look at the block structure he has just completed in another part of the classroom. He already has acquired the general request form of tapping Ms. Chan on the arm to obtain her attention, and now his team is teaching him to point to a picture of blocks in his communication book to help Ms. Chan understand the subject of Charlie's request. Ms. Chan still may not understand exactly what Charlie is communicating; she may think he's requesting blocks. So the team decides to teach yet a third response to be chained to the other two: Charlie is to be taught to tap Ms. Chan on the arm, point to the picture depicting "look," and then point to the picture of blocks. This sequence of three responses makes Charlie's request for attention very clear.

If a student has significant developmental disabilities, then the primary responsibility for maintaining a communicative interaction often is the responsibility of the social partner. One strategy to increase such students' ability to maintain an interaction is to provide them with a mechanism to remind them of a variety of topics that can be the focus of a social exchange. For example, each week Tommy visits his grandparents on Saturday morning. Tommy, who touched symbols to communicate, now can operate an electronic communication device. Prior to his visit, his mother locates the page of his device that contains picture symbols representing topics that he enjoys. This page has photos of the Cleveland Browns logo, Tommy's favorite professional wrestler, a movie theatre, and his dog. His mother places in a notebook current information regarding each of these pictures that he can share with his grandparents. His mother also reviews with Tommy a book of jokes to select four or five to enter in his electronic communication device. His grandfather particularly enjoys knock-knock jokes. Although Tommy cannot discuss any of these topics in great depth, he can keep an interaction going; the total responsibility for an exchange does not have to reside with his partner.

Interventions Associated with Sensory Stimulation

The logic of teaching a direct replacement skill for sensory or self-stimulatory behavior is the same as that for other functions (i.e., escape and access), but because consequences are not delivered by others, the assessment process looks a little different. To identify the function when the behavior is thought to be self-stimulatory, a two-step process is necessary. First, team members need to determine whether the behavior is indeed self-stimulatory or automatically reinforcing to the individual. If it is, then they need to identify which type or source of stimulation (e.g., visual, auditory, tactile, vestibular, olfactory) is reinforcing to the student. The procedures for conducting the first step of this process have been described in detail in Chapter 7 on developing hypotheses. To accomplish the second step in this two-step process, Rincover (1978) and Rincover, Cook, Peoples, and Packard (1979) offer a model of assessment procedures and recommendations for direct replacement.

To answer the question "What type of sensory stimulation (e.g., visual, auditory, tactile) is reinforcing the behavior?", team members will need to interview familiar adults and conduct observations to formulate hypotheses about potential sensory reinforcers. Team members can then test their hypotheses by implementing a procedure referred to as *sensory extinction*. For example, André's team hypothesized that his spinning objects on table surfaces was reinforced by the noise (auditory stimulation) produced. To test this hypothesis following the Rincover et al. (1978) approach to sensory extinction, Ms. Chadsey, André's teacher, covered the table with carpet, thereby eliminating the noise generated, to determine how this change in the environment would affect the object spinning.

André's spinning diminished on the carpeted table, so Ms. Chadsey removed the carpet and continued to gather data on the spinning. His spinning increased in duration when the carpet was removed from the table, so she once again covered the table to assess the effects. André's object spinning decreased and increased in a predictable fashion depending on the presence or absence of the carpet, thus confirming the hypothesis that auditory stimulation was the consequence maintaining the spinning.

One caveat with the sensory extinction assessment approach is that the precise identification of the type of sensory stimulation produced by the self-stimulatory behavior is often ambiguous and may only be identified with hypothesis testing. For instance, prior to the sensory extinction assessment, a possible hypothesis for André's object-spinning might have been the visual stimulation it produced. If André seemed to enjoy watching the object spin, then determining whether visual or auditory stimulation was the functional consequence would have been difficult (because spinning objects produce both visual and auditory feedback) without conducting the sensory extinction assessment. Although it may be theoretically possible in such a case to test each type of sensory stimulation one at a time for precise identification, in reality it may not be possible to determine precisely the types of stimulation obtained. Thus team members may need to rely on a combination of assessments (e.g., interviews, observations, hypothesis testing) to make informed guesses as to what type of stimulation, either in isolation or combination, is reinforcing the student's behavior.

Once a team forms a reasonable hypothesis about the type of stimulation that the student obtains by engaging in the behavior, a replacement skill may be selected. Before we describe replacement interventions for self-stimulatory behavior, it is important to note that our suggestions are more conceptually than empirically driven, because this function of challenging behavior has a much smaller research base than the escape and access functions. Furthermore, our recommendations are only for accessing and not for escaping sensory stimulation, because the latter has not yet been addressed by research. Having said this, we now focus on two intervention options for direct replacement. The first is to make available another, socially acceptable means of obtaining the same type of stimulation—a means that students can access themselves. In a case like André's, logic dictates finding a device that produces auditory feedback similar to that of spinning objects. (It is not yet well established whether the auditory stimulation needs to be the same or very similar to that produced by the self-stimulatory behavior; it is possible that other auditory feedback may be equally effective as a replacement.) Such a device may be a Speak-n-Spell or an Animal Noises toy for a younger student, or a music box that produces environmental sounds for an older student. As a replacement skill, students can be taught to operate these devices independently so that they can produce the sensory feedback for themselves. Employing these devices, if age-appropriate, is a type of leisure activity and a very appropriate means to obtain reinforcing sensory feedback. We need not look far to see that many typically developing children and adults listen to music (of all types) for fun and relaxation, and that some adults purchase expensive auditory systems that mimic the natural sounds of birds, the ocean, or streams.

A second option for replacing self-stimulatory behavior is to teach students to request an alternative means of obtaining the same type of sensory stimulation. Depending on students' current level of expressive communication, they can be taught either to make a request like "Sounds, please" or "Music, please," or to use a gesture or a picture symbol in order to access a tape recording or CD that contains preferred auditory sounds. In this way, the same or a similar reinforcer is accessed via an appropriate request that in the past was accessed via spinning objects on a table. When team members are applying either of these options of direct replacement, it is critical to ensure that the components of efficiency (discussed earlier in the chapter) are considered. That is, these new ways to access desired sensory stimulation need to be more efficient than engaging in self-stimulation. This may be accomplished by combining sensory extinction for self-stimulation, such as covering a table with cloth to mask the sound produced by spinning objects, with immediate and consistent access to sensory reinforcement when the student is engaging in leisure activities (Option 1) or requesting sensory devices (Option 2).

TEACHING COPING AND TOLERANCE SKILLS

Although they are indispensable features of a behavior support plan, modifying antecedents/setting events and teaching replacement skills sometimes are not sufficient and, depending on the situation, may not be appropriate. Sometimes students must be taught how to cope with difficult or unpleasant situations that are vital to the students' welfare. Earlier in the chapter, we have mentioned medical services as one such situation; however, if educational programming is functional and relevant for students, then many situations may arise daily in which teachers are providing instruction on vital skills that students find difficult or unpleasant. Examples are easy to generate: self-care skills, such as brushing teeth or combing hair; academic skills, such as reading and arithmetic; social skills, such as initiating and maintaining interaction; and employment skills, such as learning the tasks that constitute a job description.

In this section of the chapter, we describe several interventions that teach students to tolerate or cope with situations that cannot or should not be changed, because they involve skills that are vital to the students' welfare or are unavoidable realities of life (e.g., receiving corrective feedback may be unpleasant for some students, but learning how to accept feedback graciously is an important part of school, home, and community life). *Tolerance*, as used here, means teaching students to "wait" or tolerate delays in reinforcement when their requests to escape from situations or obtain materials or attention cannot or should not be immediately honored (Carr et al., 1994). *Coping* refers to teaching students how to use self-management or self-control strategies when they encounter difficult or unpleasant situations.

Teaching Tolerance by Delaying Reinforcement

Waiting and enduring difficult or unpleasant situations are critical life skills to teach students. None of us can always get what we want when we want it, and many times we must persist through important activities, even though we may dislike them. For many students with disabilities, tolerance is a skill that must be taught directly and systematically. Generally, teaching tolerance involves progressively delaying reinforcement after a student makes a request, while at the same time encouraging the student to persist through important activities by gradually increasing demands. Tolerance instruction is introduced in small increments to avoid overwhelming the student, and typically is combined with teaching a replacement skill so that the student is given control to address his or her needs. To illustrate, we provide a detailed example of teaching tolerance when a student seeks to escape an academic task, and then explain how the same steps can be applied to teach students how to wait for preferred items or activities.

Recall Asher, who worked on counting tasks for brief periods of time, but would scream and pinch his teacher after a few practice trials (Halle et al., 1995). He had no words or gestures to communicate that he wanted a break, so we prompted him to touch a "break" symbol when his interest in the counting task began to wane. As soon as he touched the symbol, we immediately removed the counting materials and assisted him to leave the table and move to a play area of the classroom.

With time, Asher touched the symbol independently and no longer screamed and pinched; however, he also was not engaging in many counting trials. Almost as soon as he arrived at his work table after a break, he touched the symbol to request another break. Although Asher learned an important new replacement skill, a new problem was introduced: He engaged in very few counting trials, and his acquisition of arithmetic skills was thus still painfully slow. Because counting was an important skill for Asher to learn, we initiated tolerance training to increase the number of counting trials Asher would "tolerate" before honoring his request for a break.

Asher typically completed two counting trials before he requested a break, so we began by placing two sets of items to be counted on his work table. When he arrived, one of three possible scenarios occurred: (1) He immediately touched the break symbol, to which we delivered a delay signal ("Do these two first [pointing to the sets], and then you can take a break"); (2) he did one trial and touched the symbol, to which we said, "Do just this one, and then you can take a break"; or (3) he did both trials and touched the symbol, to which we said enthusiastically, "Way to go, Asher; you've earned a break!"

As Asher experienced success, we placed additional sets of items to be counted on the work table. Placing sets of items on the table in advance functioned as an antecedent cue for Asher, allowing him to see and anticipate how many trials would be required before he received a break. The number of trials gradually increased by one each day, provided that problem behaviors were absent. Eventually he reached 12, which was the original number planned for the session by his teacher. The procedure was not errorless, in that occasional problem behavior occurred and we needed to strengthen his use of the replacement skill, either by requiring fewer counting trials or by freezing the required number for additional days. Asher's behavior determined the pace at which we could increase the number of trials.

An important feature of this type of intervention that needs to be considered is the relative amount of time in break versus work. During the early phases of instruction, the overall break time may be longer than the work time. As confidence grows in the success of the procedure, the duration of the break may be reduced as the number of counting trials is increased. As each break nears conclusion, it is a good idea to deliver a cue that the break is almost over. We believe that tolerance instruction was successful with Asher because the following components were introduced. First, the number of trials required before providing a break was small (the trials were easily completed) and predictable (the counting tasks to be completed were displayed on the table). Second, over time, the task requirements were increased, but only as Asher demonstrated tolerance for the increased workload. Third, returning to work from a break can be a challenging situation, but this challenge was diminished by providing longer breaks and very few required work trials during the early instruction.

One final observation from our work with Asher warrants attention. After Asher successfully completed up to 12 counting trials with no problem behavior, we began to honor his break requests immediately, without requiring additional work. Of course, this opened up the possibility that

Asher would again touch the symbol immediately upon arrival at the work table—but that did not happen, as is often the case when students learn both tolerance and control. Instead, we found that most of the time, he completed the number of trials that we had set out for him. What was most exciting, however, was that this was not his only strategy. Sometimes he would touch the symbol before completing all of the trials, and sometimes, after completing all of the trials, he opted *not* to touch the symbol at all. So we introduced additional trials one at a time, and he continued to engage in counting, until at some point he touched the symbol and we immediately provided a break. We believe that this was significant, because we literally transferred control for Asher's work requirement to him. He demonstrated that most of the time he would do what we asked (the prepared counting tasks on the table); sometimes he found the tasks more unpleasant and requested an "early" break; and occasionally it seemed as though engaging in the task was OK and he would permit additional trials beyond even the number we had planned. This type of performance is the essence of self-control: Asher regulated the number of trials he could tolerate, and he communicated with his newly acquired replacement skill, not with problem behavior.

The same strategy for teaching tolerance for delays in escaping unpleasant situations can be applied when students' requests for materials, activities, and/or attention from others cannot be honored immediately. For example, if a student wants a teacher's attention and currently asks by screaming, the very same procedures described for Asher can be implemented. First, the student is prompted to use a replacement skill to request teacher attention. Second, once the student makes some independent requests, the teacher or another adult says or signals to wait "just a moment" (the initial wait time is determined by how much time the student has typically waited in the past prior to engaging in problem behavior). Third, after waiting, the teacher immediately approaches the student and provides the attention the student wants. Over time, the prompting of the new replacement is faded, and the amount of time before attention is provided is increased.

Often when a student is being taught to tolerate delays for obtaining attention or materials, some type of interim activity or task is presented to the student, so that he or she can be productively engaged while "waiting" (see Carr et al., 1994). Usually this activity is one that is easy or enjoyable for the student, so that the unpleasant delay is moderated by something fun.

Although tolerance strategies have been repeatedly demonstrated in research and practice (Carr et al., 1994), they are not the only means for teaching students alternative skills when they encounter either difficult or unpleasant situations. There is a rich and diverse literature on teaching children and youth of all ages and disabilities to cope with such situations by employing self-management strategies, described in the next section.

Teaching Coping by Using Self-Management Strategies

Teaching tolerance depends almost entirely on teacher modifications (e.g., rearranging antecedents and consequences, such as was done with Asher), whereas coping strategies depend on teaching students new skills or strategies for controlling or regulating their own behavior during stressful or difficult situations. We generally label these skills *self-management*, because once they have been learned, they no longer require support from the teacher; students implement them independently. In fact, the recognition of a difficult situation by the student is the cue that alternative self-management strategies should be used to cope constructively with problems.

There are various approaches for teaching self-management, many of which can be combined in varying ways. These strategies, described in Table 9.2, include anger control training, relaxation training, and social problem solving. Self-management may also employ goal-setting and self-monitoring techniques, in which the student is taught to set specific behavioral goals for self-improvement and maintain a record of appropriate and problem behaviors to monitor progress.

To illustrate how self-management instruction may be used for coping, let us return to DeShawna, who shouts to obtain assistance during independent math work because she cannot solve two-digit multiplication problems. Let us assume that her teacher, Mr. Sparks, has now taught her to ask for help to directly replace shouting for assistance. However, Mr. Sparks is not available continuously to respond to DeShawna's requests, so some type of coping strategy is needed. Mr. Sparks has noticed that previously, when DeShawna screamed to obtain assistance, and now, when she makes polite requests, she quickly becomes anxious (i.e., she repeats her actions with greater intensity and stands at her seat looking around the room) if Mr. Sparks or someone else does not respond immediately. This frenzied behavior signals that teaching DeShawna to relax in such situations may be an ideal means of coping with having to wait for Mr. Sparks's help.

Many strategies exist for teaching relaxation, but two of the most popular are *diaphragmatic breathing* (Davis, Eshelman, & McKay, 1988) and *progressive muscle relaxation* (PMR; Bernstein & Borkovec, 1973). Like most self-management skills, each of these strategies requires rehearsal and practice outside of the provocative situation (e.g., math time) until the relaxation responses are acquired. Then these new responses are practiced in the actual situations that produce anxiety. Diaphragmatic or deep breathing teaches a student to breathe deeply and rhythmically by using the

TABLE 9.2. Alternative Skill Interventions for Teaching Coping and General Adaptive Skills

Anger control training

Teaches students to control anger during provoking situations. Typically involves teaching students to (1) identify triggers ("John took my favorite computer"); (2) identify physical cues ("My face is feeling hot"); (3) use self-talk reminders ("Stay calm—walk away if you have to"); (4) use anger reducers (walk away, ask for a break, count to 10), and (5) self-evaluate ("I stayed calm, even though I was very upset").

Relaxation training

Teaches students to "de-stress" when agitated or upset through deep breathing and or releasing muscle tension. Students may be taught to respond on cue (e.g., "You are getting upset. Take a few deep breaths to calm down. Ready, breathe as I count, 1 . . . [breathe], 2 . . . . [breathe], 3 . . . ") or may learn to identify the triggers and calm themselves (e.g., "This crowded room is getting me upset. I need to sit in the hall and take a few deep breaths").

Social problem solving

Teaches students to identify problem situations or triggers, generate and evaluate alternative solutions to the problem, and act on a response alternative. Typically involves teaching students to (1) state the problem ("John is teasing me"); (2) list alternatives ("I can walk away. I can report John. I can hit John"); (3) identify consequences (e.g., "If I hit John, I'll be in trouble"); and (4) choose the best alternative ("It's better to report John").

Goal setting, self-monitoring, and self-evaluation training

Teaches students to use specific techniques to set goals, monitor their own behavior, and self-reinforce or self-evaluate. Students may be taught to use these techniques singly or in combination: (1) goal setting ("When I get frustrated with my work, I will raise my hand to ask for help or ask for a break"); (2) self-monitoring (using a checklist, the student records the number of times he or she asked for help or a break); and (3) self-evaluation ("I raised my hand every time without pouting. I am doing well"). The techniques of goal setting, self-monitoring, and self-evaluation may be used to teach the student to self-manage any skill, including problem behaviors, replacement skills, and general adaptive skills.

Self-cueing

Teaches students to use external prompts such as picture checklists, audio cues (e.g., beepers) or self-statements (e.g., "First I should finish my assignment, then I can work on the computer) to prompt desired behavior. These strategies lessen teacher prompts; once learned, students direct themselves. These techniques may be applied to any skill.

diaphragm to pull inhaled air deep into the lungs. Effectiveness depends on use of the diaphragm, because this deeper breathing is incompatible with the rapid and shallow type of breathing that characterizes anxiety. Students are taught specific exercises to ensure that breathing is deep, and then self-statements (e.g., "I'm getting upset; I must breathe") to remind themselves to breathe deeply when they notice themselves getting tense in difficult situations.

PMR requires students to practice tensing and relaxing the major muscle groups of their bodies. The essence of this technique is teaching students to identify what these muscle groups "feel like" when they are tense and when they are relaxed; acquiring this discrimination is fundamental to its successful implementation. When a student is learning to relax with PMR, it is best to find a quiet place with dim light and a comfortable chair (for sitting) or mattress (for lying down). Frequent and consistent practice is necessary to learn how to induce relaxation quickly and readily in real-world situations that are associated with stress and anxiety.

Mr. Sparks may also consider teaching DeShawna to problem-solve alternative solutions for coping with waiting for assistance. If he uses this strategy, he will teach DeShawna first to identify problem situations such as needing help with multiplying two-digit math problems; then, together, they will generate and evaluate alternative solutions to the problem. Finally, they will select the best option. After they practice this sequence together, Mr. Sparks will provide less and less assistance until DeShawna can develop and act on her own problem solutions. Possible options for DeShawna may be (1) to use her newly acquired relaxation response; (2) to ask a peer who does very well in math for help; and (3) to solve the problems on the worksheet that she can do independently and ask for help at the end of the math period.

TEACHING GENERAL ADAPTIVE SKILLS

General adaptive skills constitute a broader, more complex array of skills than the first two types of alternative skills (replacement and coping/tolerance). When teaching general adaptive skills, the goal of instruction is to expand general social, communicative, or academic competence to such an extent that students can (1) prevent problem situations from occurring and (2) pursue preferences or meaningful outcomes for themselves. In other words, when including general adaptive skills in PBS, a support team attempts to shift control over prevention and lifestyle changes from adults to the student. Rather than the adults making antecedent/setting event or broad environmental changes to prevent problem behaviors, the student is taught skills that empowers him or her to circumvent problems. In addition, general competence is enhanced in ways that lead to long-lasting life-style improvements for the student—the ultimate goal of PBS.

When targeting general adaptive skills for instruction, teams should consider two guiding questions. The first is this: "What skills might we teach the student that would prevent the need for problem behavior?" Answering this question requires team members to refer back to their hypothesis to identify specific events associated with the student's problem behavior. In addition, it requires the team to think about how teaching related skills might help the student to change or avoid the instigating condition. For example, recall Juan, who screamed and pounded his desk because letter recognition tasks were too difficult. His team might consider in what ways the tasks were difficult and what skills he might be taught to make the tasks easier. Were letter recognition tasks difficult because the worksheet variations confused him? If so, would it be helpful for Juan to learn how to read directions better or learn how to respond to different types of worksheets? Were letter recognition tasks difficult because he consistently confused certain letters? If so, would it be helpful for Juan to relearn letter names? Or recall André, who spun objects for sensory stimulation when he had nothing to do. His team might consider teaching an array of appropriate leisure skills. For example, could he operate a TV, DVD player, or CD player? Could he initiate a new activity once he was finished with one, or did he wait idly for adults to offer him options? Could he be taught the skills to invite peers to play with him, rather than wait for peer initiations in order to play?

Another guiding question to ask is this: "What general skills can we teach that will lead to meaningful lifestyle improvements for the student?" The goal here is to teach skills needed for the student to pursue preferences and interests. What does the student enjoy doing? What goals are important for the student? What skills are needed to enable the student to engage skillfully in activities that he or she enjoys? When students have the skills to pursue and access activities that are meaningful to them, they are empowered to make lifestyle changes that can improve their overall quality of life. As emphasized throughout this book, goals targeted at lifestyle improvement can prevent problem behaviors by reversing or nullifying the environmental conditions that contribute to problem behaviors.

Asking these two guiding questions can lead to a broad array of possible teaching interventions, as shown in Table 9.2. At first glance, the number of possible alternatives may seem overwhelming, as almost any skill can be targeted for instruction. Teaching skills for communication, social interaction, self-care and daily living, and academics are all examples of skill areas that might be targeted for intervention. But most students will not require instruction on *every* skill. When deciding what to teach, teams will need to balance priorities between what students need to learn to do for themselves, and what antecedent or lifestyle changes are best addressed by team members making changes for students (e.g., see Chapter 11 on long-term supports).

COMBINING ALL THREE TYPES OF ALTERNATIVE SKILLS

In comprehensive support plans, interventions for teaching replacement skills, coping and tolerance skills, and general adaptive skills are often combined into one teaching plan. As shown in Table 9.1, each of the three types of alternative skills serves a different purpose, and when taught together, they can address many of the limitations inherent in focusing on only one type. The best way to explain how the three types of interventions can work together in a support plan is through illustration. Figure 9.3 depicts the instructional program developed for Jamal, which combined all three types of alternative skill interventions as part of his overall behavior support plan. (Figure 9.5, to be presented below, illustrates the combination of interventions developed for another student, Rico).

Jamal, a 7-year-old identified with Down syndrome, was a first grader in an inclusive classroom. Jamal loved interacting with his classmates, but unfortunately his silly faces and noise making—acceptable ways of playing and joking with his siblings at home—were causing disruption in school. When formulating a hypothesis for his behavior, Jamal's team concluded that he had the skills to work independently, but that he preferred clowning around or talking with his peers. Furthermore, despite Jamal's rather social nature, his team surmised that his social interaction skills were quite limited. In fact, Jamal used his silly behavior to initiate almost every interaction with his peers—a behavior that even his classmates were beginning to find annoying at times. Considering both Jamal's preferences for peer interaction and the skills he would need for successful membership in his first-grade classroom, Jamal's support plan emphasized teaching him to work quietly, while at the same time providing him with socially appropriate outlets for interacting with his peers in the classroom and school cafeteria. Jamal's team reasoned that as Jamal's general social skills increased and as he learned alternative ways of acquiring peer interaction and acceptance, his inappropriate attempts to obtain attention during independent work periods would be eliminated.

To replace his silly behaviors as a means of recruiting peer attention during classroom work periods, Jamal was reminded that he could ask permission to work with a peer at the beginning of certain independent work periods (generally, Jamal could complete assignments without acting silly as long as a peer worked alongside of him). Although Jamal's teacher, Mr. Conrad, encouraged opportunities for peer collaboration, Jamal's requests

Teaching Goals and Strategies

Student: Jamal Chamberlin

Hypothesis:

When Jamal works alone or when he is not engaged with peers during recess or lunch, he will act silly (e.g., make silly noises, facial expressions, burp, shake his butt), to gain peer attention or social interaction.

Replacement Skill:

Jamal will ask permission to work with a peer.
- At beginning of an independent work period, remind Jamal of his option to work with a peer.
- Model, if necessary (e.g., say, "Can Tiffany sit next to me?").
- Delay reminders. Praise self-initiated requests.

Jamal will appropriately initiate social conversation or play with peers during lunch and recess.
- At the start of lunch or recess, remind Jamal of his options (e.g., "Remember, you can ask a friend to look at your book [see "General Adaptive Skills," below] or play a game").
- Model, if necessary, during appropriate occasions (e.g., "Jamal, say to Jason, 'Do you want to play cards?'").
- Delay prompts and reminders. Praise self-initiations.

Coping and Tolerance Skills:

Jamal will work quietly and independently for up to 20 minutes.
- Have Jamal self-monitor working quietly.
- Slowly raise criterion for intervals of quiet work.
- Reward working quietly and completing work with praise and special stickers; hang completed worksheet in the "hall of fame" (encourage peer celebration).

General Adaptive Skills:

Jamal will use his brag book to initiate and maintain peer conversation.
- Have Jamal practice initiating, asking questions, and responding to peer questions, using the brag book in the classroom.
- Encourage Jamal to use the brag book during lunch and recess.

Jamal will learn to play a variety of age-appropriate games interesting to peers.
- Have peers teach Jamal how to play tabletop and recess games (e.g., Uno, I Spy, Trouble, tag, kickball).

FIGURE 9.3. Alternative skills teaching plan for Jamal.

to work with a peer could not always be honored. He needed to learn how to work quietly alone as well. To address this issue, Mr. Conrad taught Jamal to self-monitor "working quietly" during the classroom periods when he must work alone. Each time his wristwatch beeped, Jamal determined whether he had worked quietly. If he had, he circled a happy face on an index card to indicate an interval of quiet work (see Figure 9.4). Each week Mr. Conrad set a slightly increasing criterion for quiet intervals. When Jamal met the criterion for working quietly, Mr. Conrad placed a special sticker on his work assignment, which was then posted in the classroom "hall of fame" for a round of peer celebration and applause.

In the cafeteria, Jamal's support plan focused on teaching alternative ways of inviting peers to interact, as well as teaching him how to maintain play or social conversation once he initiated it. Jamal's team reasoned that social initiations alone would not replace silly behaviors in the long run if he had no other way of keeping his peers engaged and interested once he invited them to play. To expand his play skills, Mr. Conrad arranged for Jamal's classmates to teach him a variety of games appropriate for the cafeteria, recess, or free time in the classroom. This way, when Jamal initiated, he could invite his classmates to play games (e.g., "Do you want to play Uno?") that he knew how to play and that his peers enjoyed. With the cooperation of his mother, Jamal also was taught how to use a "brag book" to initiate and maintain conversations with peers. The brag book contained pictures or mementos (e.g., a movie ticket stub, an amusement park bracelet, a picture made in Sunday school) of some of Jamal's favorite

I am working quietly		
1	☺ Yes	☹ No
2	☺ Yes	☹ No
3	☺ Yes	☹ No
4	☺ Yes	☹ No
5	☺ Yes	☹ No

FIGURE 9.4. Jamal's self-monitoring sheet for working quietly. Numbers 1–5 represent 1-minute intervals. At the sound of each beep, Jamal recorded "yes" or "no" for working quietly.

after-school or weekend activities; his mom updated these weekly. Although Jamal's verbal language skills were limited to simple sentences, the brag book provided him with fresh topics for conversation (e.g., "I saw *Spiderman*") and a format for stimulating peer conversation (e.g., "Cool, so did I, " said Aaron, as both boys proceeded to squirt spider webs from their wrists). The brag book also aided Jamal's classmates by providing them with easily recognized symbols for comprehending the content of Jamal's initiations.

In another example, Rico, a seventh grader, had just entered an inclusive middle school classroom after spending 3 years in a self-contained class for students with emotional and behavioral disorders. Despite his sincere desire to succeed in his new school, his angry outbursts caused severe disruption and raised concern by some teachers that he would be better off back in the self-contained classroom. His angry outbursts appeared to be triggered when he was corrected or given feedback about his in-class performance in the presence of his peers. His seventh-grade team, consisting of his subject area general education teachers and a special education teacher, speculated that his angry outbursts served the dual purposes of avoiding further corrections and "saving face" (avoiding embarrassment by appearing tough).

Rico's support plan focused on teaching three types of alternative skills (see Figure 9.5). First, he was taught to request "taking time" (i.e., taking a break in the back of the classroom), which provided an immediate, more socially acceptable replacement to shouting; however, this offered only a temporary solution. Being corrected is an inescapable reality of school life. When faced with feedback, Rico needed to learn how to stay calm while continuing his work. Thus a second type of alternative skill instruction was provided: teaching Rico to control his anger. His special education teacher met with him daily during seventh period. Together, they role-played how to count silently to 10 and relax when Rico was faced with teacher corrections, and they practiced self-monitoring to help Rico transfer his anger control techniques to his general education classrooms. During each academic period, Rico recorded the number of times he felt angry, as well as the number of times he controlled his anger and remained in the classroom. His special education teacher reviewed and praised his progress during the seventh-period discussions. As an added incentive, his teacher sent weekly progress reports to his home, where he was rewarded with extra spending money for good reports.

Although teaching Rico to control his outbursts was helpful, neither of the two types of alternative skills described above addressed the underlying problem that led to teacher corrections in the first place. Rico was frequently corrected because he often was late for class, forgot things (e.g., his books, assignments, pens), and failed to complete his homework assign-

Teaching Goals and Strategies

Student: Rico Cruz

Hypothesis:

When Rico is corrected or given feedback about his social behavior in the presence of his peers, he explodes by screaming that he hates the teacher or school, in order to avoid further corrections and peer embarrassment.

Replacement Skills:

Rico will ask for time in the back of the classroom when he feels himself about to shout or scream.

- At the start of each class period or at the first sign of anger, remind Rico that he can "take time" to go to the back of the classroom and cool down if necessary.
- Rico will self-monitor, taking time without shouting or screaming.
- Praise Rico for making good choices (i.e., taking time rather than shouting). Send progress reports home.

Coping and Tolerance Skills:

Rico will control his anger and remain in his usual seat in the classroom.

- Use role play during private lessons to teach Rico to identify anger triggers and relax by counting to 10. Remind Rico that if he cannot remain calm in his usual place in the classroom, he always has the option of taking time.
- Rico will self-monitor, staying in his seat and staying calm.
- Review self-monitoring with Rico at the end of each day. Send progress reports home.

General Adaptive Skills:

Rico will use organizational and time management skills in order to come to class prepared and on time.

Rico will learn how to set goals, self-monitor, and evaluate his performance.

- During private lessons, encourage problem-solving solutions to events that lead to being corrected (e.g., coming to class late, not completing his homework, forgetting his assignments, forgetting his books and pen).
- Next, encourage Rico to set specific goals and monitor his performance in the classroom, using a self-monitoring checklist (e.g., "I arrived in class on time," "I brought in required materials"). Build upon self-monitoring for taking time and staying calm.
- Review goals and goal achievement at the end of each day. Help Rico come up with solutions to new problems.
- Reward classroom preparation and being on time with class preparation points and bonus points to exchange for homework passes.

FIGURE 9.5. Alternative skills teaching plan for Rico.

ments on time. Thus the third type of alternative skill instruction focused on teaching Rico a broader set of self-management behaviors aimed at improving his overall classroom preparation and organizational skills. The seventh-period discussions were expanded to encourage Rico (1) to identify reasons for teacher feedback or corrections (e.g., "I came to class late") and (2) to set learning goals to address the problem situation (e.g., "I'll clean out my locker, so I don't have to spend time searching for my books through the tons of paper"). Once goals were set, Rico was shown how to monitor and evaluate his progress (e.g., "I made it to every class on time; I'm doing well"). By coming to class prepared and on time, Rico earned extra class points (which were averaged into his grades) and bonus points (which, when saved, could be exchanged for an occasional homework pass).

SUMMARY

Teaching alternative skills is a vital component of a PBS plan. Alternative skills replace and thereby reduce challenging behaviors by giving students socially acceptable alternatives for addressing their wants and needs. Furthermore, alternative skills can greatly enhance students' general competence to cope constructively with difficult situations, pursue meaningful activities and social interactions, and prevent problem situations from occurring. In delineating intervention strategies, we have focused on three primary skill types: (1) replacement skills, (2) coping and tolerance skills, and (3) general adaptive skills.

Admittedly, the combination of strategies described in this chapter is not necessarily easy to implement. Teaching alternative skills requires careful planning and execution, as well as a support team who knows the student well and who is committed to teaching as its first priority. Despite the effort, the rewards are substantial. Students learn a broad array of social, communicative, self-regulatory, and general adaptive skills that will carry them through life.

COMMONLY ASKED QUESTIONS

Is there any advantage to teaching one type of alternative skill over the other? As stressed, each type of alternative skills (i.e., replacement, coping/tolerance, and general adaptive skills) addresses a specific purpose; therefore, deciding which is best will depend on what is important for the student to learn. We generally recommend that team members consider all three types of alternative skills when developing the teaching component of a behavior support plan, even though it may not be necessary to teach all three types of alternative skills.

Should we teach alternative skills in any particular order? Alternative skills are often taught in combination with one another, so skills are not taught in any particular sequence. Having said this, we do recommend that teaching a replacement skill should be a team's first priority when a student has no socially acceptable way of achieving an intended outcome (function) except through problem behavior. The student must be able to communicate, or meet his or her immediate needs, before being expected to tolerate delays or learning more complex general skills that will prevent problem situations. If teaching a replacement skill is a priority for the student, team members may choose to teach it first either alone or in combination with other alternative skills (as in Jamal's and Rico's teaching plans).

What if we are not exactly certain about the function of a student's problem behavior? Can we still teach a replacement skill? Technically speaking, the answer to this question is no. By definition, teaching a replacement skill requires the precise identification of a behavior function. However, we recognize that function is sometimes difficult to pinpoint; in such situations, it may be possible to teach a "generic" replacement skill that fits the situation and accommodates several functions. For example, in Eleni's case, it was unclear why she sometimes crumpled her assignments. Did she do it for attention or escape? Regardless, the teacher taught Eleni to raise her hand whenever she felt the urge to crumple her paper in a ball. Based on the particular circumstances, when Eleni raised her hand, the teacher responded by figuring out what Eleni needed at the time—encouragement or praise (attention) or help (escape).

It seems that coping and tolerance skills will be difficult for students to learn. Do you have any advice in this regard? Coping and tolerance skills *are* difficult for students to learn, because they are expected to deal with unpleasant or undesirable situations. Because students are not likely to be motivated and may resist learning these skills, we suggest that team members carefully reflect on the following questions: (1) Does a student really need to learn how to cope with or tolerate this particular situation, or can the situation be avoided in some way? (2) If the situation is necessary (such as learning to work independently), then how can it be made more pleasant for the student? Consider using some of the antecedent modifications described in this book, and/or using additional incentives, rewards, or strong student encouragement (e.g., "I know how hard this is for you, but you are doing great!"). (3) Does the student have the skills for making the situation less demanding or difficult? If not, consider teaching some of the general adaptive skills described in this chapter.

CASE EXAMPLES

Alternative Skill Interventions for Malik

Malik's team considered all three types of alternative skills when developing his support plan (see Figure 9.6). Although the antecedent interventions would remove many of the difficult tasks from Malik's curriculum, his teacher argued that he was bound to encounter other difficult tasks in school (including meaningful ones), and should be taught an appropriate way of leaving or terminating an activity without pushing, hitting, or throwing materials. All team members agreed. Teaching the replacement skill of saying "break" or pointing to a break card was added to Malik's support plan. To teach asking for a break, his teacher, Mrs. Nelson, planned to present Malik with some difficult tasks for a few days so that he could quickly make the association between asking for a break and getting one. At the first sign of agitation, Mrs. Nelson planned to prompt Malik by saying, "Ask for a break," while pointing to the break card. As soon as Malik said "break" or pointed to the card, the materials would be removed, and then reintroduced in a few minutes. Mrs. Nelson would introduce a few practice opportunities each day as Malik learned this new skill.

Malik's team figured that after a few days, Mrs. Nelson would no longer need to present difficult tasks to teach Malik how to ask for a break. Once he knew how to request a break, teaching could occur naturally during regularly scheduled activities if and when Malik encountered a difficult task. Mrs. Nelson and the teaching assistant would ensure that Malik's break card was available in all activities, and at the first sign of agitation, they would remind him that he could ask for one.

Of course, asking for a break would not always be appropriate. The team knew there would be times when Malik should work through difficult tasks for his own educational benefit. A second alternative skill, increasing tolerance for task difficulty, was therefore added to Malik's support plan. To teach this skill, Mrs. Nelson and the teaching assistant would incrementally ask Malik to work a little longer or complete a few more items before honoring his request for a break. Before teaching tolerance, however, the team wanted to be sure that two things were in place. First, Malik needed to ask for a break reliably during typical classroom situations. Second, Malik's curriculum was to be functional and meaningful. Teaching tolerance would work only if the curriculum was motivating enough for Malik to persist. If requests for breaks became excessive, the team members agreed to reevaluate whether they had indeed created a meaningful curriculum.

When the team members were considering general adaptive skills, communication immediately surfaced as a target. Competent communication skills are essential not only for expressing basic needs, but also for establishing friendships and meaningful relationships with others. Because a significant proportion of Malik's problem behaviors occurred when he was prompted to communicate verbally, the team rea-

Malik's Behavior Support Plan

Hypotheses:

1. When prompted through difficult work, Malik is likely to refuse/aggress, to escape the activity.
2. When asked to complete nonfunctional activities, Malik is likely to refuse/aggress, to escape the activity.
3. When required to make a transition from a highly preferred activity to a nonpreferred activity, Malik refuses/aggresses, to maintain the preferred activity and avoid the nonpreferred one.

Antecedent/setting event interventions	Alternative skills	Responses to problem behavior	Long-term supports
Eliminate letter- and number-naming activities from curriculum; avoid recall in academic activities.	***Replacement:*** Teach requests for break. Make sure Malik's break cards are available; prompt him to use cards throughout the day.		
Embed academics in functional activities; ensure meaningful outcomes.	***Tolerance skills:*** Teach working through difficult tasks; incrementally ask Malik to work a bit longer or do a few more before taking a break.		
Prompt Malik to use alternative forms of communication (pictures, gestures) when he has difficulty with verbal expression.	***General adaptive skills:*** Expand gesture and picture vocabulary. Teach incidentally through the school day. Prompt Malik to use gestures and/or pictures to expand expressions.		
Use a daily picture schedule to mark classroom activities.			
Provide a transitional warning prior to ending a preferred activity.			
When it is necessary to make a transition from a preferred to a nonpreferred activity, begin activity with a brief preferred activity (e.g., math game).			

FIGURE 9.6. Malik's alternative skills.

271

soned that he would need an augmentative system, not to replace but to supplement spoken language. The third alternative skill goal was thus to expand Malik's communication vocabulary through the use of pictures and gestures. Teaching would occur incidentally throughout the school day. Each week, the teacher would introduce new picture vocabulary cards or natural gestures that Malik could use to request materials and activities, comment about daily activities, or socialize with his peers. This way, when Malik initiated a request or an interaction (e.g., by saying "play"), his teacher could prompt him by saying, "Tell me more. What do you want to play with? Show me or point to your pictures." Words, pictures, and gestures would provide Malik with several options to become a competent communicator.

Alternative Skill Interventions for Bethany

When considering alternative skills for Bethany (see Figure 9.7), the team members agreed that they would like to see her more *engaged in academics*, which they defined as working on assigned activities, following teacher directions, and completing all assignments. The antecedent interventions (e.g., reduced written assignments, shorter tasks) were expected to make this goal more attainable; however, Bethany also needed a replacement skill during situations in which work became overwhelming for her. The team agreed that if Bethany needed something during work time, they would like to see her request assistance by raising her hand and asking for it. This was a skill that was already a part of her repertoire, but one she did not often use. Bethany suggested that reminders would help her. The team members decided that they would provide a reminder at the beginning of each academic period, and another whenever she began to disengage from an activity. Using a simple frequency count, Bethany's teacher could also monitor Bethany's requests for assistance.

With regard to general adaptive skills, the team members agreed that they would like Bethany to *interact appropriately* with her peers, which they together defined as engaging in conversation with peers that contained only kind, considerate, and appropriate topics. To address Bethany's problems with social interactions, a social skills instruction program was initiated. Bethany's teacher had noticed that several students in her class would benefit from social skills instruction. Therefore, she decided to begin social skills instruction with her entire class by holding group discussions about peer social concerns relevant for sixth graders. In addition, a cafeteria volunteer was planted close to Bethany's table and provided reminders to all of the students to be courteous to others. The volunteer also periodically provided praise when a student engaged in appropriate interactions. In helping Brittany to interact more appropriately with and tolerate unfamiliar students, the volunteer was sure to be near when new students were intentionally seated next to Bethany, so that she could monitor the situation and provide prompts and praise. In addition, to measure Bethany's appropriate interactions, the lunchtime cafeteria volunteer who had collected data during the functional assessment suggested that she use

Bethany's Behavior Support Plan

Hypotheses:
1. When Bethany is given written assignments, she engages in off-task behavior, to escape.
2. When Bethany is given lengthy assignments, she engages in off-task behavior, to escape.
3. When Bethany has visited her father over the weekend, she engages in off-task behavior, to escape work (because of fatigue).
4. When Bethany is in unstructured situations with unfamiliar peers, she engages in inappropriate interactions, to obtain their attention.

Antecedent/setting event interventions	Alternative skills	Responses to problem behavior	Long-term supports
Minimize amount of written work; provide alternative strategy for work completion (e.g., tape recorder).	*Replacement:* **When independent assignments are given, remind Bethany to request assistance when she feels overwhelmed with assignments or does not understand what she is supposed to do.**		
Break work into small increments.			
Make sure instructions are clear and explicit.	*General adaptive skills:* **Provide social skills instruction and prompt Bethany to engage in appropriate interactions.**		
Seat Bethany near classmates in cafeteria; gradually introduce new people while prompting appropriate interactions.	*Tolerance skills:* **Gradually introduce Bethany to new people.**		
Have Bethany return home earlier on Sundays after visiting her father.			

FIGURE 9.7. Bethany's alternative skills.

273

two golf counters, one in her right pocket and one in her left. That way, she could count appropriate interactions on one of the golf counters and inappropriate interactions on the other.

REFERENCES

Alberto, P. A., & Troutman, A. C. (2003). *Applied behavior analysis for teachers* (6th ed.). Upper Saddle River, NJ: Merrill/Prentice Hall.

Bambara, L. M., & Knoster, T. (1998). *Designing positive behavior support plans* (Innovations, No. 13). Washington, DC: American Association on Mental Retardation.

Bernstein, D. A., & Borkovec, T. D. (1973). *Progressive relaxation training: A manual for helping professionals.* Champaign, IL: Research Press.

Carr, E. G., & Durand, V. M. (1985). Reducing behavior problems through functional communication training. *Journal of Applied Behavior Analysis, 18,* 111–126.

Carr, E. G., Levin, L., McConnachie, G., Carlson, J. I., Kemp, D. C., & Smith, C. E. (1994). *Communication-based intervention for problem behavior: A user's guide for producing positive change.* Baltimore: Paul H. Brookes.

Davis, M., Eshelman, E. R., & McKay, M. (1988). *The relaxation and stress reduction workbook.* Oakland, CA: New Harbinger.

Durand, V. M. (1990). *Severe behavior problems: A functional communication training approach.* New York: Guilford Press.

Halle, J. W., Ostrosky, M. M., & Silliman, A. (1995). *Functional communication training: Transferring control from the teacher to the student.* Unpublished manuscript, Department of Special Education, University of Illinois.

Horner, R. H., & Day, H. M. (1991). The effects of response efficiency on functionally equivalent competing behaviors. *Journal of Applied Behavior Analysis, 24,* 719–732.

Neef, N. A., Mace, F. C., & Shade, D. (1993). Impulsivity in students with severe emotional disturbance: The interactive effects of reinforcer rate, delay, and quality. *Journal of Applied Behavior Analysis, 26,* 37–52.

Reichle, J., Drager, K., & Davis, C. (2002). Using request for assistance to obtain desired items and to gain release from nonpreferred activities: Implications for assessment and intervention. *Education and Treatment of Children, 25,* 47–66.

Rincover, A. (1978). Sensory extinction: A procedure for eliminating self-stimulatory behavior in psychotic children. *Journal of Abnormal Child Psychology, 6,* 299–310.

Rincover, A., Cook, R., Peoples, A., & Packard, D. (1979). Sensory extinction and sensory reinforcement principles for programming multiple adaptive behavior change. *Journal of Applied Behavior Analysis, 12,* 221–233.

Wacker, D. P., Steege, M. W., Northup, J., Sasso, G., Berg, W., Reimers, T., Cooper, L., Cigrand, K., & Donn, L. (1990). A component analysis of functional communication training across three topographies of severe behavior problems. *Journal of Applied Behavior Analysis, 23,* 417–429.

CHAPTER 10

◆ ◆ ◆

Responding to Problem Behavior

◆

LEE KERN

Chapters 8 and 9 have described antecedent/setting event interventions and alternative skill instruction. As we have discussed, these components are critical to a comprehensive positive behavior support (PBS) plan because they can prevent problem behavior from occurring and teach alternative and more appropriate behaviors. Well-designed antecedent/setting event and alternative skill interventions can dramatically reduce problem behavior. However, in spite of the hope of every support team, unfortunately even the most carefully designed PBS plan does not always eliminate problem behaviors completely. This is not good news. It is very discouraging to spend days, weeks, or even months developing a plan, only to find that problem behaviors still occur. However, when problem behaviors come to the attention of support teams and are serious enough to warrant a comprehensive behavior support plan, they have usually been practiced over an extended period of time and have, in some way, met the needs of the individual. Given this history, it is unreasonable to anticipate that problem behaviors will readily vanish. As such, comprehensive support plans are remiss if they do not include carefully considered strategies for responding to problem behaviors.

This chapter addresses the third component of a PBS plan: *responses to problem behavior*, also called *response interventions*. Various response approaches are described, along with considerations for selecting a specific intervention approach. In addition, background information is provided that may be important to take into account when team members are contemplating the most fitting approach that is effective, yet consistent with the values of PBS. It should be noted that this chapter focuses exclusively on responses or consequences for *problem* behavior. It is just as important to assure that responses for alternative behaviors are equally well planned and implemented, so that those behaviors will be strengthened and increased. For a review of strategies for doing so, see Chapter 9. In the current chapter, we focus only on reductive approaches for unwanted behavior.

HOW RESPONSES INFLUENCE PROBLEM BEHAVIOR

As we have discussed throughout this book, environmental events have a great deal of influence on behavior. Chapter 9 has illustrated the ways that responses to alternative appropriate behaviors can be designed to teach or strengthen those behaviors. Specifically, when something desirable follows a behavior, this behavior is likely to occur again in the future. In just the same way, events can be planned so that unwanted behaviors are *less* likely to occur in the future. That is, in order to reduce an unwanted behavior, it is critical that pleasurable or desirable events *do not* follow that behavior. As discussed in Chapter 9, alternative skills must become more effective or efficient in producing desired outcomes. Likewise, problem behaviors must become *ineffective or inefficient* at producing the desired outcome.

School staff members frequently spend a great deal of time and effort planning the way their systems will respond to problem behavior; they assume that there are common events that all students will find unpleasant, and that these events will stop the problem behavior. For example, schoolwide or classwide systems of behavior support generally respond to problem behavior in a uniform way. Chapter 13 describes the manner in which schoolwide systems establish a set of rules for which infractions are met with predetermined responses applied across the entire student body. Similarly, classroom teachers often develop rules for expected conduct within their own classrooms, along with consequences for rule breaches. This is an effective approach for most of the students within a given school. However, for various reasons, some students will be unresponsive to this universally applied approach. In cases where problem behaviors continue to occur in spite of universal interventions, strategies for responding to problem behavior must be crafted with a great deal of care.

Responding effectively to problem behavior is critically important because it often happens that school staff members respond to a student's problem behavior in ways that have the inadvertent outcome of actually increasing that behavior. For example, consider Rich, a seventh-grade student with a history of academic difficulty. Rich's disruptive classroom behavior has accelerated rapidly during his current school year. In order to maintain an environment where *all* students can learn, the schoolwide system states that disruptive classroom behavior results in an immediate office referral, accompanied by after-school detention to make up missed work. On the face of it, this appears to be a reasonable approach. However, in Rich's case, his disruptive behavior is a result of being embarrassed with his own inability to complete the assigned work. He is perfectly happy to be sent to the office, where he can escape the embarrassment of his peers' seeing him as "stupid," as he perceives himself in these situations. Furthermore, during after-school detention he is generally given individual assistance, which he desperately needs to be able to complete his work. In Rich's case, continued application of this standard consequence is likely to strengthen his disruptive classroom behavior, as long as it enables him to avoid embarrassment and to access assistance with his difficult work.

The example of Rich underscores the importance of carefully crafting responses to problem behavior within the context of a behavior support plan. The fact that a particular response is effective for most students in a school does not mean that it will necessarily be effective for the small group of students with the most intransigent behavior problems. The usual responses to problem behavior may have an unintended effect. For example, a student who has a history of difficulty with academic assignments may find suspension rewarding. Suspension allows the student to escape the many difficult academic expectations placed on him or her throughout the day. Thus it is critical to select responses carefully, so that they actually weaken the behavior. That is, the response that follows the problem behavior must not be one that enables the student to gain the intended outcome. Fortunately, there are many, many different ways of responding to problem behavior. Considerations for assuring that responses are effective are discussed later in this chapter.

In addition to selecting a response that will be effective, it is important to bear in mind an array of other issues, such as compatibility of the response with the values of key support team members, the long-term impact of the response, and the potential for undesirable side effects that may be caused by the response. These issues are also discussed in subsequent sections of the current chapter.

At this point, it is important to underscore that interventions relying exclusively on response strategies will not be effective over the long term for students with ongoing behavior problems. We have learned the shortcomings of consequences alone from many, many years of experience. Depending only on response strategies for behavior change neglects the long-term and more general needs of these students, and thus has only a temporary effect. It is critical for responses to problem behavior to be judiciously selected and applied, so that they complement the overall efforts of a support plan.

ETHICAL ISSUES

A great deal of debate has surrounded the issue of appropriate and ethical, yet effective, responses to problem behavior. Concern emerged as early as 1970 about a number of issues related to what many viewed as extremely punitive responses to the problem behaviors of people with disabilities. Among the many issues raised were the extreme types of procedures used (and, in some cases, the high frequency of their use), the inconsequential behaviors that were subject to very punitive procedures, and the limited training of many care providers who were implementing the procedures. Coupled with these concerns was the more fundamental question of whether there are ethical grounds for regularly applying procedures that result in pain, humiliation, and stigmatization. In fact, many of the procedures that were seemingly acceptable for individuals with disabilities had been long before outlawed for other groups within established social institutions, including students in public schools and inmates within the penal system.

The heightened concern coincided with the premise (which had growing scientific support in the research literature) that many, if not most, extreme forms of problem behavior have the specific purpose of attempting to communicate a need, in the absence of other conventional forms of communication (e.g., language). Thus, in addition to moral concerns, ethical violations occur when punitive interventions fail to appreciate the function of problem behavior, particularly when a student has no alternative means for meeting his or her needs. These matters converged to launch a movement expressly determined to eliminate the use of aversive procedures for individuals with disabilities. Groups supporting the *nonaversive movement* (as it came to be known) not only argued against the use of aversive procedures, on ethical grounds; they also determined that the evidence for its effectiveness was tenuous, and that the circumstances of its use were questionable.

The nonaversive movement was in stark contrast to conventional thought, which held that an intervention should be judged effective if it results in a decrease in a particular problem behavior. Many supporters of the new movement, however, argued that various dimensions of evaluating intervention effectiveness have been neglected when it comes to punitive responses to problem behavior (Guess, Helmstetter, Turnbull, & Knowlton, 1987). More specifically, they have rightfully argued that much of the evidence that punitive approaches are successful is based on measurement of their effectiveness over only very short periods of time. A quick fix is not analogous to a long-term solution.

Opponents of punitive approaches also point out the many unwanted side effects of extreme procedures. These generally come in the form of counteraggression, or acts that seek revenge on the perpetrator. In fact, it has been shown that schools that are highly punitive actually have higher rates of vandalism and other destructive acts, compared with schools that are positive and supportive (Mayer & Butterworth, 1979; Mayer, Butterworth, Nafpaktitis, & Sulzer-Azaroff, 1983).

Finally, concern has been raised about the individuals who are frequently positioned to implement punitive procedures. Often individuals with severe problem behaviors are assigned one-to-one teaching assistants or other care providers who may not have training or knowledge of effective ways to teach skills and build repertoires of appropriate and functional behavior. Furthermore, it is well documented that the potential for abuse or overapplication of such procedures is very real, regardless of staff members' training or experience (Guess et al., 1987).

Beyond these specific concerns about the use of aversive procedures, it is equally important to keep in mind the values of PBS, which have been expressed throughout this book. To recap, PBS should be based on an understanding of the individuals and his or her problem behaviors (including what those problem behaviors are meant to communicate), and must involve approaches that teach new behavior, are effective over the long term, and respect an individual's rights. These values are inconsistent with the application of highly punitive procedures. As we will describe in this chapter, there are many ways to respond to problem behavior that need not be hurtful, humiliating, or stigmatizing.

THE GOALS OF RESPONSE INTERVENTIONS

When team members convene to determine how to respond to a student's problem behavior, four goals should be considered (see Table 10.1). It may not always be possible to accomplish all four goals with equal consistency in a student's support plan. Likewise, the urgency or relevance of each may not be parallel for a given student. Nonetheless, each may have a bearing on the type of intervention selected.

The first and foremost goal is to reduce positive or desirable outcomes for problem behavior. As long as problem behavior is reinforced in some way, it will continue to occur. Determining how to avoid reinforcing problem behavior requires an understanding of why problem behavior occurs, or exactly what its purpose, outcome, or function is for the individual. Although it is important for students to learn that problem behavior will

TABLE 10.1. Major Goals of Response Interventions

1. Reduce desirable outcomes for problem behavior.
2. Prevent escalation of problem behavior.
3. Provide natural or logical consequences.
4. Teach alternative appropriate behavior.

not produce a desirable result, it is equally important to simultaneously teach alternative skills so that desirable results can be obtained in appropriate and acceptable ways, as discussed in Chapter 9. Ultimately, the message should be that problem behavior is no longer an effective and efficient way to achieve the desired outcomes; rather, an alternative behavior is needed.

The second important goal of response interventions is to prevent escalation of the problem behavior so that harm to the student and others is avoided. Many responses or consequences do just the opposite: They actually cause behavior to accelerate or provoke more severe problem behaviors. Physical intervention is one such example. Frequently, physically restraining a student (e.g., physically escorting him or her out of the classroom) can result in avoidant, protective, or combative behaviors (such as hitting, kicking, or biting). Consequently, staff or student injury may result—not from the initial problem, but rather from the imposed consequence. Similarly, yelling or severely reprimanding a student for a behavior can lead to escalation of behavior to avoid embarrassment or perceived loss of control. Usually a calm, quiet, yet persistent response will deescalate a volatile situation. Responding in ways that will prevent continued problems requires an individualized approach, based on an understanding of what escalates and what deescalates each student's behavior.

A third goal of response interventions is to introduce the student to natural or logical consequences. Consequences that bear a close relationship to problem behavior and are likely to naturally occur help students to understand rules both in and outside of school, as well as to make the connection between the violations of rules or expectations and forthcoming results. For example, rather than imposing an arbitrary consequence for destroying a piece of school equipment, such as suspension, a natural and logical consequence would be to have the student work after school or on weekends to earn money to replace the item. This response teaches not only rules, but also the value of property—an important lesson for life outside of school.

A final goal of response interventions, whenever possible, is to encourage alternative and more appropriate ways to behave. Often simply redirecting a student to engage in desired behavior is sufficient to stop a problem and provides the opportunity to teach the student the expected behavior, which (ideally) will be remembered. At other times, requesting the student to engage in a problem-solving sequence or activity may be used to generate alternative behaviors or provide opportunities for practicing (e.g., through role play) more appropriate behaviors.

CONSIDERATIONS FOR RESPONDING TO PROBLEM BEHAVIOR

When team members are selecting responses to problem behavior, a number of considerations that will help them accomplish the goals described above, while also assuring that the response is compatible with both their own values and the ongoing demands of the environment. The first consideration is whether the response will decrease the problem behavior. This requires that the response is linked to the function the behavior serves. As stated earlier, if others respond to problem behavior in ways that meet the needs the individual is seeking to meet, the problem behavior will most certainly continue. Instead, it is important to find a way to respond to problem behavior that will make the problem behavior ineffective for obtaining the desired outcome. Doing so requires understanding the function of the behavior and assuring that the function is not met. To illustrate, in Ricardo's classroom, students who were disruptive had to "take time" in a chair in the corner of the room. Ricardo, however, would not take time as required. Instead, he would make loud noises and stand or jump on the chair, requiring the teaching staff to intervene. To avoid this escalation, Ricardo's teacher modified the response so that he was taken outside of the classroom with a classroom aide to complete his time. After several weeks, the classroom staff noted that Ricardo's disruptive behavior had actually increased. The classroom staff found that Ricardo's disruption was a way for him to get the attention of his teaching staff. The consequence habitually provided him with one-to-one adult attention. Modifying the response so that it was linked to the function of attention—that is, completely ignoring the disruption, as well as providing lavish attention for appropriate behavior—resulted in its rapid decrease.

Certain types of responses can also increase appropriate behavior. For example, appropriate alternative responses can be prompted following problem behavior. An advantage of responses that teach is that they are used during naturally occurring situations; therefore, they increase the likelihood of generalization by instructing the student exactly when the alternative behavior should occur.

Another consideration is possible side effects the response might have. Embarrassment and humiliation are among the more evident side effects of aversive approaches, and can diminish feelings of self-worth. Yet there are many equally concerning but less apparent side effects. Harsh punishment can cause students to fear or avoid those who deliver it or situations where it might occur. This outcome becomes serious when it infringes on the desire to attend and participate in school activities. Also concerning is that students often respond to an overly punitive school system by increasing aggressive, destructive, and nonproductive behaviors aimed at the school and its members. This does not bode well for systems already plagued with high rates of violence. Finally, responses such as removal from class or suspension from school may interfere with students' academic progress. In the long run, this type of response may actually contribute to problem behavior, as there is a well-established relationship between academic difficulty and problem behavior.

Applicability and acceptability of the response across settings should be considered as well. Applying some responses, such as time out, may be difficult across settings, such as a grocery store full of interesting stimuli. Furthermore, certain responses may not be acceptable to team members or others. Acceptability is characterized by how the response may be viewed by others, such as parents, teachers, peers, and the student him- or herself. Responses that cause stigma are unacceptable. Stigma may result when a response would not be considered appropriate if used with nondisabled peers. The response should also respect the age of the target person. Sending a 13-year-old student to stand in the corner would not be considered age-appropriate.

Another consideration is the *contextual fit* of the response. This means that a given response must be sensitive to the values of support team members. If a response is one that a teacher is uncomfortable administering, or a parent is opposed to, then it does not offer a good contextual fit. Also, the response must be easy to administer within ongoing routines. Removal from the classroom would not be a good response in situations where staffing is limited. Existing resources, including personnel, effort, and time, must be considered.

Finally, what a student can draw from the response or comprehend as a result of it should be considered. Restitution, in the form of asking an individual to pay for a window he or she broke, will be meaningful only if the student understands the value of money. Knowledge of an individual's history, learning experiences, and cognitive understanding will help guide a decision about whether the individual can take away meaning from the response.

Table 10.2 proposes key questions and related considerations for selecting responses to problem behavior.

TABLE 10.2. Key Questions and Considerations for Selecting Responses to Problem Behavior

Questions	Considerations
• Will the response decrease the problem behavior?	• Is the response linked to behavioral function? • Are reinforcing outcomes for problem behavior reduced?
• Will the response teach appropriate behavior?	• Is there a way to prompt alternative or replacement behavior? • Does the response allow modeling of appropriate behavior? • Does the response teach general societal rules and expectations?
• Will the response have any unwanted side effects?	• Could the response escalate the behavior? • Could the response result in unwanted long-term problems? • Will the response cause negative reactions by peers?
• Can the response be applied across settings?	• Can the response be easily implemented across environments? • Will the response cause any stigmatization in natural settings?
• Is the response age-appropriate and respectful?	• Would the response be appropriate for a nondisabled same-age peer? • Is the response free from stigmatization and humiliation?
• Does the response offer a good contextual fit?	• Does the response reflect the values of support team members? • Is the response feasible to implement within the ongoing routine?
• Is the response matched to the cognitive understanding of the student?	• Does the response result in an outcome that is meaningful for the focus individual?

TYPES OF RESPONSES TO PROBLEM BEHAVIOR

Overview

Responses to problem behavior fall along a continuum with respect to acceptability and degree of intrusiveness. Many responses are considered so intrusive and socially unacceptable that they have been outlawed by various states, institutions (e.g., schools), and/or other service-providing agencies. For example, many states prohibit the use of electric shock for behavior problems. Physical or corporal punishment is currently outlawed in schools in about half of the states within the United States. It is also not permissible to withhold basic human rights, such as food, water, or sleep.

Many other procedures, such as exposure to noxious substances (e.g., ammonia), water mist to the face, and the presentation of unpleasant noise (e.g., white noise), although not banned, are widely viewed as painful, humiliating, or stigmatizing. These types of highly punitive procedures are not acceptable; nor are they necessary when responses to problem behavior are well planned and used in conjunction with other support plan components (i.e., antecedent/setting event interventions, alternative skill instruction, and long-term supports). The following sections describe procedures that can contribute to the overall effectiveness of a comprehensive behavior support plan, but fall at the less aversive end of the continuum of acceptability. A caveat is that an intervention's acceptability is a very individual and personal decision. A procedure considered very mild by one person may be considered highly offensive by another. Thus all team members should sanction the decision to use any given response.

In the following sections, five broad categories of response intervention are described: *instructional approaches*, *extinction*, *differential reinforcement*, *negative punishment*, and *positive punishment*. Each category has its own strengths and weaknesses. It is imperative that less aversive approaches be considered prior to more aversive ones. In addition, response selection must be carefully weighed in the context of behavior function and team preference. Table 10.3 provides a description of the response strategies described.

Instructional Approaches

Many responses seek to direct the student to engage in an alternative behavior. A common strategy is to praise or comment on the appropriate behavior of another student in the class. For example, if Heather is making noises during work time, the teaching assistant might remark, "Harry, you're working very quietly; thank you for following the class rules." This statement is intended to remind Heather that working quietly is the expectation. A response of this type is most likely to be effective with students who value praise. That is, they will be motivated to engage in the stated behavior so that they too can obtain teacher praise. Praising others is well matched to behavior that serves an attention function, because the underlying message is that appropriate behavior will receive attention. Furthermore, attention is not provided to the student who is engaging in the inappropriate behavior, thereby avoiding the possibility of reinforcing behavior that is maintained by attention. In addition to behaviors with an attention function, this strategy can be structured to address behaviors with alternative functions. For example, the statement "I appreciate how Timmy is sharing his materials" may provide a relevant prompt for another student engaging in inappropriate behavior to obtain a desired item, while the

TABLE 10.3. Description of Response Strategies

Strategy	How it works	Examples	Cautions
Instructional procedure	Teaches an alternative behavior	Peer praise Prompting Discussion Problem solving Restitution	Attention provided for problem behavior Skills must be a part of behavioral repertoire
Extinction	Discontinues reinforcement for inappropriate behavior	Planned ignoring	Increase in frequency of behavior Escalation in severity of behavior
Differential reinforcement	Provides reinforcement for appropriate behavior	Scheduled attention	Reinforcement may not be delivered when student wants or needs it
Negative punishment	Removes preferred items or activities	Time owed Removal of privileges/ preferred activities Time out	Escalation in severity of behavior
Positive punishment	Provides something unpleasant	Feedback Reprimand Phone call home	Counteraggression Escalation in severity of behavior

prompt "Jean, thank you for raising your hand to ask for help" is matched to an escape function by suggesting an appropriate alternative for another student's escape behavior. When this strategy for responding to problem behavior is used, it is important to keep in mind that the target student must have the designated behavior in his or her repertoire. The statement "Nathan is playing nicely with his peers" will be inconsequential for a target student who lacks appropriate play skills.

In the same way that prompts are directed at another student, they also can be directed at the student engaging in problem behavior. Because the content of the prompt states expected behavior, this approach is often referred to as *redirection*. The statement redirects the student to engage in an appropriate behavior, as in the prompt "Jennifer, if you need help, you can bring me your 'help' card," delivered to a student engaging in hand biting during a task. The prompt should be issued when the staff member is in close proximity to the student, to avoid stigma, and it should be delivered in a neutral manner and respectful tone. A caveat is that because a prompt necessarily provides attention, it thus has the potential of reinforcing inappropriate behavior that serves the purpose of gaining attention. Making the prompt very brief can reduce this risk.

In some cases, a lengthier discussion with a student about alternative behaviors is appropriate. Another individual, such as a parent or school counselor, can be part of such a discussion or conference. This may provide an opportunity to develop a plan to avoid similar problems in the future, and to solicit the cooperation of the other individual in implementing the plan. An advantage to this approach is that the discussion can be held outside the location where problem behavior has occurred, and at a time removed from the problem. This change of setting may help to deescalate a volatile situation. Another advantage is that an individual who is uninvolved in the problematic situation can be designated to carry out the conference. This neutral person may also help to defuse the situation, whereas a prompt or other intervention imposed by the teacher who angered the student may cause further escalation. A major concern with this response is the rich attention that it can provide. This can be exacerbated if the individual designated to join in the conference is a highly preferred person. Although the student may prefer to leave the setting and discourse with a more preferred person, a situation should not be created in which the student receives high-quality attention only after engaging in problem behavior.

Problem solving offers a structured format for the discussion and is specifically focused on teaching a student to generate and select a more appropriate response to a problematic situation. It should be noted that this type of problem solving is initiated following problem behavior. This differs from the type of problem-solving sequence described in Chapter 9, Alternative Skills, which provides general instruction when problem behaviors are not present. However, the ultimate goal of both is to teach an alternative behavior. Problem-solving training should occur prior to implementing this approach; such training usually includes didactic instruction and modeling to teach problem-solving sequences that can be used during situations of conflict. A typical problem-solving sequence requires the student to (1) identify the problematic situation; (2) generate alternative, more appropriate behaviors in response to the situation; (3) select one from among the alternative behaviors; and (4) role-play the alternative appropriate behavior. Following this didactic instruction, the student is prompted and reminded to apply these problem-solving strategies at signs of problem behaviors. There are many problem-solving sequences described in the literature, including those accompanied by acronyms to remind students of each step in the sequence. These can be adapted to address the needs and abilities of students at a variety of ages.

Amish, Gesten, Smith, Clark, and Stark (1988) describe a six-step problem-solving approach for students of elementary school age. The first step is for a student to state how he or she feels and determine what the problem is. The second step is to decide on a goal. The third step is to stop and think before acting. Step 4 is to think of as many solutions as possible. Step 5 is to think about what will probably happen next. The final step is to select a good solution and try it. Initially, an instructor may need to guide a student through this sequence, using prompting procedures and direct questions (e.g., "What is the problem?" "What are some things you can do?"). However, for such a sequence to be useful when problems arise, the student must eventually learn to apply it independently.

Although problem-solving sequences are usually taught by adults, peers can also successfully teach them. As with any approach that requires prompting or one-to-one implementation, the risk that attention will reinforce the problem behavior is a concern. This approach should be used judiciously in response to behavior that serves an attention function, and the effects should be carefully monitored when it is used.

Generalization is an additional concern. Because the alternative behaviors are taught and practiced outside the natural environment, it is important to monitor whether the student is able to produce those behaviors when they are needed. Many students are unable to generate an alternative behavior in the heat of a situation, in spite of accurate modeling. This is why prompting students to use the problem-solving sequence when problems actually arise is important. A final caveat is that problem solving appears to be less effective for students with cognitive limitations.

An alternative form of instructional intervention is *restitution*. The purpose of restitution is for the individual to learn how to repair the damage caused by the behavior. It should not be delivered in a way that is punitive, but rather to teach the student that misbehavior must be corrected. For example, if a student's disruptive behavior results in books being destroyed, an appropriate type of restitution would be working after school to pay for replacement of the books. Writing a letter of apology would be an appropriate form of restitution for making a disrespectful comment to a peer. As always, function should be considered when team members are selecting the type of restitution. An inappropriate comment that functioned to gain attention would be better repaired through a written letter than through a face-to-face apology, which would risk providing additional attention. Restitution has the advantage of teaching natural contingencies similar to those encountered outside of school.

Extinction

Extinction is a procedure in which reinforcement for inappropriate behavior is discontinued. This approach is based on the concept that behavior continues because it is reinforced in some way. It has been well established that problem behavior usually results in a response that provides something desirable for the target person, such as attention or escape. The purpose of extinction is to discontinue that reinforcement. Planned ignoring is an example of the application of extinction. For instance, Alexi often emits shrill and loud screams when asked to complete self-care activities. Because these ear-piercing screams are disruptive to the classroom environment, her teacher usually assists her with the self-care activity as soon as they begin. Although this quiets her, it also reinforces the behavior of screaming, because she has learned that it is a sure way to get assistance. In order to discontinue this reinforcement, her teacher will completely ignore the screaming and continue to request that she complete self-care independently. The message to Alexi is that her screaming is no longer a way to get help with self-care. However, note that when extinction is used in demand situations, it is important to assure that the individual is able to complete the requested task. For example, ignoring a student's protests and tantrums, and insisting that his or her math be completed before recess, are not appropriate if the student does not have the skills to complete the assignment.

Extinction is well matched to behavior that serves an attention function, because attention is withheld. However, it is important that extinction is applied only to the problem behavior. In other words, the individual should not be ignored altogether. Appropriate behaviors, such as working, should be specifically reinforced. Only the problem behavior is ignored. Extinction is not advised if the problem behavior has the potential to cause harm to the individual or another. A risk of extinction is that about half of the time the frequency or topography of the behavior escalates before it decreases; this is referred to as an *extinction burst*. This happens when an individual accelerates the rate or severity of behavior in an effort to obtain the reinforcement that occurred previously. It should also be reiterated that extinction, along with all consequence-based approaches, should only be implemented in conjunction with other approaches, especially replacement behavior instruction. The student must have alternative means for achieving the desired outcome; otherwise, extinction will not be effective over the long term.

Differential Reinforcement

Differential reinforcement strategies represent a class of procedures that uses reinforcement to decrease undesirable behaviors. One example is *differential reinforcement of other behavior* (DRO). To implement DRO, reinforcement matched to behavioral function (e.g., attention) is provided if the undesirable target behavior does not occur during a specified period of time. For example, Ms. Detrich approaches and interacts with Stacy every 5 minutes, provided that Stacy has not engaged in self-injury, which has been determined to have an attention function. Another variation is *differential reinforcement of low-rate behavior* (DRL). This procedure is used when the goal is to decrease, but not eliminate, a particular target behavior. Lance provides an example of a situation where DRL may be effective. Mrs. Pitt allows students to leave class to use the bathroom as needed during the morning language arts block. She has noticed that Lance leaves at least five times each day. She determines that he does not like language arts, and leaves for a break from assignments. She will inform Lance that if he uses the bathroom fewer than three times during the morning block, she will allow him to have free time at the end of the period. She will gradually decrease the number of bathroom visits he can make in order to receive free time, until he is making only one, consistent with his classmates. Other variations of differential reinforcement include *differential reinforcement of incompatible behavior* (DRI), whereby behavior that is topographically incompatible with the target behavior, such as manipulating a toy rather than hand mouthing, is reinforced; and *differential reinforcement of alternative behavior* (DRA), in which behaviors dissimilar to (but not necessarily incompatible with) problem behavior is reinforced, as in the case of hand raising rather than talking out to obtain teacher attention. As with other reductive procedures, differential reinforcement does not teach alternative skills; thus it should not be implemented in isolation.

Negative Punishment

Removal of preferred items, privileges, or activities following problem behavior falls into the category of negative punishment. Negative punishment procedures differ from instructional procedures because they do not directly teach an alternative behavior. However, when well planned, they are instructional in a different way. Specifically, negative punishment should be designed to teach the logical or natural outcomes of engaging in socially unacceptable behavior. As such, the student learns that an inappropriate behavior results in the loss of something valued. For example, time owed is a natural and logical consequence for failure to complete work. In this case, the rule "Your work must be completed before recess" should be made clear to the student prior to work time. Any student who fails to complete the assignment because of off-task behavior will owe time during recess. As this example illustrates, the lost activity or item should be directly linked to the behavior, so that it teaches what can be reasonably expected in the world at large. Time wasted during nonpreferred activities results in time taken away during preferred activities. Likewise, withholding a person's pay for failing to complete a job, or prohibiting use of a toy for using it in an acceptable manner, is a logical and likely consequence.

When team members are matching a consequence to a behavior, function should also be considered. If the function of off-task behavior or failure to complete work is to obtain attention, then owed time should not be a situation where the individual will receive attention. A caution with this approach is that removing something preferred may anger a student and lead to the escalation of problem behavior. This can be reduced by clearly informing the student of the consequence for misbehavior ahead of time.

Time out is an example of negative punishment that is frequently used in schools. The effectiveness of time out rests on removing a student from a reinforcing activity for a period of time; hence it should be considered time out from reinforcement. Frequently, however, it is misapplied by removing a student from a nonpreferred activity. In this context, problem behavior is inadvertently reinforced by allowing the student to escape. As such, time out is typically not well matched to problem behavior that serves an escape function. It can be a successful intervention for attention-seeking problem behavior. Time out should always be used judiciously, since it removes a student from opportunities to learn and socialize.

Positive Punishment

The converse of negative punishment is positive punishment. Rather than removing something desirable, it consists of adding something undesirable; hence the term *positive* is used. An example of a usually mild form of positive punishment is feedback, such as a statement or a gentle reprimand. The simple statement "That's not acceptable" or "There is no talking in class" may be adequate to stop an undesired behavior. Very brief statements or reprimands such as these will reduce the likelihood of providing additional attention when the problem behavior is attention seeking. Another form of positive punishment might be a phone call home to report the behavior. Like negative punishment, however, positive punishment has the potential of causing an escalation in behavior and should be selected with care.

CRISIS MANAGEMENT

In some cases, a student's behavior may escalate to the point where there is risk of serious damage to him- or herself, others, or valuable property. Such a situation constitutes a *crisis* and its management must be different from the response interventions described above. In these situations, it is important to develop a crisis management plan. It should be kept in mind that the single purpose of a crisis intervention is protection of people and major property. Thus it is a distinct component of a behavior support plan. Unlike response interventions, a crisis management plan is not expected to reduce future occurrences of problem behavior. In fact, concerns about whether a crisis management response may reinforce undesired behaviors are suspended in order to do what is necessary to protect the student and others.

When team members are determining whether a crisis management plan is needed, there are many considerations (see Table 10.4). First, it is important to examine the actual potential of serious harm or damage. There should be team consensus that a student's behavior is likely to escalate to a level that defines a crisis, warranting the use of protective procedures. Many students threaten to hurt someone or posture in menacing ways, but are very unlikely to carry out those threats. Furthermore, although the issue has not been widely studied, preliminary data indicate that crisis management procedures often may be overused and unnecessarily used (George, 2000). This is a concern for two reasons: (1) crisis interventions are usually labor-intensive to implement; and (2) when physical intervention is required, it entails a risk of injury to both staff and students, in spite of extensive and requisite staff training. This is because physical intervention, such as restraint, typically results in defensive behavior on the part of a student, designed to protect him- or herself and evade the restraint. Not only are staff members at risk of being injured by a flailing or

---

TABLE 10.4. Key Questions for Developing a Crisis Management Plan

Before
- Is the behavior likely to cause injury or property damage?
  - If yes, crisis management is needed.

During
- What procedures are needed to maintain safety?
  - Will procedures deescalate student's behavior?
  - Will procedures cause disruption?
- When will plan be implemented?
  - What precursors signal that plan should be activated?
  - Will timing avoid serious injury?
- How many people are needed to implement plan?
  - How will staff be alerted to assist?
- What behaviors signal that crisis has ended?
  - How can we be sure dangerous behavior is over?

After
- How will student be reintroduced into ongoing routine?
  - What supports are needed for rapid return?
- How will use of crisis procedures be documented?
- Will team convene to review plan?

fighting student, but also the combative behaviors tend to result in increasingly forceful or imprecise implementation of the procedure by the staff—which can lead and has led to student injury, including death from asphyxiation in many documented cases. We caution support teams to carefully consider the real potential for serious harm or damage before deciding that a crisis management procedure is needed.

A second area of consideration is the choice of procedures needed to maintain a safe environment. It is important to select procedures that will deescalate, rather than escalate, the student's behavior. As noted above, physical intervention, such as restraint, causes an escalation in behavior for some students. In such a case, alternatives should be identified. Many procedures can deescalate behavior while at the same time protecting the student and others from harm. These include providing the student with time alone, taking a walk with the student, placing a pillow between the head of a self-injurious student and a hard surface, and clearing the room.

An additional consideration is the amount of disruption the procedure will cause. Although clearing the room may eliminate the need for physical intervention, it disrupts the entire class. Furthermore, additional staff members may be needed to move peers who are nonambulatory. This leaves fewer staff members to assist the student in crisis. For some students, gently escorting them out of the classroom to a quiet place may be preferred.

After the team has identified the type of procedure to use, the next decision is when to implement the plan. Many times a crisis can be avoided by implementing response procedures at the sign of precursors to severe behaviors. Determining when to intervene requires understanding the student's pattern of problem behavior (as described in the section below).

The team also must determine how many people will be required to implement the plan, who those people will be, and how they will be alerted that they are needed for assistance. For example, Evan's crisis management procedure was to escort him out of the classroom to a quiet room down the hallway. Two people were required to escort him, one on each side, because this minimized his disruptions along the way. Because there were only two adult staff members in Evan's class, the aide from the classroom next door was designated to assist with the procedure. At the first sign of a precursor to severe behavior, a responsible student was instructed to go next door and tell Ms. Stone she was needed immediately. This readied the necessary personnel, whether or not the plan was actually implemented.

A final decision is how to determine when a crisis has ended. Because crises usually call for the involvement of a number of staff members and are disruptive to ongoing activities, usual activities should be resumed as soon as possible. This requires also having a plan for reintroducing the student into the typical routine. For some students, the resolution of dangerous behaviors requires a long duration of calm, while others may show continued indicators of agitation or anger without a likelihood of serious behaviors. Similarly, some students can be reintroduced into the routine rapidly, whereas others will require a gradual reintroduction (such as a duration of time with no demands followed by the gradual increase of demands, along with teacher assistance and encouragement).

Whenever a crisis management plan is activated, not only should its use be documented, but the environmental events that led to the crisis should also be noted. This will sometimes help to avert future crises. For example, a review of the documentation may allow staff members to identify antecedents to a crisis, which can be modified to reduce the likelihood of future crises.

A final note about crisis management procedures is that they should be required very infrequently. If they are needed on an ongoing basis, then the support plan is inadequate. Frequent use indicates that the support team should reconvene to modify or strengthen the support plan. Figure 10.1 provides an example of a crisis management plan.

UNDERSTANDING A STUDENT'S
PROBLEM BEHAVIOR CYCLE

Each student has a unique pattern of problem behavior. Familiarity with the pattern helps to determine the type of response that should be used and the time(s) when it will be most effective. It is important to implement the least intrusive response that will deescalate the behavior and ensure safety. Many times a carefully selected response to escalating behavior can divert a crisis. Thus responses may differ, depending on the student's behaviors. In addition, the timing of a response can make it either more or less effective. A great deal of research on response procedures has shown that it is important for the response to come in close proximity to the behavior problem. This is perhaps most important for younger students and those with cognitive challenges, who must clearly understand the direct relationship between the behavior and the resulting consequence. However, particular types of responses may be ineffective if implemented while an individual is still angry, upset, or agitated. Colvin (1993) has described an acting-out cycle that begins with a trigger, followed by the escalation of problem behavior. If not interrupted in some way, the behavior may escalate into a crisis situation. Eventually, there is a recovery phase, where problem behavior deescalates and the individual is again calm.

Two different acting-out cycles are shown in Figure 10.2. The top left panel shows the progression of Renee's acting-out cycle. Renee's cycle shows a slow escalation, peaking with behavior that is not very intense, with a quick recovery. The illustration in the right panel shows the specific

Crisis Management Plan

Student: Kate   **Date:** January 14, 2003

Reason for plan: To avoid escalation of Kate's problem behavior to a point where she will be aggressive toward peers and staff.

Acting-out cycle: When Kate is in a demand situation, she will refuse to complete her work. She then begins to engage in minor property destruction (crumpling paper, breaking pencil). This escalates to overturning her desk, throwing furniture, and aggressing toward peers and staff.

Who will implement plan: Mrs. Roman (classroom teacher) OR Mr. Winters (classroom aide) AND Dr. Laird (school psychologist).

Procedures:

1. When Kate refuses to complete her work, prompt her to request a break or help by stating, "Kate, you can ask for a break, or you can ask for help." Provide this prompt once every minute. If she requests a break or help, provide it immediately.

2. If Kate begins to engage in minor property destruction, stay close beside her and between Kate and other students. Remove all materials from her vicinity that she could throw (e.g., books, her desk). Request another staff member to page Dr. Laird. When Dr. Laird arrives, prompt Kate to leave the classroom by stating, "Kate, you need to go to the counseling office to calm yourself." Continue to prompt her in this way approximately once every minute.

3. When Kate is transitioning, be sure each staff member is beside her. Block any attempts to aggress. Once she reaches the counseling office, instruct her to let you know when she is ready to problem-solve. Follow problem-solving protocol.

4. When she has completed problem solving, retrieve her work. Ask Kate to begin her work.

5. When Kate has completed 5 minutes of work without complaining or making disparaging comments, she can be returned to class without the threat of serious behaviors. Escort Kate back to class. Make sure that a classroom staff member is nearby. For the first 30 minutes, prompt Kate approximately every 5 minutes to take a break or ask for help if she needs it.

FIGURE 10.1. Kate's crisis management plan.

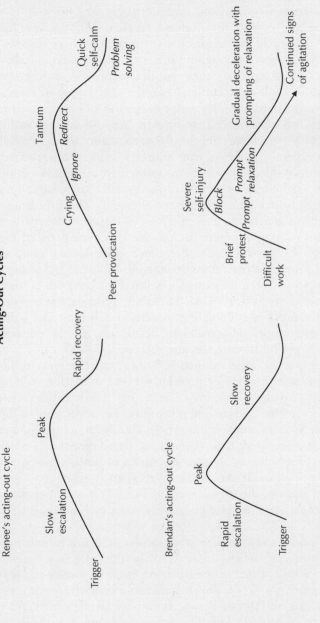

FIGURE 10.2. Two examples of acting-out cycles. (Staff members' responses are given in italics.)

behaviors that occur during the cycle. Renee's acting out usually begins when a peer makes a comment toward her that she considers disparaging. In the past, Renee would cry and have tantrums until her mother stepped in to intervene and protect her. Renee's teacher, Mr. Chavez, has worked extensively on teaching her alternative responses to comments by other children. His responses throughout the cycle can be seen in italics. Because Mr. Chavez wants Renee to learn that her inappropriate responses will no longer produce adult intervention, he ignores her crying. If crying escalates into a tantrum, he provides a prompt in the form of redirection to another area of the classroom. These unobtrusive responses are possible because Renee's behavior problems are not dangerous and are only mildly disruptive. Renee generally complies with redirection and is able to compose herself quickly once she is away from the immediate vicinity of her peer. When she is calm, she completes problem solving with Mr. Chavez and the peer who was involved in the problematic incident. The problem-solving sequence involves generating and role-playing appropriate interactions.

Brendan's acting-out cycle, seen in the lower left panel of Figure 10.2, is very different from Renee's. Brendan's cycle shows rapid escalation, peaking with much more intense behavior, followed by a very slow and gradual recovery. The right panel shows that his behavior is triggered by a request to complete difficult work. He briefly protests, but his reaction usually escalates rapidly, culminating in serious self-injurious behavior. His self-injurious episodes then gradually decelerate, and he remains agitated for a lengthy period of time. Because of the seriousness of his cycle, staff members' responses (again shown in italics) must be very different from those with Renee. Because of Brendan's rapid escalation, a staff member immediately provides a prompt to begin his relaxation exercises. This is occasionally effective at avoiding self-injury. However, more often the episode quickly leads to severe self-injury, including punching his cheeks, temples, and ears. To avoid tissue damage, staffers immediately block the self-injury by holding pillows between his fists and head. Simultaneously, they begin prompting Brendan to engage in relaxation exercises. Although he is still slow to recover, the exercises are the quickest way they have found to help him deescalate. Prompting relaxation continues until his agitation subsides.

It is important to note in these examples that each response is delivered at a time in the cycle when it is most likely to be effective. Problem solving with Renee would be ineffective when she is in the middle of, or recovering from, a tantrum. She is best able to generate alternative behaviors when she has fully recovered. Prompting with Brendan must be issued immediately at the first sign of protest. Although prompting does not consistently avert self-injury, when it is effective, it must be immediate because of his behavior's rapid escalation. Furthermore, prompting for relaxation begins immediately and continues throughout the cycle, to curtail the episode as quickly as possible.

In addition to the timing of the response, the consistency of implementation is important. Individuals with disabilities often receive services from many different staff members, such as counselors, school psychologists, speech teachers, physical therapists, teaching assistants, and teachers. If staff members respond differently to problem behavior, particularly in ways that reinforce the behavior, it will be much more difficult to eliminate. In addition, consistent implementation of a crisis management plan is critical for safety reasons.

SUMMARY

A strategy for responding to problem behavior is a critical part of a comprehensive support plan. Selecting an appropriate response must embrace ethical considerations as well as local values and policies. Furthermore, effective responses take into account a variety of student-related issues, such as the function of the behavior, the likelihood of escalation, and the long-term impact of the response. Just as antecedent/setting event interventions and instruction in alternative skills are carefully planned and connected to assessment information, so must response interventions be. Effective responses can teach or reinforce new behaviors, deescalate problem behavior, and minimize environmental disruption.

COMMONLY ASKED QUESTIONS

When we punish students in our class, it usually stops the behavior right away. Why do we need to do anything else? Mild punishment can be effective with students who engage in very minor problem behaviors. But in the case of serious and ongoing behavior problems, punishment usually only stops it temporarily. To decrease such behaviors over the long term, additional intervention components are needed, including teaching alternative behaviors and making antecedent/setting event modifications.

Will a severe form of response be more effective than a mild one? Severe responses to problem behavior are not necessarily more effective than mild forms. Less intrusive approaches should always be used first. This also will diminish the likelihood of unwanted side effects.

Shouldn't we implement a severe consequence, so that students learn they are accountable for their behavior? Implementing severe consequences alone to teach accountability assumes that students already have a repertoire of alternative skills and can readily implement those skills when needed in difficult situations. This is not the case for most students with ongoing challenging behaviors. Although it is important to teach students to be accountable for their actions, they must simultaneously be taught how to behave in more appropriate ways, as described in Chapter 9. In addition, educators are obligated to assure that the environment is structured to support students (see Chapter 8).

Our school requires certain responses to misbehaviors as listed in our district's discipline code. How do we go about making exceptions? Making accommodations and adaptations to support students with disabilities in general education settings is supported by the Individuals with Disabilities Education Act (IDEA). This includes making exceptions for students with behavioral difficulties. And, as discussed in this chapter, there are many reasons why responses to problem behavior should be individualized. Having said this, we acknowledge that it is another matter to get the team, administration, and other school personnel on board with this understanding. While making decisions about what to do, team members will need to consider what is required by a school's or district's discipline code and what is effective. In addition, whenever interventions differ from standard practice, involving the building principal and perhaps other district administrators (e.g., the director or supervisor of special education) in the teaming process is critical to finding an effective solution with which all team members can agree.

CASE EXAMPLES

Responses to Problem Behavior for Malik

Malik's team anticipated that with the antecedent changes made in Malik's curriculum and with the introduction of alternative forms of communication, problem behaviors would occur very seldom if they happened at all. Nevertheless, the team members considered how they should respond to instances of problem behavior in effective and instructive ways if problem behaviors indeed occurred, and what to do in crisis situations if Malik's challenging behaviors ever threatened the safety of others (see Figure 10.3).

Malik's team came up with several strategies. First, if during a difficult task Malik began to refuse or attempted to hit or throw objects, he would simply be directed to use his break card. The team believed that this would be the most effective solution, because using the break card would achieve the same outcome as

Malik's Behavior Support Plan

Hypotheses:

1. When prompted through difficult work, Malik is likely to refuse/aggress, to escape the activity.
2. When asked to complete nonfunctional activities, Malik is likely to refuse/aggress, to escape the activity.
3. When required to make a transition from a highly preferred activity to a nonpreferred activity, Malik refuses/aggresses, to maintain the preferred activity and avoid the nonpreferred one.

Antecedent/setting event interventions	Alternative skills	Responses to problem behavior	Long-term supports
Eliminate letter- and number naming activities from curriculum; avoid recall in academic activities.	*Replacement:* Teach requests for break. Make sure Malik's break cards are available; prompt him to use cards throughout the day.	**During difficult tasks, at the first signs of problem behavior, prompt Malik to use his break card.**	
Embed academics in functional activities; ensure meaningful outcomes	*Tolerance skills:* Teach working through difficult tasks; incrementally ask Malik to work a bit longer or do a few more before taking a break.	**During transitions, do any of the following:**	
Prompt Malik to use alternative forms of communication (pictures, gestures) when he has difficulty with verbal expression.	*General adaptive skills:* Expand gesture and picture vocabulary. Teach incidentally through the school day. Prompt Malik to use gestures and/or pictures to expand expressions.	• **Use his picture schedule to show Malik he can return to the activity on another day.**	
Use a daily picture schedule to mark classroom activities.		• **Tell Malik what the upcoming activity will be.**	
Provide a transitional warning prior to ending a preferred activity.		• **Praise other students for lining up.**	
When it is necessary to make a transition from a preferred to a nonpreferred activity, begin activity with a brief preferred activity (e.g., math game).		**Crisis management:**	
		• **Remove throwable materials.**	
		• **Block blows; protect others.**	
		• **Escort Malik to a quiet location in the building.**	
		• **Bring him back to the classroom as soon as he is calm.**	

FIGURE 10.3. Responses to problem behavior for Malik.

refusing, hitting, or throwing objects. In other words, problem behavior should immediately stop, because Malik was being directed to use an effective alternative. Once more, through redirection, Malik would learn an important lesson: that requesting a break would work to escape an activity, but not problem behavior.

The second response strategy was aimed at transitions. If Malik refused to make a transition, the team agreed to employ any combination of the following three approaches, depending on the activity: (1) show Malik on his picture schedule that he can return to the activity on another day; (2) remind Malik of what the upcoming activity will be (e.g., Math Bingo); and (3) ignore Malik's refusals while praising the other students for lining up. The team believed that these strategies should be successful because the reasons for difficult transitions (e.g., moving from preferred to nonpreferred activities) would be eliminated by the antecedent strategies of building preferred activities into Malik's school day.

Because Malik's problem behaviors could very quickly escalate to throwing objects, destroying materials, and hitting his teachers and classmates, a crisis intervention plan was needed. If Malik's problem behaviors escalated to the point of threatening others or damaging classroom materials, the teacher or teaching assistant would take the following actions. First, all materials within arms' reach of Malik would be removed (e.g., books, art materials, tables, and chairs would be pushed away). Second, the teacher or assistant would block any blows aimed at them or the other students. Third, either the teacher or assistant would escort Malik out of the classroom to a quiet location in the school building. When he was calm, Malik would be encouraged to join in the regularly scheduled activities.

Responses to Problem Behavior for Bethany

The responses to Bethany's problem behavior during academic activities were linked to teaching alternative skills (see Figure 10.4). That is, the responses were instructional and intended to teach Bethany to engage in an alternative appropriate behavior, rather than off-task problem behavior. Thus the first tactic following initial signs of off-task behavior was to prompt her to request help. But Bethany's team was not sure that she could easily determine why she might need help. It could be that she was becoming fatigued by a long assignment, was having difficulty with a task requiring fine motor skills, or did not understand the assignment instructions. The team decided that brainstorming with her might assist her to self-identify in the future why she needed help. Thus, if Bethany was not able to explain why she needed help following a teacher prompt, the teacher was to approach her and prompt her to generate ideas about why she was not completing her work. If Bethany indicated that she was becoming fatigued with the task, the staff was to offer her an alternative option. Likewise, if she indicated she was having difficulty with a fine motor task, another medium could be identified. Bethany agreed that this would help her, and that she would work hard with the staff to try to figure out why she was having academic difficulty.

Bethany's Behavior Support Plan

Hypotheses:

1. When Bethany is given written assignments, she engages in off-task behavior, to escape.
2. When Bethany is given lengthy assignments, she engages in off-task behavior, to escape.
3. When Bethany has visited her father over the weekend, she engages in off-task behavior, to escape work (because of fatigue).
4. When Bethany is in unstructured situations with unfamiliar peers, she engages in inappropriate interactions, to obtain their attention.

Antecedent/setting event interventions	Alternative skills	Responses to problem behavior	Long-term supports
Minimize amount of written work; provide alternative strategy for work completion (e.g., tape recorder).	*Replacement:* When independent assignments are given, teach Bethany to request assistance when she feels overwhelmed with assignments or does not understand what she is supposed to do.	**At the first sign of off-task behavior, prompt Bethany to request help; if behavior continues, brainstorm with Bethany to determine why the assignment is problematic.**	
Break work into small increments.			
Make sure instructions are clear and explicit.			
Seat Bethany near classmates in cafeteria; gradually introduce new people while prompting appropriate interactions.	*General adaptive skills:* Provide social skills instruction, and prompt Bethany to engage in appropriate interactions.	**Require Bethany to apologize to peers for inappropriate comments.**	
Have Bethany return home earlier on Sundays after visiting her father.	*Tolerance skills:* Gradually introduce Bethany to new people.	**Provide all feedback quietly and discreetly.**	

FIGURE 10.4. Responses to problem behavior for Bethany.

Because the team had previously determined that the function of Bethany's off-task behavior was escape from the assignment, not attention, there was little risk that the staff attention this response provided would encourage the response. Rather, the team viewed it as a way to identify and resolve the problem quickly, so that Bethany could resume the academic lesson in one format or another.

With respect to Bethany's inappropriate comments to peers, Bethany suggested that she should apologize when she insulted someone or hurt their feelings. The team agreed that this was not only a natural consequence, but also was likely to repair any damage made by the inappropriate comment.

Finally, Bethany stated that she felt embarrassed by teacher feedback. Her team suggested that any corrections or prompts could be provided quietly and discreetly. This was acceptable to Bethany. Her teachers also agreed that this would be respectful and likely to avoid further stigma.

REFERENCES

Amish, P. L., Gesten, E. L., Smith, J. K., Clark, H. B., & Stark, C. (1988). Social problem-solving training for severely emotionally and behaviorally disturbed children. *Behavior Disorders, 13,* 175–186.

Colvin, B. (1993). *Managing acting out behavior.* Eugene, OR: Behavior Associates.

George, M. (2000). Establishing and promoting disciplinary practices at the building level that ensure safe, effective, and nurturing school environments. In L. M. Bullock & R. A. Gable (Eds.), *Positive academic and behavioral supports: Creating safe, effective, nurturing schools for all students* (pp. 11–15). Reston, VA: Council for Children with Behavioral Disorders.

Guess, D., Helmstetter, E., Turnbull, R. H., & Knowlton, S. (1987). *Use of aversive procedures with persons who are disabled: An historical review and critical analysis.* Seattle, WA: The Association for Persons with Severe Handicaps.

Mayer, G. R., & Butterworth, T. (1979). A preventive approach to school violence and vandalism: An experimental study. *Personnel and Guidance Journal, 57,* 436–441.

Mayer, G. R., Butterworth, T., Nafpaktitis, M., & Sulzer-Azaroff, B. (1983). Preventing school vandalism and improving discipline: A three year study. *Journal of Applied Behavior Analysis, 16,* 355–369.

CHAPTER 11

◆ ◆ ◆

Long-Term Supports
and Ongoing Evaluation

◆

TIM KNOSTER
DON KINCAID

The preceding five chapters have focused primarily on strategies to identify and create interventions and supports for variables closely related to problem behaviors. Specifically, along with assessment approaches, the three positive behavior support (PBS) plan components described have been antecedent/setting event interventions, instruction in alternative skills, and response interventions. Though important, these three components generally are not sufficient to achieve meaningful outcomes and maintain long-term change. To fully assure a valued quality of life and continued progress over long periods of time, additional support and planning will need to be considered. Thus long-term supports constitute the fourth essential component of a comprehensive support plan.

The purpose of this chapter is to provide guidance for the design and implementation of long-term supports. Included is an overview of factors that contribute to a valued and satisfying quality of life. In addition, this chapter provides a perspective on important issues concerning ongoing evaluation; it thus builds upon and expands the measurement strategies described in Chapter 5. Finally, this chapter offers considerations for reviewing progress over the long term and modifying the support plan if needed.

DESCRIPTION OF LONG-TERM SUPPORTS

Providing a meaningful educational program for a student with a history of problem behavior is a challenging task. In order to realize durable, positive change for such a student, a team will need to (1) design interventions and supports that address the student's immediate needs through antecedent modifications, teaching alternative skills, and responding appropriately, as described in previous chapters; and (2) develop long-term supports that address broader quality-of-life factors for the long-term prevention of problem behavior.

Long-term supports, the fourth component of a comprehensive PBS plan, consist of two distinct yet related types of approaches: *lifestyle changes* and *strategies to sustain support*. Both of these approaches are essential for achieving and maintaining positive, meaningful outcomes for all involved in the process (i.e., the student and his or her family, school staff, other support team members).

Lifestyle Changes

Lifestyle refers to the rhythm and routines (ebb and flow) of daily life. There are many factors that influence lifestyle, including where a student lives, what school the student attends, what the student does to have fun, with whom the student interacts, and how the rhythm and routines of the student's day contribute to his or her personal satisfaction and enjoyment. In short, such factors directly contribute to the student's quality of life as seen from the student's perspective. Lifestyle provides the larger context or "big picture" within which a support team generates goals and selects supportive interventions. Particularly relevant to children and adolescents with long histories of problem behavior, lifestyle changes include interventions and supports to make their lives more satisfying. Ultimately, lifestyle changes contribute to long-term prevention of problem behavior as a result of general improvements in an individual's quality of life (Bambara & Knoster, 1995, 1998).

Long-term prevention through lifestyle changes can be achieved by addressing two primary sets of issues. First, a student who is dissatisfied with his or her quality of life (e.g., experiences loneliness and exclusion, has limited opportunity for age-appropriate choice and control over decisions, has few opportunities to engage in activities of personal interest) is more likely to engage in problem behavior than a student who is generally satisfied in this regard. Such dissatisfaction may be, in fact, the most significant issue that a team will need to address. No matter how well other support components are designed and delivered, enduring behavior change may not be realized if quality-of-life factors are not effectively addressed and dissatisfaction with them persists.

Second, students in general learn best in settings and activities that they find enjoyable and meaningful. Meaningful contexts can enhance a student's acquisition of, and fluency in, both academic and social skills. Unfortunately, students who engage in problem behavior can experience limited access to typical school, home, and community settings and activities that they find enjoyable and meaningful. And the more persistent the problem behavior becomes, the longer the limited access to such environments continues. Student dissatisfaction typically grows as this cycle continues. Furthermore, in an effort to control persistent problem behavior, it is not uncommon to see increasingly intrusive behavior management procedures put into practice. As a result, students with problem behavior may experience increasingly fewer opportunities to have choice and a voice in daily decisions that are made concerning their educational programs; they are also more likely to be assigned to more restrictive educational placements. Lifestyle changes are necessary to create motivating contexts for learning and to reverse the cycle of student dissatisfaction that can result from intrusive and restrictive approaches.

To illustrate the importance of lifestyle changes, consider the following example. Kellen was a 17-year-old student with moderate cognitive disabilities who received his educational program at his local high school in the morning, and at a prevocational sheltered workshop with other students with disabilities in the afternoon. The workshop component of his program was a new feature added in the current school year and was part of his transition plan. Kellen was a physically capable young man with a variety of interests (e.g., helping his dad around the house fixing things, going to the mall, and hanging out at the video store with his brother and some of the other kids from the neighborhood). Kellen wanted to find a job where he could do lots of different things during the day and be outdoors. He was also very motivated to "get a job fixing things" and "start making some cash." He was able to speak and could maintain conversation with his peers; however, he struggled at times with expressing himself in a clear and concise manner. Despite Kellen's many strengths and interests, his "bad" reputation had been growing over the school year among school staff as a result of increasing levels of problem behavior (e.g., verbal defiance and refusal to comply with staff direction at the workshop). Somewhat familiar with PBS, the staff members attempted different adjustments in Kellen's workshop routine, but little positive change in behavior resulted. They tried changing his work station from one day to the next, grouping him with different peers with disabilities at the work stations, and increasing the level of verbal praise for a job well done. Despite these efforts, the team's and Kellen's difficulties continued until one day in a team meeting, a staff member relayed a conversation he had had with Kellen about his behavior and getting and holding a job. This report of Kellen's comments made it clear that he had no interest in being at the workshop, because "the jobs we do here are dumb," "we are always stuck inside," and "none of my friends do this kind of stuff." At first Kellen's support team was shocked. Although the team members had in good faith tried adjusting his program to make it more enjoyable for him, they missed the bigger picture with Kellen: what *Kellen* was interested in doing and with whom he wanted to work. Minor adjustments in his work routine to address problem behavior were ineffective, because Kellen was unhappy with the workshop setting. In response, and to their credit, Kellen's team members revisited his transition plan and changed his work setting to a construction site with a local contractor. Although his neighborhood friends did not work with the same contractor during the same time as Kellen, some of them held similar after-school and/ or summer jobs in the local community. Not surprisingly, Kellen's behavior took a very dramatic change for the better in a very short period of time. Had this major lifestyle change not been considered, it is unlikely that Kellen's behavior would have improved.

Considerations for Choosing Lifestyle Changes

Selecting appropriate lifestyle interventions/supports to create constructive changes requires the team to conduct one or more assessments of the student's current lifestyle, as well as his or her interests and preferences. In addition, the team may need to develop an action plan to address the multiple lifestyle interventions that may be implemented.

Perhaps one of the most effective ways to promote lifestyle changes is through the use of *person-centered planning* (PCP) activities. As indicated in Chapter 1, a variety of structured PCP processes exist, including Personal Futures Planning (Mount, 1987; Mount & Zwernik, 1988), Lifestyle Planning (O'Brien, Mount, & O'Brien, 1990), Planning Alternative Tomorrows with Hope (PATH; Pearpoint, O'Brien, & Forest, 1996), Essential Lifestyle Planning (Smull, 1997), and Making Action Plans (MAPS; Vandercook, York, & Forest, 1989). All assist a team in better understanding the student, his or her history, the current environment, and the student's dreams for the future. A PCP process may occur at several times throughout the five-step PBS process for an individual student. Perhaps the most logical place for PCP to begin is in Step 2—when the team is conducting a functional assessment, during which broad information about the student and his or her environment is gathered. This broad information provides the foundation and context for more clearly understanding the student and his or her problem behaviors. The process may also need to be repeated periodically (every 3, 6, or 12 months), based on the students' progress. PCP is not a discrete activity. It should be ongoing, taking place as the support plan is continually revisited and revised, depending on the student's progress and environmental changes.

During the PCP process, a facilitator assists the team in gathering information through a series of "frames." Some of the frames assess the student's environment; others assist the team with developing a vision for the student; and still other frames assist the team in planning for the future. Possible themes for these frames include the following:

Assessment
- Identifying who are the important people in the student's life.
- Identifying where the student goes and what he or she does in a typical day.
- Discussing significant health concerns.
- Reviewing positive and negative issues from the individual's history.
- Examining the types of choices available to the student in the home, school, and community.
- Discussing the behaviors that cause the student to gain or lose respect among peers and adults.
- Identifying strategies that are effective and ineffective in supporting the student.

Vision
- Developing a long-term vision for the future for school, home, and/ or community life.
- Identifying goals for the future that are positive and possible.
- Clarifying the hopes and fears of the team members.

Planning
- Assessing barriers and opportunities that might have an impact on the success of the team.
- Assisting the team to determine critical themes identified in the process that must be addressed in the future.
- Developing an action plan for achieving short- and long-term goals.
- Supporting the team members in making a commitment to some first steps in pursuing identified goals.

As a result of the PCP process and follow-up activities, the team can come to consensus on a positive vision for the student's future that can be attained by committing to and implementing long-term supports, including both lifestyle changes and strategies to sustain the support plan. Without a PCP approach, a student-centered support team may inadvertently narrow its focus to address only the short-term outcome of decreasing problem behavior (as in Kellen's situation). Understanding a student's life in the broad context of home, school, and community naturally leads to considering a variety of lifestyle changes that can influence the student's overall quality of life.

If one of the structured PCP processes listed above (PATH, MAPS, etc.) is used, it may require considerable time and commitment from a team. If using a structured PCP process is not possible, team members should still attend to numerous lifestyle factors that may affect the effectiveness of the support plan. Table 11.1 lists key lifestyle factors, considerations for the team, and sample lifestyle goals that may be included in a PBS plan. These lifestyle factors are reviewed below.

Important Lifestyle Factors

Choices. Numerous research studies indicate that opportunities to make choices can have a positive impact on students' problem behavior (Cole & Levinson, 2002; Munk & Repp, 1994; Peterson, Caniglia, & Royster, 2001; Seybert, Dunlap, & Ferro, 1996; Vaughn & Horner, 1997). Often, however, students with problem behavior are provided with limited or no opportunities to make choices either inside or outside the school environments, particularly when behavior management strategies focus on behavior control. As a result, students may be denied opportunities to make simple choices such as what to eat, what activities to engage in, and with whom to work; thus they become increasingly unprepared to make important large choices later in life, such as where they want to live, what they want to do, and with whom they want to establish relationships. Specific examples of choice making as an antecedent strategy are presented in Chapter 8. Table 11.1 illustrates broader lifestyle opportunities for student choice and decision making.

School and Community Inclusion. Although many families and school systems work together to support inclusive educational settings, other families are faced with the formidable task of creating inclusive communities for their children during and after their formal schooling. Severe problem behaviors typically inhibit both school and community inclusion, and restrict a family's access to traditional community activities. A comprehensive PCP process extends beyond the school environment to address issues affecting the family, student, and community. An effective PCP/PBS process should provide families and educators with strategies for establishing and maintaining supports in inclusive school and community settings.

Relationships. At the heart of a high-quality life are positive interpersonal relationships with peers and adults. Members of the team may differ in the perceived value of social relationships. With today's increasing focus on high-stakes testing, it is not unusual to see schools emphasize a need for immediate behavior change, because a student's current behaviors are interfering with his or her academic progress. Although parents may share the

TABLE 11.1. Examples of Lifestyle Factors, Team Considerations, and Sample Lifestyle Goals

Lifestyle component	Team considerations	Sample lifestyle goals
Choice	How often, when, and where does the student get to make choices?	• Embed choice-making opportunities in all routines (choice of materials, location, activities, etc.).
	To what extent do daily routines and school activities reflect student interests and preferences?	• Incorporate student interests into curriculum and academic activities.
	How much say does the student have in daily decision making? In the school curriculum?	• Involve student in individualized education program (IEP) planning meetings to express interests and personal goals.
School and community inclusion	To what extent is the student included in typical school activities in typical school classrooms and settings?	• Increase participation in general education classes. • Enroll student in after-school clubs and activities.
	To what extent does the student participate in age-appropriate community activities?	• Identify a new community activity of interest for the student to explore each month.
Relationships	To what extent does the student have healthy, satisfying relationships and friendships with other students and adults?	• Identify peers within the classroom with whom the student shares common interests.
	How can we promote opportunities for the development of more healthy relationships with peers and adults?	• Plan opportunities for peers and adults to interact with the student around areas of his or her strengths or interests. • Encourage student to invite neighborhood friends for sleepovers and afternoon movies.
Valued roles	Are there areas where the student can make a contribution to his or her family, school and community?	• List possible "helper" activities for the student in each environment. • Encourage the student to volunteer with local community activities (festivals, fundraising, etc.).
	Are there specific responsibilities that the student can assume in the school and the classroom?	• Help the student select valued roles that are important to him or her in each environment.

(continued)

TABLE 11.1. *(continued)*

Lifestyle component	Team considerations	Sample lifestyle goals
General health and well-being	Are there short- or long-term health issues that need to be addressed for this student?	• Identify possible health issues and assist the student to self-manage such issues.
	How will we know whether the student is pleased with his or her classroom, supports, life, etc.?	• Get frequent feedback from the student and others about satisfaction with school, home, and community.
	How can we promote a safe environment for the student while also providing him or her with the dignity of risk?	• Teach the student necessary safety skills, including how to ask for assistance from friends, team members, and others.

school's concern on this issue, they (at a minimum) may also place equal emphasis on social issues and the importance of peer relationships. Parents may indicate that a primary goal for their child is to "have at least one friend at school" or "to have someone call her on the phone to just talk like most other teenagers do." Simply being physically present in the inclusive school and community environment is typically insufficient by itself to build meaningful and sustainable relationships. Likewise, simply participating in school activities and doing regular things with other students do not always result in long-term connectedness. In response to this reality, parents often want the school program to facilitate real connections between their child and other children that will result in long-term, supportive friendships. However, developing "friendships" is often not a spontaneous process. Rather, for students with histories of problem behavior, it typically requires structured opportunities in tandem with creativity and a long-term commitment by the team. Some sample goals and related activities to facilitate relationships are provided in Table 11.1.

Valued Roles. We all often define ourselves by our valued roles. We are teachers, parents, athletes, friends, spouses or partners, and so forth. Often, however, students with problem behavior are viewed by others in a negative light (e.g., "This kid is my worst nightmare"). One of the critical outcomes for such children in schools is to acquire opportunities to develop positive roles, such as being student helpers, friends, peer tutors, or dance club members. Valued roles help to create a sense of belonging for these students and can ease negative perceptions that can lead to continued isolation and rejection. These valued roles in childhood also may lead to valued roles into adulthood.

General Health and Well-Being. Parents indicate that health and safety issues are heightened as a child moves into adulthood (Brotherson, 1988; Nehring, 1990). Thus parents frequently ask, "What will happen to him when I am gone?" "Who will be there for my daughter?" "Who will his friends be?" or "Will she have a good life?" Addressing the issues of choice, school and community inclusion, relationships, and valued roles can help alleviate (to some degree) such concerns. However, the team may need to spend time problem-solving lifestyle factors that have an impact on more global and long-term issues, such as the student's health, safety, and happiness.

Strategies to Sustain Support

Strategies to sustain support are as important as lifestyle changes in maintaining the long-term effectiveness of a PBS plan. Strategies to sustain support involve providing support both for the student and for members of the team. School and community environments are often in a constant state of flux, with changes occurring on a regular and sometimes unpredictable basis. Most students with histories of problem behavior will need continuity across settings and people, and ongoing assistance over time to maintain and generalize (to new settings and people) newly acquired social skills. Along the same line, team members will typically need parallel forms of assistance in order to facilitate ongoing support for the student.

Ongoing Support for the Student

Planning for long-term student support requires the team to consider strategies that will have an impact student behavior over several years, or that will prepare the team and the student to face challenges that may not yet be present in the student's life. When generating long-term student supports, team members should consider how to (1) teach the student to maintain and generalize new alternative skills, (2) prepare others to support the student, and (3) address environmental changes.

Teach the Student to Maintain and Generalize Skills. Maintenance is a term used to describe a student's ability to continue to exhibit learned skills across time, generally within a similar environment (Ferro & Dunlap, 1993). *Generalization* is understood as the student's use of existing skills in new environments (Dunlap, 1993; Ferro & Dunlap, 1993). Long-term planning by the support team will need to address issues of both maintenance and generalization.

One of the most effective methods to promote the maintenance of new skills is to teach the student to use self-management strategies. In Chapter 9, self-management strategies for teaching coping and general adaptive skills have been introduced. Many of these self-management strategies, such as goal setting, self-monitoring, and self-cueing, may be used to help students maintain newly learned alternative skills over time. Self-management strategies have been shown to be effective in maintaining a wide-range of positive behaviors, such as academic engagement (McDougall & Brady, 1998), schedule following (Clees, 1994), transitioning between tasks (Newman, 1995), adhering to self-care routines (Pierce & Schreibman, 1994), and playing appropriately (Stahmer & Schreibman, 1992). Self-management strategies also have been used to help students maintain reduced levels of problem behaviors, such as stereotypical repetitive behaviors (McAdam, 1993) and stuttering (Ingham, 1982). Early in the process of teaching alternative skills, support teams should consider teaching self-management techniques as a means of helping students to maintain behavior change outside the initial teaching arrangement. Examples of self-management techniques include (but are not limited to) using a checklist to self-monitor assignment completion and/or using picture cues to solicit teacher praise when a student is performing well on tasks.

But before skill maintenance is considered, students must be able to apply newly learned skills to match new settings and situations; again, this is referred to as *generalization*. For instance, a student initially may be taught important social skills involved in initiating conversations at home and in school. However, the student may need additional instruction to exhibit these skills in new community and work settings. The student may also need to learn more subtle social distinctions in those environments, such as when it is appropriate to talk, how to initiate conversations with unfamiliar people, what to do if an individual is not willing to talk, and how to expand on topics for discussion with people whom the student meets regularly. In another example, a child may be instructed to verbally express an opinion as to what game he or she would like to play after dinner with a parent at home. However, at school the student may need instruction as to when it is appropriate to express such preferences and how to read the social cues of others in the classroom (teachers, other staff members, and peers).

Planning opportunities to apply and adapt alternative skills in new situations is an important priority for support teams concerned about producing positive long-term outcomes. Thus an important generalization strategy to consider when team members are selecting alternative skills is to ensure that the skills are a "good fit" to the school, home, and community settings in which they will be used. Good-fit skills are appropriate to the setting; understood by a range of social partners; and likely to be naturally reinforced or responded to by peers and adults in home, school, and community settings.

Prepare Others to Support the Student. The support team must also make efforts to teach other students and teachers how to support the student more effectively. Despite the team's efforts to select good-fit alternative skills, many adults and peers may not know the best ways of interacting with the student or of implementing behavior supports without being taught directly. This may be especially true when the methods of support are not typical, but unique to a particular student. When designing long-term supports, a team should consider whether others know how to prevent problem behaviors, encourage alternative skills, and respond to instances of problem behavior should they occur. In addition, the team should consider whether others understand how the student communicates and how to welcome and include the student in typical school, community, or home activities.

One strategy to consider is involving other students early in the support process. Developing a Circle of Friends (Frederickson & Turner, 2002) is an effective way for encouraging peers to include the focus student in their social activities and for establishing friendships. Using this strategy, peers learn how to interact with the student in positive and sensitive ways. As students move through their school years, they may not maintain the same "circle of friends." Therefore, teams will need to occasionally assess peer relationships to determine whether new peers need to be added into the student's circle.

Although it is possible that a student will maintain a consistent set of friends, it is inevitable that he or she will experience a wide array of teachers from year to year. Thus it is essential that the support team consider strategies to involve future teachers proactively in the long-term planning process. We have found that it is valuable to identify future teachers for the focus student for the upcoming year (when possible) during the spring of the existing school year, and to invite them to a fun activity to get to know the student and team. The team's documentation of the PCP process, the functional assessment, the behavior support plan, and other relevant information should also be shared and discussed with future teachers during this activity. In addition, the team may assist with identifying the teacher or teachers who may be most receptive to supporting the student, or who present a style of interaction and teaching that best meets the student's current and long-term needs.

Address Environmental Change. Changes in all of our lives are sometimes accidental and sometimes planned. Successful PBS teams will understand that accidental changes may require extemporaneous problem solving. These changes may result in significant differences in team membership and adjustments in a behavior support plan, such as the identified goals for the student. For example, an unexpected leave of absence by a teacher will result in a team membership change and may require adjustments to the support plan to accommodate differences in the new teacher's teaching style and preferences.

Other more predictable changes, such as moving from the local elementary school to middle school or moving into a more inclusive classroom setting, can (and should) include proactive planning. Important planning will include making sure that antecedent modifications and long-term adaptations are in place as the student makes the transition. To operate successfully, the team will need to have the capacity to have a vision for the future while also living in the immediacy of today.

All three strategies for sustaining student support will require teams to make student-specific decisions based on a variety of considerations. It is impossible to create an exhaustive list of such decisions, due to the individualized nature of decision making; however, Table 11.2 presents considerations for support teams, with general examples of strategies that may be written into students' support plans.

Supports for Team Members

Supporting team members has been discussed in Chapter 4. It is essential that team members openly and honestly discuss and establish supports for themselves, so that they are in a position to meet the needs of the student. One of the best ways to ensure that team needs are implemented is to write team supports directly into the student's behavior support plan. The types of supports will vary, depending on (1) the team's experience with PBS and (2) the context or settings within which the team is supporting the student. Examples of team supports include changing staffing patterns to better implement antecedent interventions more effectively, training staff members to identify and teach alternative skills, and scheduling dates and times for regular team meetings to review progress and modify the support plan over time. Although the types of supports that are needed by team members will vary from team to team as well within a team over time, cost is not typically prohibitive. For example, sometimes supporting team members may be as inexpensive as providing a friendly face and an open ear for a team member to vent his or her frustration after a particularly difficult experience, as discussed in Chapter 4. Table 11.3 provides examples of various team supports that may be included in a student's support plan.

Team membership is likely to change over time, for a variety of reasons (e.g., naturally occurring transitions from grade to grade or school to school, staff reassignments, personal reasons). Strategies to sustain support enable the team to continue functioning in a competent manner, despite changes in team membership. Staff turnover is one reason why it is essential to have the team (as a unit) involved with each of the five steps in the PBS process. Continued team involvement in all steps will help to promote a good contextual

TABLE 11.2. Examples of Team Considerations in Planning Long-Term Supports

Concern	Team consideration	Examples of strategies
Teach the student to maintain and generalize newly learned alternative skills	How can we respond to Bob so that he continues to raise his hand to gain teacher attention in Mrs. Smith's classroom over time?	After consistently responding to Bob's hand raising, teach him to wait for Mrs. Smith when she is busy with other students.
	How can we teach Bob to raise his hand to gain teacher attention with other teachers in different classrooms?	After Bob consistently raises his hand, teach him to do so in other settings. Introduce self-monitoring to remind him to use the skill across different settings.
Prepare others to support the student	What do new teachers and other students who are unfamiliar with Jaron need to know to support him to use his "Play with me" statement on the playground?	Teach other students about Jaron's limited expressive language and his use of one simple statement to indicate that he wants to play. Also, share this information with staff who monitor playground activities.
	How will we address transitions with Jaron to new play settings, such as the local recreation center?	Meet and share relevant information with staff (and other kids) at new locations.
Address environmental changes	What long-term adaptations will Sheila require to work successfully and get along with coworkers on various job sites?	Ensure that Sheila has her picture board available in all locations, and make sure coworkers understand her picture system. Also, schedule opportunities for social interactions with others during breaks.

fit (i.e., make sure that the support strategies are reasonable for the situation and setting); it will also build in redundancy among team members (i.e., provide a shared experience base across team members), to minimize the potentially adverse impact of turnover on the support team.

In summary, long-term supports, whether they focus on the student or on the support team members, are part of an ongoing PBS approach. Teams will need to meet on a scheduled basis to determine whether progress is being made and what long-term supports are needed to ensure durable outcomes.

To make rational decisions, a support team should monitor a student's progress in a variety of ways. The next section discusses how team members can use outcome data to evaluate whether the team is being successful in its PBS efforts.

TABLE 11.3. Examples of Team Supports

Types of supports	Examples
• Training in the PBS process and technical skills	Attend inservice training on PBS. Provide on-site technical assistance.
• Enhancing communication among team members and providing positive reinforcement for the team	Send e-mail progress notes and words of support to one another.
• Providing of respite (when needed)	Provide a teacher with a break after difficult times with the student.
• Establishing clear expectations among team members coupled with shared accountability	Create an action plan with a "to do" list for team members.
• Establishing a clear team process to discuss issues and resolve differences	Establish and follow an agreed-upon protocol for team meetings and problem solving.

EVALUATING AND MONITORING PROGRESS

Once a behavior support plan is implemented, a team will be immediately faced with determining effectiveness—addressing such questions as "Is progress being made?" and "Are we being successful?" Answers to these questions can directly translate into modifications to the support plan, as warranted in Step 5 of the PBS process (implementing, evaluating, and modifying the plan). Support plans are effective when they produce meaningful outcomes. Because problem behaviors can significantly interfere with an individual's quality of life (e.g., relationships, access to preferred activities, inclusion), effectiveness must be evaluated in terms of personally meaningful results (Bambara & Knoster, 1998; Meyer & Janney, 1989). Personally meaningful results should comprehensively reflect the student's, the student's family members', and other team members' perspective on what is important. In other words, has sufficient progress been made to satisfy the team members and the student? To answer this question, support teams will need to consider collecting outcome information (data) to monitor progress by a number of means. It is very important to collect and analyze information pertaining to three types of meaningful outcomes: (1) increases in alternative skills, (2) reductions in problem behavior, and (3) improvement in quality of life. Chapter 5 details data collection strategies for tracking changes in alternative skills and problem behaviors. In the following discussion, we introduce quality-of-life measures and discuss data-based decision making across the three outcomes.

Lifestyle Outcome Measures

As important as it is to evaluate increases in the acquisition and use of alternative skills and reductions in problem behavior, it is equally important to assess positive changes in quality of life for the student, his or her family, and other relevant parties involved in the student's life. Over the last several decades, health and human service agencies have embraced the concept of *quality of life* as an overarching principle of service delivery (Schalock, Bonham, & Marchand, 2000). In this sense, quality of life guides service delivery and helps educators and other service providers to focus on goals that are important to the student and his or her family. Quality of life also has become a critical principle that is used to measure the improvements made in an individual's life as a result of PBS (Kincaid, Knoster, Harrower, Shannon, & Bustamante, 2002).

Essential domains for assessing quality of life have been identified in the literature by various sources (Felce & Perry, 1995, 1996; Schalock et al., 2000). In particular, the Tri-State Consortium on Positive Behavior Support (a federally funded project for training schools in PBS) has defined measures to assess the impact of PBS on overall quality of life, and has identified five pertinent to assessing changes in quality of life: (1) interpersonal relationships, (2) self-determination, (3) social inclusion, (4) personal development, and (5) emotional well-being. Table 11.4 lists components for each of these five.

Assessing quality of life can be challenging for a school-based support team. At a minimum, it will require assessment of progress toward both short-term outcomes (i.e., reductions in problem behaviors, increases in alternative skills) and longer-term outcomes (e.g., development of friendships). As such, team members should gather information concerning targeted outcomes in a manner that yields useful data for decision making without significantly interfering with the typical ebb and flow of school, home, and community routines (i.e., selecting data collection procedures that provide a good contextual fit). Time sampling (described in Chapter 5) is an example. Whereas increases in alternative skills and reduction in problem behavior lend themselves to quantitative procedures, it is likely that support teams will find qualitative procedures valuable in terms of assessing impact on quality of life. Some students may be able to provide information themselves about their satisfaction in important domains, such as friendships. At other times, particularly for students without extensive verbal language, this will depend on the observation of others. For example, a parent may provide information about a child's enthusiasm while participating in leisure activities.

In an ideal world, a support team will see dramatic outcomes in positive behavior change and improved quality of life for all involved in the

TABLE 11.4. Five Subscales on Quality of Life Used by the Tri-State Consortium on Positive Behavior Support

Dimension	Component parts of each subscale
Interpersonal relationships	• Relationships with family members and peers • Time spent interacting with peers • Affection when interacting with peers
Self-determination	• Participation in school and community activities • Ability to make decisions and express preferences • Satisfaction with living conditions
Social inclusion	• Relationships with members of the community and school • Response child receives from peers • Ability to engage in leisure activities
Personal development	• Access to personally stimulating activities • Willingness to attempt new tasks/activities • Ability to learn new skills
Emotional well-being	• Self-confidence • Emotional stability • Satisfaction with level of independence and general happiness

process within a short time frame. Although some support teams may realize such outcomes in a very brief time frame, others will not be as fortunate. As such, effective support teams demonstrate the capacity to plan and monitor student progress in both the short and long terms.

Developing a Plan to Monitor Progress

As discussed, meaningful outcomes include reductions in problem behavior, increases in use of socially acceptable alternative skills, and general improvement in quality of life. To monitor progress toward these outcomes, a support team will need to develop an evaluation plan. For each of the three outcomes, team members should address two major questions. The first is this: "What do we expect to happen as a result of implementing the behavior support plan?" For example, what types of problem behavior will be reduced, and to what level of acceptability? What alternative skills should the student use, and in what situations? What quality-of-life changes are expected as a result of the support plan? Once the team agrees on expected outcomes, the next question to ask is "How will we measure this?" Teams may measure outcomes by choosing from a variety of tools introduced in Chapter 5, including direct, indirect, and subjective (satisfaction) ratings of progress. Table 11.5 provides some team examples of expected outcomes and measures.

TABLE 11.5. Examples of Meaningful Outcomes

Meaningful outcomes	What do we expect to happen?	How will we measure this?
Long-term and acceptable reductions in problem behavior	Bob's shouting out in class will stay at zero throughout the remainder of the school year.	Review frequency counts of Bob's shouting monthly.
	Jaron's grabbing/taking play items on the playground will be reduced to no more than once a month.	Review incident accounts completed by the playground monitor weekly.
	Sheila's self-injury (hand biting) will be reduced to less than once a week.	Review frequency counts of hand biting every 3 days; check for red marks at the end of each day.
Increases in alternative skills	Bob will raise his hand in class to gain the teacher's attention instead of shouting.	Obtain sample by counting hand raising in two periods each week.
	Jaron will state " Play with me" instead of grabbing/taking play items from others on the playground.	Ask playground attendant to monitor and record Jaron's use of "Play with me" statement with others; review weekly.
	Sheila will seek help by pressing the "help" button on her microswitch.	Review frequency counts of "help" requests during instruction daily.
Improvement in quality of life	Bob will meet his long-term academic progress goals and achieve passing grades in general education classes.	Review teacher anecdotal progress notes monthly; review homework and test scores weekly.
	Jaron will be included by peers in games on the playground.	Review teacher and paraprofessional anecdotal notes of Jaron's being included by others in games weekly.
	Sheila will work alongside new coworkers at her job site, completing job requirements, requesting assistance when needed, and socializing with others during breaks.	Call floor manager once a week to ascertain her perceptions; obtain and review relevant records monthly.

Evaluating Progress and Making Decisions

Although reaching agreement on expected outcomes and measures is important, understanding how to make decisions using this information is essential for determining whether progress is being made or whether there is a need to make changes in the support plan. Based on the information collected, a team may decide to reevaluate components of the plan, to strengthen or add supportive interventions, and/or to expand the scope of the current plan to new settings or situations. When making such decisions, team members are likely to encounter one of three types of data patterns.

In Pattern 1, despite good-faith efforts, the student may experience few or to no reductions in problem behaviors, and/or minimal increases in using socially acceptable alternative skills. In other words, what the team has been doing has yet to be sufficiently successful. This can occur for a number of reasons. It may be that additional time is required for the supports to be effective. Alternatively, only some of the support plan components may be effective, requiring additional review and evaluation of each component. It may also be that there is a mismatch between the functional assessment information and the support plan. This situation will require modifications to the support plan. When little progress is seen, the team should discuss the considerations described in Table 11.6.

Pattern 2 occurs when a student exhibits a moderate reduction in problem behavior, along with modest increases in socially acceptable alternative skills, but this progress is considered insufficient. In other words, progress is noted, but not to the level expected by the team. In this situation, the considerations indicated in Table 11.6 continue to be relevant. In addition, the team may need to reassess the goals or expectations it has identified for a student; perhaps they are not attainable or realistic within the identified time frame. To illustrate, a goal for a 14-year-old student who has a well-documented history of profanity and noncompliance might be expected to have "no instances of cursing or noncompliance for an entire week following 3 months of intervention." A relevant consideration for this student's support team might be to question whether such a goal is attainable and/or reasonable, given the student's history of problem behavior prior to intervention. Perhaps a 90% reduction in problem behavior would be satisfactory after 3 months.

In Pattern 3, a student may exhibit significant reductions in problem behaviors and improvements in socially acceptable alternative skills. Improvements in quality of life are noted as well. In this instance, the team should turn its focus to addressing the issues of maintenance and generalization. In addition, the team may consider fading particular supports to facilitate age-appropriate levels of independence and decision making (i.e., self-determination) by the student. Also of great importance, the team members should take time to *celebrate* their accomplishments to date!

COMMON CHALLENGES CONFRONTED BY TEAMS

A team is likely to face a series of critical challenges throughout the support process that can affect student progress, decision making, and long-term outcomes. For the most part, these challenges will generally fall within

TABLE 11.6. Considerations for Determining Whether Support Plans Need to Be Revised

Considerations	Possible decision by the team
Has sufficient time been allotted for the support plan to take effect? • Is more time needed for student growth?	Review strategies and determine time line for additional review after more time has been allowed.
Is the support plan being implemented as planned? • Are all components are being implemented consistently across team members?	Observe to see whether all components are being implemented; review strategies with team members; offer training if necessary; make strategies easier to implement.
Are all components necessary? Effective? • Are some components of the plan are working? • Do any components need modification?	Review each component of the support plan; maintain effective components; strengthen or revise ineffective components.
Is the support plan linked to hypotheses for problem behavior? • Is there is a mismatch between the hypotheses and supports?	Review the interventions to determine how they address the setting events, antecedents, and function of problem behavior; revise if necessary.
Are the hypotheses still relevant? • Have the conditions related to problem behavior changed? • Are new data needed to better inform the plan?	Return to the functional assessment process; gather additional information and modify, or formulate new hypotheses as warranted.
Have student preferences and quality of life been sufficiently addressed? • Did the support plan miss the "big picture" of student satisfaction with settings and activities?	Review the student's satisfaction through student interviews or conduct a person-centered planning; emphasize lifestyle changes if needed.

three domains: (1) the system, (2) the student, and/or (3) the team. Earlier in this chapter, we have discussed two particular issues that are important: naturally occurring transitions for students, and changes in the support team's membership. Likewise, we have discussed how changes in the life circumstances of the student require adaptations in support provided by the team. The possible changes in life circumstances that could have an impact on a child and team are too numerous to list. However, we have found that a family's relocation, a student's health, the employment status of family members, and domestic violence are common impediments to the maintenance of a successful student-centered team process. It is important for the team to remember that no matter how well it may "engineer" support for a student, there are issues within the student's family, society, and school that may impede or completely derail their best efforts at a given point in time.

Situations related to the team's functioning may be more amenable to change than system- or student-oriented issues. For instance, team members frequently have differences of opinions about quality-of-life issues. They may disagree about the most important issues or goals to pursue at a particular moment in time. They also may disagree about when they think the support process is complete. Some team members may be satisfied with simple reductions in problem behavior, while others may want to continue the support process until long-term quality-of-life changes are evident. Differences in opinion among team members are most likely to occur in the event that the support team has not reached consensus on the vision and desired results of the PBS process. In an instance where team functioning is of concern, the team may want to revisit the planning and vision stages of the teaming process to maintain (or acquire) a consensus about their expectations, where they are going, and how they are going to get there.

SUMMARY

In this chapter, we have described long-term supports as the fourth component of a comprehensive behavior support plan. Long-term supports consist of two distinct yet related types of strategies: lifestyle changes and strategies to sustain support. Lifestyle changes address the student's perspective concerning satisfaction with a number of lifestyle components (i.e., choice, school and community inclusion, relationships, valued roles, and general health and well-being). For example, it is important to ask whether the student finds his or her educational experience enjoyable and meaningful. Strategies to sustain support address the long-term support needs of both the student and members of the team. Also in this chapter, we have provided guidance on how to monitor meaningful outcomes throughout the PBS process. Specifically, a support team should be looking for reductions in problem behavior, increases in socially acceptable alternative skills, and positive impact on the quality of life for all involved in the process.

COMMONLY ASKED QUESTIONS

Are long-term supports identified and implemented all at once? No, not necessarily. Developing a support plan with an eye toward long-term outcomes is an evolving process. Long-term supports, including lifestyle changes, are often added to a support plan as a team implements other components. For example, the team may first teach alternative skills in one setting, and then, as part of its long-term planning, consider whether additional instruction is needed in other settings. Or the team may make antecedent adaptations in one classroom, and, once these have proved successful, consider how the same modifications can be carried out in additional classrooms. In other words, whereas some long-term supports may be implemented at once as part of an initial behavior support plan, other strategies will evolve over time as support components are implemented and progress is made.

Do we really have to implement lifestyle changes if we have seen reductions in problem behavior? In a word, yes. Remember that lifestyle provides the larger context within which to view student-centered PBS. If a student is dissatisfied with his or her quality of life, it is more likely that the student will engage in problem behavior in the future, even if the team has realized short-term reductions in problem behavior.

Do we really need to measure progress beyond reductions in problem behavior? The old adage of "what is important gets counted" applies to this question. PBS is first and foremost a teaching approach. As such, the primary emphasis is on teaching socially acceptable alternative ways for students to meet their needs and to replace problem behaviors. This is precisely the reason why it is critical for support teams to measure not only reductions in problem behavior, but also increases in alternative skills and the impact on quality of life.

At what stage in the PBS process is it necessary to identify the needs of support team members? Simply stated, it is critical to provide necessary supports throughout the entire process and within each step of the PBS process. Addressing the needs of support team members will increase the likelihood that members will work together and communicate effectively and efficiently. Equally, addressing the needs of team members when the team is designing and implementing supportive interventions is important to ensure a good contextual fit and to increase the likelihood that the support plan will be competently implemented over the long term. Therefore, the needs of team members should be monitored within the context of team meetings over time, with supportive strategies used where warranted with individual members.

What happens if a team member appears resistant to meeting the needs of the student within the least restrictive environment (e.g., the current educational placement)? Some team members may have different agendas. For instance, a teacher may want the student with a disability to be removed from his or her general education class. Under the Individuals with Disabilities Education Act (IDEA), the student's team must provide educational services in the least restrictive setting. In such a situation, the team would be well served by addressing this question: "What will it take in order to provide the IEP, including the behavior support plan, within the least restrictive environment?" Explicitly identifying and operationally defining relevant barriers to implementation, and determining the supports needed by team members to deliver an appropriate program, are important prerequisites. In a practical sense, it is unlikely that a support team will realize durable positive outcomes if the needs of team members are not addressed adequately. As such, it is imperative for the team to specifically identify and address the needs of all team members (including the one team member who appears resistant) in order to realize durable, positive outcomes.

How do we best ensure that the student behaves appropriately throughout the entire school day, as well as in the community? Although team members will want to provide prevention strategies on an ongoing basis (thus minimizing the likelihood of problem behavior by addressing the antecedents and setting events for problem behavior), the two key issues here in terms of durable behavior change by the student are maintenance and generalization of the newly acquired alternative skills. In order to maintain the use of the alternative skills over time, it is essential to continue to reinforce their use over time. In addition, it is important to teach specifically for generalization by providing direct instruction of the appropriate behavior(s) across relevant settings that have been identified by the team, and to reinforce the use of the alternative skills in those settings.

CASE EXAMPLES

Malik's Long-Term Supports

The members of Malik's team understood the importance of developing long-term supports, but found it difficult to plan for the future without knowing whether their hypotheses were correct or whether the first three plan components would indeed be successful. In addition, they found it difficult to consider lifestyle changes, because they were unsure about what aspects of school Malik would like. Despite his teacher's reassurance that she would continue to work with Malik, his grandmother feared that he would again be kicked out of school and placed in an even more restrictive setting. Thus, focusing on more immediate concerns, the team decided to implement the first three components of the support plan, and then evaluate Malik's progress over the next 2 months before considering long-term supports. The team also thought this would be more feasible and manageable for them to implement than considering all four components at once.

Meaningful outcomes	What do we expect to happen?	How will we measure this?
Long-term and acceptable reductions in problem behaviors	Malik will make transitions from activity to activity with minimal or no resistance, and no problem behaviors.	Count the number of positive and negative (those with problem behaviors) transitions each day. Review data weekly.
	Malik will exhibit no signs of problem behavior when he encounters a difficult task.	Count the frequency of problem behaviors associated with difficult tasks each day on an ABC log. Review weekly.
Increases in alternative skills	Malik will say "break" or use his break card instead of throwing things, hitting, or biting others when he encounters a difficult task.	Count the number of times that Malik asks for a break during regularly scheduled activities each day, until satisfied with progress; review weekly.
	During difficult but meaningful and important activities, Malik will work for increasingly longer periods of time.	For relevant activities, record the number of items completed and/or time on task. Compare growth each week, until satisfied with progress.
	Malik will use a combination of speech, pictures, and gestures to communicate; gesture and picture vocabulary will increase.	Maintain record of new vocabulary introduced. Every 3 weeks, record Malik's use of new picture or gesture vocabulary across 1 school day. Review data monthly.
Improvements in quality of life	Malik will participate more in school activities.	Using Malik's picture schedule, mark off the number of activities participated in each day; review weekly until satisfied with progress.
	Malik will enjoy and be happy in school.	Indicate in the school–home daily communication book whether Malik seems happy and which activities he enjoys. Use observed preferences to modify curriculum.
	Malik's teachers and grandparents will be satisfied with his progress.	Discuss satisfaction at each team meeting.

FIGURE 11.1. Malik's evaluation plan.

To evaluate the success of Malik's support plan, the team monitored important outcomes in three critical areas: reductions in problem behavior, increases in alternative skills, and improvements in quality of life (see Figure 11.1). Not surprisingly, the team's outcomes matched the original team goals—an indication that these measures of success indeed reflected meaningful outcomes. Mr. Rodriguez, the behavior support specialist, helped the teaching staff come up with classroom-friendly ways of recording problem behaviors and alternative skills. At the end of each week, Mr. Rodriguez helped summarize the data, and the entire team reviewed the summary information at its bimonthly meetings to evaluate progress. Interestingly, the team members elected to record the frequency of problem behavior on an ABC (antecedent–behavior–consequence) chart, so that they could constantly analyze the antecedent triggers and presumed functions of problem behavior, and thus could modify their hypotheses and support plan as needed.

After 2 months, the team was ready to add long-term supports to Malik's plan (see Figure 11.2). Because Malik seemed happy at home, lifestyle changes focused primarily on school—in particular, on making permanent changes in Malik's curriculum and transitioning him back to his neighborhood school. Malik's support plan was successful. His challenging behaviors decreased substantially and did not pose a threat to others. His communication and participation in school activities increased, and perhaps most importantly, he seemed to begin enjoying school. Considering lifestyle changes forced the team to think about what to do next. Revising Malik's curriculum emerged as a priority. The teaching staff and Malik's grandparents agreed that his current curriculum was largely constructed to avoid problem behaviors, and did not, in any cohesive way, prepare Malik to gain critical skills needed for his future. But what was his future? What did he need to learn? Traditional academics did not seem appropriate, but what did? A critical support added to Malik's plan was to develop an individualized curriculum identifying essential goals for the next 5 years, based on a preferred vision for the future. To do this, the team would engage in personal futures planning to paint a vision, and then assess the critical skill areas Malik would need to participate in that future. Malik's grandmother insisted that being included in his neighborhood school was part of his future, and asked that the school's transition coordinator be part of the planning. Planning for transition would begin immediately. A final consideration for lifestyle changes was the extent to which Malik has the opportunities to interact with nondisabled peers. This was a critical concern—not only because he would once again return to a regular school, but because the opportunities would be needed for life. In addition, Jenna and Thomas would not always be there to occupy his time. To address this issue, Malik's grandmother agreed that she would enroll Malik in after-school activities such as Boy Scouts.

After identifying lifestyle changes, the team considered strategies to sustain positive outcomes over time. Three were added to the support plan. First, the team recognized that all future teachers would need to understand critical components of Malik's behavior support plan. The transition coordinator agreed to facilitate this

Malik's Behavior Support Plan

Hypotheses:

1. When prompted through difficult work, Malik is likely to refuse/aggress, to escape the activity.
2. When asked to complete nonfunctional activities, Malik is likely to refuse/aggress, escape the activity.
3. When required to make a transition from a highly preferred activity to a nonpreferred activity, Malik refuses/aggresses, to maintain the preferred activity and avoid the nonpreferred one.

Antecedent/setting event interventions	Alternative skills	Responses to problem behavior	Long-term supports
Eliminate letter- and number-naming activities from curriculum; avoid recall in academic activities. Embed academics in functional activities; ensure meaningful outcomes. Prompt Malik to use alternative forms of communication (pictures, gestures) when he has difficulty with verbal expression. Use a daily picture schedule to mark classroom activities. Provide a transitional warning prior to ending a preferred activity. When it is necessary to transition from a preferred to a nonpreferred activity, begin activity with a brief preferred activity (e.g., math game).	*Replacement:* Teach requests for break. Make sure Malik's break cards are available; prompt him to use cards throughout the day. *Tolerance skills:* Teach working through difficult tasks; incrementally ask Malik to work a bit longer or do a few more before taking a break. *General adaptive skills:* Expand gesture and picture vocabulary. Teach incidentally through the school day. Prompt Malik to use gestures and/or pictures to expand expressions.	During difficult tasks, at the first signs of problem behavior, prompt Malik to use his break card. During transitions, do any of the following: • Use his picture schedule to show Malik he can return to the activity on another day. • Tell Malik what the upcoming activity will be. • Praise other students for lining up. Crisis management: • Remove throwable materials. • Block blows, protect others. • Escort Malik to a quiet location in the building. • Bring him back to the classroom as soon as he is calm.	*Lifestyle changes:* • **Develop an individualized curriculum that identifies essential goals, based on a preferred vision of Malik's future.** • **Begin planning for transition back to his elementary school; invite transition coordinator to team meetings.** • **Enroll Malik in after-school activities (e.g., Boy Scouts).** *Strategies to sustain support:* • **Teach future teachers about Malik's support plan; invite them to planning sessions.** • **Provide opportunities for Mrs. Nelson to learn more about embedding academic skills in meaningful activities.** • **Encourage Malik to use augmentative communication systems at home and in the community.**

FIGURE 11.2. Malik's long-term supports.

327

activity. Second, Mrs. Nelson asked for support for herself. Because she did not feel confident that she knew the best ways to embed academics in functional activities, she requested more guidance. Her building principal arranged for her to take personal inservice days to work with teachers from other schools who were skilled in this area. And, third, to ensure that Malik's communication skills would continue to expand and that be used across settings, Malik's grandparents agreed to encourage Malik to use his augmentative systems in at home and in the community.

Bethany's Long-Term Supports

The long-term supports planned by Behtany's team are shown in Figure 11.3. Bethany's mother felt that it was important to make lifestyle changes outside of school as soon as possible. She believed that the changes would make Bethany happier. Also, she felt that this would help alleviate her worries about Bethany's being unsupervised when she herself had to work late. The first thing the team did was to facilitate Bethany's enrollment in an after-school sports program. Bethany's favorite sport was volleyball, so the team searched for a volleyball league. The team located a league that practiced at the local YMCA, two blocks from the school, so Bethany could walk there after school. The league practiced on Tuesday and Thursday afternoons.

Bethany's special education teacher was able to arrange for her to have a Big Sister. The Big Sister identified was a college student named Alicia. Because Alicia was busy with classes and studying during the week, she scheduled Friday afternoons to spend with Bethany. Ms. DeLope was thrilled that a college student was identified and hoped Alicia could encourage Bethany to become serious about her schoolwork.

The only remaining days that Bethany was left alone and unsupervised were Monday and Wednesday. Mrs. Lane, the DeLopes' next-door neighbor, offered to have Bethany watch her 3-year-old for a few hours after school on these two days. Mrs. Lane usually hired a baby sitter for half a day on Wednesday afternoons so she could complete housework and run errands. Mrs. Lane suggested she could hire Bethany instead and would be willing to give her a small amount of pay. Ms. DeLope was delighted with this arrangement, and also was eager to have Bethany earn and handle money.

Finally, the general education teacher identified a "study buddy" whom Bethany could phone if she needed help with her homework in the evenings. This student, Claire, was very studious and enthusiastic about serving in this role. In fact, Claire took the initiative to suggest that she call Bethany in the evenings for the next few weeks, just to make sure she understood the homework.

After identifying lifestyle changes, the team determined ways to sustain support over time. Because Bethany would be making the transition to middle school the following school year, her current team planned to meet with her future teachers prior to the beginning of the school year to describe Bethany's support plan. In

Bethany's Behavior Support Plan

Hypotheses:

1. When Bethany is given written assignments, she engages in off-task behavior, to escape.
2. When Bethany is given lengthy assignments, she engages in off-task behavior, to escape.
3. When Bethany has visited her father over the weekend, she engages in off-task behavior, to escape work (because of fatigue).
4. When Bethany is in unstructured situations with unfamiliar peers, she engages in inappropriate interactions, to obtain their attention.

Antecedent/setting event interventions	Alternative skills	Responses to problem behavior	Long-term supports
Minimize amount of written work; provide alternative strategy for work completion (e.g., tape recorder).

Break work into small increments.

Make sure instructions are clear and explicit.

Seat Bethany near classmates in cafeteria; gradually introduce new people while prompting appropriate interactions.

Have Bethany return home earlier on Sundays after visiting her father. | *Replacement:* When independent assignments are given, teach Bethany to request assistance when she feels overwhelmed with assignments or does not understand what she is supposed to do.

General adaptive skills: Provide social skills instruction, and prompt Bethany to engage in appropriate interactions.

Tolerance skills: Gradually introduce Bethany to new people. | At the first sign of off-task behavior, prompt Bethany to request help; if behavior continues, brainstorm with Bethany to determine why the assignment is problematic.

Require Bethany to apologize to peers for inappropriate comments.

Provide all feedback quietly and discreetly. | *Lifestyle changes:*
• **Enroll Bethany in an after-school sports program.**
• **Identify a Big Sister for Bethany who can spend time with her and serve as a role model.**
• **Arrange for Bethany to stay at Mrs. Lane's house and babysit after school until her mother arrives home.**
• **Pair Bethany with a "study buddy" whom she can phone for homework help.**

Strategies to sustain support:
• **Make sure future teachers implement classroom supports.**
• **Identify support group for Bethany's mother.** |

FIGURE 11.3. Bethany's long-term supports.

329

addition, the school psychologist suggested that Ms. DeLope join a support group. She was familiar with a local group of parents with adolescent children that convened once a month. The group was very positive and proactive; its members could help Ms. DeLope (and Bethany) prepare for the transition to middle school, identify after-school activities for Bethany after her transition, and address general issues pertaining to adolescents.

Bethany's team felt confident that they had developed a support plan that reflected the functional assessment information and would provide the supports she needed in both the short and long terms. Although the team members had already come up with a way to measure short-term gains in Bethany's academic engagement and social skills, they recognized that they needed a way to monitor her progress over the long term (see Figure 11.4). It was important not only to continue measuring her engagement and social skills in a way that could be easily sustained over the long term, but also to monitor her general satisfaction and well-being. They decided to continue the direct observation of Bethany's engagement they had designed for the classroom, with the teacher monitoring her behavior every 10 minutes, but to fade the number of observations after Bethany showed adequate improvement. Once their data indicated that the support plan was effective, they would fade data collection to monthly observations. Data collection in the cafeteria, whereby the volunteer observed during two 5-minute intervals, would be continued over time, but faded to a less frequent schedule in the same way as the classroom observations. Finally, to monitor Bethany's general satisfaction with her quality of life, the school psychologist suggested scheduling weekly sessions to discuss how she was doing. The school psychologist also got permission from Bethany and her mother to have monthly contact with Bethany's volleyball coach, her Big Sister, and Mrs. Lane, to get their opinions of Bethany's progress.

Meaningful outcomes	What do we expect to happen?	How will we measure this?
Long-term and acceptable reductions in problem behaviors	Bethany will decrease off-task behaviors during academics to less than 10%.	Momentary time sampling of engagement every 10 minutes daily until goal reached; then fade to monthly observations thereafter.
	Bethany will engage in no inappropriate interactions with peers.	Two 5-minute observations, using a frequency count during lunchtime, daily until goal reached; then fade to monthly observations thereafter.
Increases in alternative skills	Bethany will engage in academic activities and request assistance as needed.	Record daily frequency of hand raising, until satisfied with progress.
	Bethany will complete all homework assignments.	Teacher will determine number of assignments completed and missing, and report to Ms. DeLope biweekly.
	Bethany will engage in appropriate interactions with new peers.	See above.
Improvements in quality of life	Bethany will participate in sporting or other activities she enjoys.	School psychologist will monitor during scheduled meetings with Bethany and will contact volleyball coach and Ms. DeLope monthly.
	Bethany will develop friendships.	School psychologist will ask Bethany to self-report and will contact Ms. DeLope and Big Sister monthly.
	Bethany will be responsible with her "job."	School psychologist will contact Mrs. Lane monthly.

FIGURE 11.4. Bethany's evaluation plan.

REFERENCES

Bambara, L. M., & Knoster, T. (1995). *Guidelines on effective behavioral support.* Harrisburg: Pennsylvania Department of Education.

Bambara, L. M., & Knoster, T. P. (1998). *Designing positive behavior support plans* (Innovations, No. 13). Washington, DC: American Association on Mental Retardation.

Brotherson, M. J. (1988). Transition into adulthood: Parental planning for sons and daughters with disabilities. *Education and Training in Mental Retardation, 23,* 165–174.

Clees, T. J. (1994). Self-recording of students' daily schedules of teachers' expectancies: Perspectives on reactivity, stimulus control, and generalization. *Exceptionality, 5,* 113–129.

Cole, C. L., & Levinson, T. R. (2002). Effects of within-activity choices on the challenging behavior of children with severe developmental disabilities. *Journal of Positive Behavior Interventions, 4,* 29–37.

Dunlap, G. (1993). Promoting generalization: Current status and functional considerations. In R. Van Houten & S. Axelrod (Eds.), *Behavior analysis and treatment* (pp. 269–296). New York: Plenum Press.

Felce, D., & Perry, J. (1995). Quality of life: Its definition and measurement. *Research in Developmental Disabilities, 16,* 51–74.

Felce, D., & Perry, J. (1996). Assessment of quality of life. In R. L. Schalock (Ed.), *Quality of life: Vol. 1. Conceptualization and measurement* (pp. 91–104). Washington, DC: American Association on Mental Retardation.

Ferro, J., & Dunlap, G. (1993). Generalization and maintenance. In M. Smith (Ed.), *Behavior modification for exceptional children and youth* (pp. 190–211). Boston: Andover.

Frederickson, N., & Turner, J. (2002). Utilizing the classroom peer group to address children's social needs: An evaluation of the Circle of Friends intervention approach. *Journal of Special Education, 36,* 234–245.

Ingham, R. J. (1982). The effects of self-evaluation training on maintenance and generalization during stuttering treatment. *Journal of Speech and Hearing Disorders, 47,* 271–280.

Kincaid, D., Knoster, T., Harrower, J., Shannon, P., & Bustamante, S. (2002). Measuring the impact of positive behavior support. *Journal of Positive Behavior Interventions, 4,* 109–118.

McAdam, D. B. (1993). Self-monitoring and verbal feedback to reduce stereotypic body rocking in a congenitally blind adult. *Review, 24,* 163–172.

McDougall, D., & Brady, M. P. (1998). Initiating and fading self-management interventions to increase math fluency in general education classes. *Exceptional Children, 64,* 151–166.

Meyer, L., & Janney, R. (1989). User-friendly measures of meaningful outcomes: Evaluating behavioral interventions. *Journal of The Association for Persons with Severe Handicaps, 14,* 263–270.

Mount, B. (1987). Person futures planning: Finding directions for change. *Dissertation Abstracts International, 48*(8), 2158A. (UMI No. AAT 8724642)

Mount, B., & Zwernik, K. (1988). *It's never too early, it's never too late: A booklet about personal futures planning for persons with developmental disabilities, their families and friends, case managers, service providers, and advocates* (Publication No. 42-88-109). St. Paul, MN: Governor's Council on Developmental Disabilities.

Munk, D. D., & Repp, A. C. (1994). The relationship between instructional variables and problem behavior: A review. *Exceptional Children, 60,* 390–401.

Nehring, W. M. (1990). *Transition needs for children with chronic illness into adulthood: Alleviating the concerns of families with information and knowledge.* Lanham, MD: Education Research Information Center. (ERIC Document Reproduction Service No. ED326025)

Newman, B. (1995). Self-management of schedule following in three teenagers with autism. *Behavioral Disorders, 20,* 190–196.

O'Brien, J., Mount, B., & O'Brien, C. (1990). *The personal profile.* Lithonia, GA: Responsive Systems Associates.

Pearpoint, J., O'Brien, J., & Forest, M. (1996). *Planning alternative tomorrows with hope: A workbook for planning possible and positive futures.* Toronto: Inclusion Press.

Peterson, S., Caniglia, C., & Royster, A. J. (2001). Application of choice-making intervention for a student with multiply maintained problem behavior. *Focus on Autism and Other Developmental Disabilities, 16,* 240–246.

Pierce, K. L., & Schreibman, L. (1994). Teaching daily living skills to children with autism in unsupervised settings through pictorial self-management. *Journal of Applied Behavior Analysis, 27,* 471–481.

Schalock, R. L., Bonham, G. S., & Marchand, C. B. (2000). Consumer based quality of life assessment: A path model of perceived satisfaction. *Evaluation and Program Planning, 23,* 77–87.

Seybert, S., Dunlap, G., & Ferro, J. (1996). The effects of choice-making on the problem behaviors of high school students with intellectual disabilities. *Journal of Behavioral Education, 6,* 49–65.

Smull, M. (1997). *A blueprint for essential lifestyle planning.* Napa, CA: Allen, Shea.

Stahmer, A. C., & Schreibman, L. (1992). Teaching children with autism appropriate play in unsupervised environments using a self-management treatment package. *Journal of Applied Behavior Analysis, 25,* 447–459.

Vandercook, T., York, J., & Forest, M. (1989). The McGill Action Planning System (MAPS): A strategy for building the vision. *Journal of The Association for Persons with Severe Handicaps, 14,* 205–215.

Vaughn, B. J., & Horner, R. H. (1997). Identifying instructional tasks that occasion problem behaviors and assessing the effects of student versus teacher choice among these tasks. *Journal of Applied Behavior Analysis, 30,* 299–312.

CHAPTER 12

◆ ◆ ◆

Extending Behavior Support in Home and Community Settings

◆

LYNN KERN KOEGEL
ROBERT L. KOEGEL
MENDY BOETTCHER
LAUREN BROOKMAN-FRAZEE

CASE HISTORIES

We begin this chapter by introducing two new case examples.

Juanita

Juanita was a 5-year-old Hispanic girl diagnosed with autism. Her symptoms were archetypal—delayed communication, social isolation, and repetitive play with a limited number of toys. Juanita's mother attended parent education classes, where she learned procedures to encourage Juanita to communicate her needs. As a result of her mother's diligence in prompting expressive words, Juanita's disruptive behaviors greatly decreased, and she was able to use short phrases to express her needs and desires. Juanita demonstrated steady and consistent progress, but all of that changed when her little sister was born. Juanita took little interest in her sister throughout the day, but her mother reported that every meal was interrupted by disruptive and aggressive behavior. She said that family meals were miserable and they had not been able to enjoy a meal for months.

Jimmy

Jimmy, a 4-year-old European American boy, was also diagnosed with autism. Jimmy's father worked outside of the home, and his mother stayed at home with him. Like Juanita's mother, Jimmy's mother participated in a parent education program and learned how to prompt communication throughout the day. As a result, Jimmy's behavior problems decreased, and he regularly used short phrases to communicate his needs and wants. However, when Jimmy's brother was born, there was a significant increase in his problem behavior. Although he had had tantrums in the past, he had never been aggressive until the baby was born. At first, Jimmy appeared to be bothered by the infant's crying—a sound that many people find annoying. He covered his ears and left the room. This adaptive response seemed to work fine in most situations.

As the baby grew, Jimmy continued to use his adaptive strategies, but not all of them worked in every situation. For example, car rides with both children were a problem. Jimmy found the crying unbearable, and since he was unable to leave the car, he began lashing out at the infant. He pinched and hit his brother. Of course, that did not stop the crying; it only made it worse. Jimmy's mother threatened him, yelled at him, and reprimanded him, but nothing worked. At times she reported that she even had to pull the car over to calm the baby down after Jimmy hit him. Further and more intense aggression was observed when the baby brother began to crawl. Fascinated with toys, on occasion he took one of Jimmy's. Jimmy pushed his brother to keep him away from the toys, and shortly afterward he began pushing the baby every time he got near the toy area.

These examples illustrate the diverse challenges experienced by families of children with disabilities. Working with such families in home and community settings necessitates considering a number of variables in order to assure that supports are acceptable, they can be implemented easily, and that they are effective in both the short and long terms. This chapter discusses a number of important variables that improve the likelihood of "goodness of fit" when teams are providing comprehensive support to families of children with disabilities in home and community settings. Home–school coordination is desirable and beneficial for all children, with and without disabilities. However, the need for a behavior support plan in the home depends on many variables, such as the settings where problem behaviors occur, the intensity of the problem behavior, the skill and consistency of parents in delivering interventions, and so forth. Following a discussion of family support and general areas to consider in working with families, specific steps for developing a plan for home and community settings are discussed. Finally, the cases of Juanita and Jimmy—two young children for whom we developed home-based support plans—are described further.

UNDERSTANDING THE CONTEXT OF FAMILY SUPPORT

Overview of Family Support Issues

Over the years, the literature in the areas of disabilities and positive behavior support (PBS) suggests that family members are crucial components who must be considered in the development and implementation of support programs for children with disabilities (Dunlap & Robbins, 1991; Dunst & Trivette, 1994; Dunst, Trivette, & Deal, 1994; Lucyshyn, Albin, & Nixon, 1997; Prizant & Wetherby, 1989; Singer & Irvin, 1991; Turnbull, Blue-Banning, Turbiville, & Park, 1999; Vaughn, Clarke, & Dunlap, 1997). Recommendations for family support have been made by many family support movements, such as the Family Resource Coalition; by the U.S. Department of Health and Human Services; and in laws dating back to the Education of the Handicapped Act Amendments of 1986 (P.L. 99-457; Dunst & Trivette, 1994). In addition, most well-established intervention programs, such as those for children with autism, have a family component, which usually involves some form of parent education and other types of family support. Some examples of programs and models with this component include the Treatment and Education of Autistic and related Communication handicapped CHildren (TEACCH) program (Schopler, 1989), the early intervention model used by Prizant and Wetherby (1989), the May Center's model (Campbell et al., 1998), Pivotal Response Intervention (Koegel, Koegel, Harrower, & Carter, 1999), and Learning Experiences: An Alternative Program for Preschoolers and Parents (LEAP; Strain & Hoyson, 2000). Furthermore, a survey of "experts" in the field of autism found that family support and family and child involvement in community programs emerged as areas that are important to address in intervention and research (Pfeiffer & Nelson, 1992). Clearly, comprehensive programming across settings is needed.

Lucyshyn and Albin (1993) have proposed several family support best-practice themes, which are also endorsed elsewhere in the literature. These include (1) the importance of understanding the ecology of the family; (2) the development of collaborative partnerships between parents and professionals (Dunlap & Robbins, 1991; Turnbull et al., 1999); (3) the identification of family strengths and the child's positive contributions; (4) the development of standards and practices that strengthen family members and build on their existing skills and resources (Dunst, Trivette, & Deal, 1994; Lucyshyn et al., 1997); and (5) the identification of sources of stress for the family (Singer & Irvin, 1991). Many researchers have noted the importance of such practices in enabling and empowering families (Dunst & Trivette, 1994; Dunst et al., 1994; Robbins, Dunlap, & Plienis, 1991; Ruef, Turnbull, Turnbull, & Poston, 1999; Singer & Irvin, 1991; Turnbull et al., 1999). Specifically, family empowerment is an important area of focus in this literature (Dunst et al., 1994). Enabling the family in this manner emphasizes the importance of viewing the family members as members of the support team and as "experts" in their own right. In short, PBS also focuses on support for the family, not just the child. This in turn helps family members support their child in meaningful and productive ways.

Variables Affecting Family Members' Response and Adjustment to Disability

The literature on family support interventions posits that a family's overall response to the circumstances presented by having a child with a disability will result from the interaction of many variables (Robbins et al., 1991; Turnbull & Ruef, 1997). These variables may include "social dynamics with the family unit, cognitive appraisal and coping strategies, practical resources, and social support from outside the family" (Singer & Irvin, 1991, p. 291). Therefore, intervention must take all these variables into account, and must have a family-oriented focus (as opposed to an individual-child-oriented focus), if it is to be successful in reducing family stress, enhancing coping, promoting skill development, and empowering families in general. Incorporation of ecocultural theory (Gallimore, Weisner, Kaufman, & Bernheimer, 1989) is important as well, since consideration of variables related to culture, values, and family priorities is crucial in developing support plans that exemplify "goodness of fit." That is, effective family support considers the particular family's unique environment, as well as its cultural values. This will enhance the success of child interventions.

A particularly critical area that warrants consideration is the family members' emotional reaction to having a child with a disability. Family members, by necessity, make adjustments in their daily routines to accommodate the special needs of a child with a disability. Regardless of how they may negotiate the logistics of their daily routines, however, they often experience a number of negative emotional responses to caring for such a child. Family members (including siblings) of persons with a variety of disabilities may experience higher than average incidences of family stress and depression (Bristol, Gallagher, & Holt, 1993; Singer & Irvin, 1991). Many sources of stress are associated with raising a child with special needs, all of which may influence family members' adjustment to the disability. Receiving the initial diagnosis of a disability can be both surprising and stressful for parents. An added source of stress may be uncertainty about the cause of the disability. Furthermore, child characteristics may affect stress levels in parents. For example, more severe disabilities require a greater amount of effort on the part of care providers, thereby influencing stress. Many parents also report a critical lack of trained personnel with whom they feel comfortable leaving their children, which in itself often causes clinical levels of stress among parents (Koegel et al., 2002; Moes, 1995; Moes, Koegel, Schreibman, & Loos, 1992). When one considers the increased responsibilities involved in caring for a child with disabilities, coupled with the lack of acceptance that still persists in mainstream American society, it is no wonder that many primary caregivers in particular report higher levels of stress related to their children's symptoms, increased levels of isolation, greater health issues such as fatigue and illness, and more depression than parents of typically developing children do.

Community reactions to persons with disabilities also influence the context in which the family lives. Generally, the more severe a child's symptoms, the more isolated parents are likely to be from the community, because people do not typically know how to react to an individual with a severe disability. Turnbull and Ruef (1997) examined parents' perspectives on lifestyle issues and support for children with problem behavior, in relation to inclusion issues. The parent interviews revealed several themes regarding inclusion of their child across environments. For instance, parents reported that it was nearly impossible for them to participate in preferred religious activities, for reasons including attitudes and competencies of religious staff, the formal and structured nature of the services, and difficulty in obtaining age-appropriate groupings. Religious involvement can be a source of community support; however, when participation is difficult, it may lead to more social isolation.

In addition, when looking specifically at family members' relationships with the child, parents consistently commented on sibling relationships. Parents reported that specific challenges included lack of a close bond between the child with problem behavior and his or her siblings, frustration or embarrassment, and resentment about the amount of time and attention devoted to the sibling with problem behavior.

Still another source of stress concerns transition issues as a child moves into adulthood. Parents of a child with a disability may be concerned about their child's move out of the house, self-sufficiency, and marriage. The caregiving responsibilities of these parents are more likely to continue into adulthood. This leads to concern about what will happen to the child after the parents are unable to care for him or her.

Parent and Family Empowerment

The concept of *parent and family empowerment* is an important goal and outcome of support programs (Mahoney et al., 1999; Turnbull & Turnbull, 2000). Although *empowerment* has traditionally referred to advocacy, the term now refers to parents' and other family members' collaboratively participating in their child's behavior support. An empowered parent is one who demonstrates confidence and effectiveness in teaching his or her child, successfully manages daily routines, interacts well with school personnel and other service providers, and is able to obtain services for the child (Koren, DeChillo, & Friesen, 1992). Conversely, an unempowered parent may exhibit behaviors and attitudes that reflect frustration, stress, depression, helplessness, and overall dependence on professionals. Interventions aimed to empower parents enable them to acquire competencies to solve problems, meet their needs, and attain family goals. Some hypothesize that empowering parents will lead to greater child gains. In fact, studies have shown that interventions that utilize parent participation, wherein parents take an active role in intervention implementation, result in greater child improvement and increased generalization of treatment gains (Koegel, Koegel, & Schreibman, 1991).

Parent–Professional Partnerships

The *parent–professional partnership* model of support is an approach that aims to empower parents. Such a partnership includes jointly developing a support plan that will fit into the family's daily routines, as well as an emphasis on family choice and decision making. That is, not only are parents (or other primary caregivers) involved in developing the supports, but they are also the ultimate decision makers in goals and implementation (Allen & Petr, 1996). It is hypothesized that interventions developed in this way are more likely to be competently and consistently implemented. Dunst and Paget (1991) have defined a parent–professional partnership as a relationship between family members and professionals who work collaboratively, using agreed-upon roles and common goals. Lucyshyn, Horner, Dunlap, Albin, and Ben (2002) have provided a comprehensive definition of collaborative partnerships with families in the context of PBS interventions:

> [Such a partnership involves] the establishment of a truly respectful, trusting, caring, and reciprocal relationship in which interventionists and family members believe in each other's ability to make important contributions to the support process; share their knowledge and expertise; and mutually influence the selection of goals, and design of behavior support plans. . . . the traditional expert–client dichotomy is transferred into an equal partnership in which fam-

ily members and practitioners offer complementary expertise, solve problems together. . . . (p. 12)

Overall, this type of partnership involves professionals supporting parents in problem solving related to the child, rather than directly solving problems for the parents. Whereas parent educators should be responsible for assuring that parents have specific skills and techniques designated to help their child, the parents are responsible for choosing how the techniques are applied in their particular family (Turnbull et al., 1999; Turnbull & Turnbull, 2000). In a partnership between parents and professionals, the professionals may be the "experts" in particular procedures, while the parents are the "experts" on their own child and should be responsible in deciding how the procedures are incorporated into the family's daily routines. Table 12.1 provides examples of ways that professionals can structure their interactions with parents so that they reflect a true partnership, rather than being directed by the professionals.

Now that we have discussed general issues regarding parenting of a child with disabilities, there are a number of considerations that will enhance the PBS process and the effectiveness of a support plan. These are presented below, followed by specific suggestions for developing home-based support programs.

CONSIDERATIONS FOR FACILITATING COLLABORATION WITH FAMILIES IN PBS PROGRAMS

Consideration 1: Has an Alliance with the Family Been Established?

Establishing an alliance with the family is critical before a behavior support plan can be implemented (Dunlap & Robbins, 1991; Dunst & Trivette, 1994; Lucyshyn & Albin, 1993). This process necessitates ongoing and open communication with and feedback from the family. Finding a good match between professionals and family members is also an important consideration. Specifically, cultural and linguistic issues should be considered; matching people who are of similar cultural and linguistic backgrounds is likely to result in a more appropriate support plan. When this is not possible, the professionals should educate themselves regarding the culture of the family (see Consideration 4, below). Similarly, some families have a preference for male or female professionals. Finally, personality matches have been reported to be important to families. Some family members report that their child responds better to very animated, outgoing persons

TABLE 12.1. Examples of Professional Directed Interaction versus Parent–Professional Partnership in Parent Education

Goal	Professional directed interaction	Parent–professional partnership
Identification of naturally occurring opportunities for language during parent education session	Professional: "It looks like John is interested in playing with the ball. Let's try having him say 'ball' for you to throw it to him."	Professional: "It looks like John is interested in playing with the ball. What opportunity for language would you like to target in this activity?" If the parent needs more specific suggestions, the clinician may add: "There are a number of choices, such as . . . what would you like to try?"
Identification of naturally occurring opportunities in the family's daily routines	Professional: "You can use the same techniques at home by having Katie make a verbal attempt for 'juice' before giving her juice when she expresses interest."	Professional: "It is useful for you to identify opportunities for Katie to make verbal attempts throughout the day. Can you identify any opportunities that would fit in your daily routines?"
Setting of parent education session	Professional: "I think that it will be helpful for us to have a few sessions at home, since that is where you spend most of the time with your child."	Professional: " Where do you think it would be most helpful for the sessions to occur?" Or "We have a couple of options for the setting of our sessions . . . which of these would be most useful to you?"
Identification of target behaviors	Professional: "I think that we should first work on labels of your child's most highly desired activities, such as . . . "	Professional: "Do you have any words that your family finds particularly important for your child to learn?" Or "We often start by targeting . . . which of these would be the most appropriate and useful for your family and your routines?"
Points targeted for feedback	Professional: "Let's focus on maintenance tasks today."	Professional: "Which of the points in the manual that we have covered would you like to focus on today?"

who enjoy gross motor activities, while others report that they prefer calmer and quieter individuals. In short, establishing an alliance with the family so that a program provides a good "match" for a family is likely to enhance the overall effectiveness of the program (Koegel et al., 2002).

Consideration 2: Does the Team Understand the Family's Priorities?

Goals for intervention should be based on the family's priorities combined with the assessment information, and should be mutually agreed upon by professionals and family members. Mutual goals are most likely to be pursued by the family members, since they will be motivated to attain these goals. Likewise, professionals are most likely to be invested in certain goals if they see them as important for the child or individual with a disability.

Research has repeatedly shown that supports addressing goals that are not coordinated with the family members, or that the family members do not consider to be of value, will not be implemented or maintained over time (Steibel, 1999). Support plans that are not coordinated across environments can be ineffective. For example, Dunlap, Koegel, and Koegel (1984) demonstrated that toilet training pursued in individual settings (e.g., school or home) without systematic efforts to coordinate training across environments were minimally effective. In contrast, programs that offer a continuity of intervention across environments may enjoy rapid and durable success. Again, this points to the importance of developing goals as a team, so that there is "buy-in" from all participants.

Consideration 3: Can Supports Be Incorporated into Family Routines?

It is critical that the support strategies to be carried out by family members can be incorporated into existing family routines. Parents of children with disabilities report increased stress and difficulty implementing support strategies that require them to set aside time to work with their children in a one-on-one format. In contrast, when interventions can be incorporated into daily routines, families report a reduction in their stress levels and increases in teaching episodes (Koegel & Koegel, 1995; Moes & Frea, 2000; Steibel, 1999). However, this process necessitates extensive and ongoing collaboration and alliance with a family. An alliance must be established wherein the professionals and the family members are able to determine the family's values and priorities, have a good feel for the family's daily activities, and develop a plan that does not result in added stress and is coordinated across all care providers.

Consideration 4: Does the Team Understand the Family's Culture?

An important aspect of PBS is to consider the child in the context of his or her family, community, and culture (Koegel, Koegel, & Smith, 1997). In order to conduct a culturally appropriate assessment, it may be important to include (in addition to the immediate family) the extended family, as well as any others (godparents, etc.) who play an important role in the child's life. It is essential to determine the presenting problem *in the eyes of the family*. What are the family's expectations for the child? In addition, when a team is designing support plans, it is critical to assess individual needs of the family related to resources and constraints. For example, does the family have special language needs? Is a translator needed so that all identified participants can be included in the intervention planning? Is transportation needed? Families' cultural values have largely been ignored in behavior intervention programs, and most parent education programs have been developed and evaluated primarily with families of European American backgrounds (Forehand & Kotchick, 1996). Again, goals will be more likely to be implemented and maintained over time if each family's unique cultural needs are considered.

Another important area relating to cultural values is the perception of the presence of a "disability." In other words, many cultures do not perceive a "disability" in an extremely negative light, and therefore may not experience the sense of need or urgency for intervention services (Santarelli, Koegel, Casas, & Koegel, 2001). This is in contrast to the issues of stress described above (it should be noted that the research cited in the earlier description was again conducted primarily with European American families). Although early intervention is recommended, the degree of the problem and parental motivation for intervention may vary with the stress level of a family, and culture may play a large role in a family's stress level.

Consideration 5: Have the Family's Strengths Been Assessed?

In addition to assessing the specific goals for the family and possible constraints on implementing the support plan, it is useful to identify strengths that can be used as a foundation for the support plan. For example, does the family have a strong social support network? Does the family participate in community activities? Does the family have strong collaborative relationships with other treatment providers? What are strengths that individual family members can contribute? For instance, one child we worked with had great needs in social areas. We developed an intervention program that focused on developing relationships outside the school setting.

The family invited children over for regular play dates. However, within a short period of time, the father (who was the primary after-school care provider) began canceling the play dates. Upon closer inspection, we learned that he did not enjoy the activities in which the children engaged after school. Once we collaboratively developed a list of activities with him—which included outdoor activities he preferred and was good at, such as rock climbing at a local gym, hiking, going to the park, and bike riding—he resumed the play dates.

DEVELOPING AND IMPLEMENTING A SUPPORT PLAN

Intervention within a PBS framework is comprehensive and long-term (see Chapter 1; see also Horner & Carr, 1997). Risley (1996) has noted that behavior change that leaves a child in an isolated or restricted life is a hollow accomplishment. Thus the need for comprehensive, family-centered support is clear. A support plan must facilitate the individual's participation in a variety of family and community settings. Because community inclusion, contextual fit for families, family empowerment, and improvement in quality of life are key features of PBS, a comprehensive approach with these goals is necessary to fulfill the mission of this model.

Within the five broad steps of the PBS process as described in this book, there are several smaller strategies with particular emphasis on family contexts, which we have outlined in the sections to follow. These substeps include (1) assessment of behavior and context; (2) collaboratively developing and evaluating the interventions and goals; (3) assessment of the parent–professional partnership; (4) evaluating the goodness of fit of interventions; (5) considering the social validity and long-term importance of the goals; (6) follow-up and ongoing program assessment/monitoring; and (7) assessment of the fit of interventions within the family's daily life.

Step 1: Assessment of Behavior and Context

Importance of Assessment

Assessment in the context of family and community takes on a larger unit of analysis and a greater number of settings (Carr et al., 1999, 2002; Lucyshyn, Olson, & Horner, 1995). This broader scope of assessment is important for understanding the complex roles of the family and community. In addition to traditional functional assessment methods, Carr et al. (2002) propose that one important tool may be focus group methodology (not just the use of experts) for assessment of key variables. That is, in carrying out assessment, just as with intervention, it is important to develop a partnership among all involved members of the intervention team, such that each can learn from the others. In contrast to more traditional methods of assessment (in which an "expert" gives tests or does observations and presents data to others involved), PBS emphasizes the need for assessment tools that are more user-friendly and pragmatic, so that reliance on "experts" will decrease and the use of assessments by other stakeholders will increase. Some examples of these procedures are discussed below.

Collecting Functional Assessment and Baseline Data

With any behavior support plan, it is important first to collect data on the behavior for the purpose of establishing how often the behavior occurs, where it occurs, under what circumstances, and for what purpose (as described in Chapters 5 and 6). These data are important for several reasons. First, the literature notes that successful intervention planning is always based on functional assessment data (Dunlap, Kern-Dunlap, Clarke, & Robbins, 1991; Groden, Groden, & Stevenson, 1997; Horner, 2000; Horner & Carr, 1997; Lucyshyn & Albin, 1993; Lucyshyn et al., 1997). Second, during the later steps of reevaluating the intervention and its progress, it is important to have baseline data to which the intervention data can be compared, so that progress can be monitored systematically rather than haphazardly.

There are many ways to collect baseline data. Frequency data (how many times the behavior occurs in a time period) and percent occurrence (of specified time intervals, how many contain the behavior) are two of the most common. Whichever method is chosen, it is worthwhile to consider how functional assessment procedures can be incorporated into the process, so that collecting baseline data and completing behavioral assessments can be done simultaneously, if possible. Maximizing efficiency in this manner is important, because data collection can be intrusive and labor-intensive for families. Checklists (e.g., Frea, Koegel, & Koegel, 1994) are an example of one way in which both frequency and functional assessment data can be collected at the same time. If behaviors recorded over a specified time period are noted on this checklist, along with the antecedents and consequences of those behaviors, these data can be used both as assessment data (to determine functions of behaviors) and as baseline data (to evaluate current rates for future comparison with intervention rates).

Functional assessment places the focus on environmental events and considers carefully the role that such events play in eliciting, reinforcing, and maintaining problem behavior (Horner & Carr, 1997). Thus, challenging behavior is not viewed as a result of something within the individual;

rather, it is seen as the "result of challenging social situations for which the problem behavior itself represents an attempted solution" (Horner & Carr, 1997, p. 85). This focus on assessment leads to the emphasis on redesigning environments and teaching skills to the individual, as opposed to controlling/managing the person and his or her behaviors. In this way, these data can be used to directly inform support planning. All members of the team or partnership can and should be involved in carrying out these and similar procedures. It is important to note that such procedures are easily learned by "nonexpert" individuals, such as family members, and should be taught when appropriate.

Ecocultural Assessment

Another important aspect of assessment when working in parent–professional partnerships is consideration of ecocultural variables occurring in the natural context in which the individual functions (Lucyshyn & Albin, 1993; Lucyshyn et al., 1995, 1997). These assessments are geared toward understanding the child from both a developmental and an ecological perspective (Fox, Dunlap, & Philbrick, 1997). Specifically, if interventions are to take ecocultural factors into account, careful assessment of such factors must be considered. Ecocultural variables that may be important to assess include socioeconomic status (SES), family values, beliefs about parenting, philosophies on education and inclusion, number of family members living in the household, constraints on the parents' time, and many more. Some formalized measures for assessment in this area, such as the Ecocultural Family Interview (EFI; Weiner, Koots, Bernheimer, & Arzubiaga, 1997), have been developed for use in this area (Albin, Lucyshyn, Horner, & Flannery, 1996). Additional measures have been developed for use in assessing "goodness of fit" once intervention plans have been formulated (Koegel, Koegel, & Dunlap, 1996). These are discussed in the section on evaluating the fit of intervention within daily routines.

Step 2: Collaboratively Developing and Evaluating the Interventions and Goals

Once the assessment has been completed, these data can be used to inform support planning. The specifics of supports are beyond the scope of this chapter and are described in detail elsewhere in this book; however, some broad categories of interventions typical for home and community settings are outlined in Table 12.2.

After the support plan is up and running, regular, planned reevaluation of specific interventions and goals is necessary to assure that they are still relevant and important to both the family and the individual with the

TABLE 12.2. Specific Types of PBS Interventions Relevant for the Home and Community

Type of supports	Examples	Citations
Antecedent modifications	• Modified routines • Scheduled activities • Self-help strategies (e.g., scheduled bedtime activities) • Strategic placement of items in environment	Dunlap et al. (1991); Horner & Carr (1997); Koegel, Steibel, & Koegel (1998); Lucyshyn et al. (1995)
Skill building or teaching alternative skills	• Functional communication training • Play skills • Social interaction skills • Self-care • Mobility • Problem solving • Regulation of personal physiology	Carr et al. (1999); Dunlap & Robbins (1991); Fox et al. (1997); Horner & Carr (1997); Lucyshyn & Albin (1993); Lucyshyn et al. (1997); Wetherby & Prizant (1992)
Response interventions	• Systematic reinforcement of appropriate behavior • Redirect to appropriate behavior	Horner & Carr (1997); Lucyshyn & Albin (1993); Lucyshyn et al. (1997)
Long-term family support	• Facilitation of social inclusion/ participation in family activities • Education/information sharing • Respite care • Training in behavioral techniques • Counseling/emotional support • Advocacy • Personal futures planning	Fox et al. (1997); Lucyshyn & Albin (1993); Lucyshyn et al. (1997)

disability. Adjustments to plans may be needed to increase the feasibility of implementation. That is, the "kinks" may need to be addressed in any plan. One very helpful way to accomplish this goal is to have regularly scheduled meetings with *all* members of the child's team (see Chapters 4 and 11). These meetings should ideally be scheduled to accommodate all stakeholders, particularly the family. It is suggested that a plan be made in advance for regularly scheduled meetings, rather than the "wait and see" method that so many teams rely on. It is our experience that if the team decides to wait and see how the intervention goes before calling a meeting, the meeting only gets called once a behavioral crisis has occurred. At this point the focus of the meeting becomes crisis intervention, rather than evaluation of many important variables (such as progress, goodness of fit, ongoing relevance of goals, etc.). By having a meeting schedule, team members can evaluate these important variables on an ongoing basis and can deal with problem behaviors proactively (i.e., before they occur), rather than only after a crisis has occurred. The next four steps (Steps 3–6) include areas that may be helpful to address during these ongoing scheduled team meetings.

Step 3: Assessment of the Parent–Professional Partnership

Once a behavior support program is implemented, assessment of the ongoing parent–professional partnership continues to be of critical concern. Below are some questions compiled from the literature that may help in evaluating whether a partnership has been established with the parents or other primary caregivers (Dunlap & Robbins, 1991; Dunst, Trivette, & Deal, 1994; Lucyshyn & Albin, 1993; Singer & Irvin, 1991; Turnbull et al., 1999):

1. Are the parents being viewed as the "experts" regarding their child?
2. Are the family members being regarded as resources and sources of strength for the child, rather than as persons who do not contribute to or who hinder intervention?
3. Are the goals in line with what the family members have expressed is important to them over time? Does the family agree with all of the goals? Does the family have goals that are not being addressed?
4. Are the intervention settings important to the family? Are there any settings that are not being addressed?
5. Do the family members continue to view the goals as "doable" within their daily routines? Does incorporation of these goals into daily routines increase or decrease family stress?
6. Are there any areas/sources of family stress that are not being addressed (e.g., need for respite, desire for a certain type of service, parent education, etc.)?
7. Is the emphasis on "fixing" the ecology rather than the child or family, and thereby on empowering the family?
8. Are cultural and SES factors being taken into consideration (e.g., language barriers, need for transportation, location of meetings, the family's view of the disability, etc.)?

Step 4: Evaluating the "Goodness of Fit" of Interventions

As discussed elsewhere in this chapter and book, contextual fit affects the likelihood that an intervention will be implemented successfully (Horner, 2000; Lucyshyn et al., 1997). Horner (2000) has suggested that support is less likely to be carried out if family or staff members consider it to (1) be cruel/dehumanizing, (2) be unlikely to be effective, (3) include procedures that they do not know how to perform, (4) require time and equipment that they do not have, or (5) place them at risk of reprimand or abandonment by supervisors. In addition, support must "work" for everyone involved, and the goal in support planning is to devise a plan that is technically sound and is also a good "fit" with the values, skills, and resources of people within a particular setting (Horner, 2000). When team members are evaluating the goodness of fit of interventions, it may be helpful to consider some or all of these areas.

It is also important to evaluate the extent to which supports can feasibly be incorporated into the family's daily routines. In particular, will incorporation of supports into routines constitute a burden for the family? If an intervention procedure is considered a burden, it has likely not been well incorporated into their routine. This area is discussed further in Step 7.

Step 5: Considering the Social Validity and Long-Term Importance of the Goals

PBS plans and in-home programs always need to consider the "big picture." It is often stated that quality of life as an outcome measure (rather than changes in discrete behavioral variables) is a major and important focus of PBS (see Chapter 11; see also Carr et al., 2002). Although professionals may be helping parents learn procedures of presenting clear instructions and reinforcement, they also need to think on the global level. Questions Risley (1996) has discussed as important include the following:

- How are the child and family doing overall and over time?
- Are all family members happy, satisfied, and safe?
- Does the person have a stable home? Does the person have family and friends on which to base her or his life and future, and after whom to model her or his ways?
- Is the child independent, productive, and included in family activities?
- Is the child a participating member of the family?
- Is the person continuing to develop new interests, new friends, and new skills?

Team members often focus on individual target behaviors, such as reductions in self-injury, rather than considering the relative degree of importance of what they are teaching. The importance of such thinking in the long term is critical.

Step 6: Follow-Up and Ongoing Program Assessment/Monitoring

As discussed above under Step 2, it is important to continue monitoring the program once the initial intervention has been implemented. In addition to following the guidelines for setting up regular team meetings, several other important steps may be helpful. First, continuing assessment of the areas mentioned thus far (the partnership, goodness of fit of interventions, long-term importance/social validity of goals) will be important in maintaining a viable, successful intervention program. It is also important to note that periodically the team may need to return to Step 1 (assessment). Often as individuals make progress, new behaviors emerge, skills are acquired or are no longer relevant (e.g., using picture cards once a child learns to talk), environmental changes occur (e.g., a family move or the birth of a new sibling), and many other variables change (and therefore cause changes to antecedents and consequences). All such changes necessitate ongoing assessment. At these times it may not be enough to meet and discuss progress, goals, and the like, because further systematic assessment may be required. It is important to emphasize that these steps are actually a cycle that will need to be repeated periodically with involvement from all members of the team.

Step 7: Assessment of the Fit of Interventions within the Family's Daily Life

When team members are designing intervention programs, it is important to assess the fit of interventions and supports into the family's daily lives. Are the family members likely to implement behavior plans when the professionals are not present? The perceived demands of programs will influence the family's likelihood of following through with plans. This can be evaluated behaviorally, by assessing whether the family is actually implementing the support plan, and through discussions during ongoing interactions. In addition, if goals are developed with consideration for the family members' cultural values and their priorities for their child, the likelihood of long-term maintenance is improved (Koegel, Steibel, & Koegel, 1998).

JUANITA'S IN-HOME BEHAVIOR SUPPORT PLAN

We now return to Juanita to illustrate how a support plan was developed for her home. The first step in Juanita's program was to assess the situation and to evaluate rates of the problem behavior, prior to implementing the support plan. According to Juanita's mother, dinnertime was a problem. In addition, the family members expressed that they did not feel comfortable having someone in the home during family dinners. In respecting the family's wishes for privacy during the dinner hour, we attempted to collect data without being there in person. The family members expressed their willingness to set up a video camera and turn it on prior to each meal, so data from each videotape were analyzed the following day.

The videotape analysis indicated that Juanita's aggressive behavior had a number of antecedents or triggers. The first trigger occurred during "down time." Juanita's mother seated the two children at the table while she finished her last-minute meal preparations and placed the food on the table. During this period of time, there was a high likelihood of aggression and disruption. Second, Juanita's baby sister had a metal tray on her highchair, which she frequently banged with her spoon. This noise always caused Juanita to become aggressive toward her sister. Third, the baby had begun to make communicative noises, which regularly caused aggression also. Another thing we noted was the proximity of the two children. During meals, Juanita's mother placed her next to her baby sister's high chair.

Mealtime therefore required a multicomponent intervention. First were some antecedent interventions. During discussions in our initial meeting to develop a plan, the family members indicated that in their garage they had another highchair with a plastic tray. The family replaced the metal tray with the plastic tray, which greatly reduced the noise that irritated Juanita. Second, when Juanita's mother realized that "down time" was a problem, she felt that it would be easy to wait until dinner was served to bring the children to the table. This eliminated a period of time when aggression was frequent. Juanita's parents also moved the high chair to the other side of the table, so that it was not physically possible for Juanita to assault the baby.

Second, a teaching component was implemented. In order to deal with the baby's communicative noises, Juanita was taught to respond differently to the vocalizations. Her parents prompted her to try to figure out what the baby was saying, instead of hitting the baby when she vocalized. The parents actually came up with many humorous examples, such as "Juanita, do you think Bonita is saying, 'I don't want Barney for dinner'?" We continued to analyze the videotapes after the support plan was in place, and after a short period of time, the aggression was completely eliminated. Furthermore, the intervention seemed to result in a lifestyle change for the family: We noted that the father was not home for dinner during many of the baseline tapes, but that after the aggression was eliminated, the father was always home and eating with the family at the table. Likewise, the family showed negative and neutral affect during baseline sessions, but showed positive affect during meals after the aggression had been eliminated.

JIMMY'S IN-HOME AND COMMUNITY BEHAVIOR SUPPORT PLAN[1]

Jimmy's mother reported that his aggressive behavior occurred during play-time and in the car. During playtime, the mother felt that someone entering the home and observing, to assist with the assessment, would not be disruptive to him. During car rides, Jimmy's mother felt that she could collect data herself. These data yielded information regarding what maintained the behavior problems.

During the playtime observations, a specific and regular cycle emerged. First, Jimmy's mother set out toys on the floor for him; second, the baby brother crawled over toward the toys; third, Jimmy pushed his baby brother so hard that he fell over, almost always hitting his head on the floor. Fourth, following each incident the mother took Jimmy's crying baby brother away from the toys, reprimanded Jimmy, then left him to play with the toys alone while she comforted the baby. In short, the aggression was serving the useful and desired function for Jimmy of getting rid of his brother and having the toys all to himself.

Analysis of the data sheets that Jimmy's mother filled out after car rides indicated that the problem behavior occurred only in the afternoons, when Jimmy's mother picked him up from preschool. The baby was placed in a car seat, which was buckled in the back seat. Often the baby began to cry, at which time Jimmy would lash out and hit him repeatedly. This caused the baby to cry more; once the baby had been hit, he would continue crying until the mother stopped the car to comfort him or until they arrived at their home.

Now it was time for us to develop a program with the parents, as a team. Each setting required a different intervention, and Jimmy's mother in particular was more than willing to participate actively in a program, as she feared for the safety of the baby. We met as a team and discussed a behavior support plan.

First was the playtime. The parents' goal was to decrease Jimmy's aggression while also developing a good sibling relationship. Therefore, the program jointly created was twofold. One part of the program involved first providing Jimmy with personal space so that his toys would not be taken by the baby. This antecedent change was made by having the parents place a small table in their living room during playtime—one that was low enough for Jimmy to play on, but high enough that the baby could not reach the top. Jimmy's mother then placed the desired toys on the table. Although this greatly reduced the behavior problems, we also wanted to respect the family's desire to create a bond between the children, so the

---

[1]See data for playtime in Koegel et al. (1998).

family gathered a small basket of baby toys—toys in which Jimmy had no interest, but were of great interest to the baby. Whenever the baby crawled over toward Jimmy, the parents prompted him to give the baby a toy from the basket. This served the function of decreasing the baby's interest in Jimmy's toys and providing an initial way of creating positive interactions between Jimmy and his brother. Finally, because it was important for Jimmy to have a replacement behavior for the aggression, he was prompted to say, "Mom, take Noah." After the prompt, Jimmy's mother immediately picked the baby up so that he was not near the play area. Initially, his mother prompted this functionally equivalent response on a regular basis before the baby got close to the play area (i.e., during noncrisis times); she did this until Jimmy began to use the phrase spontaneously. These three intervention components resulted in rapid and steady decreases in aggression during playtime.

Intervention for the car rides was perhaps more straightforward. We approached this from two perspectives. First, logistically, the children had to ride together on a regular (daily) basis; however, we were able to make antecedent changes by placing the car seat far enough away from Jimmy to immediately increase the baby's safety. Still, the crying could not be completely eliminated, and Jimmy did continue to scream, cover his ears, kick the back seat of the car, and try to reach out to hit the baby every time he cried. From Jimmy's perspective, the crying was quite irritating, so the parents bought Jimmy a tape player with earphones and some of his favorite tapes. Then, when Jimmy began to become upset at the baby's crying, his mother prompted him to listen to a tape. Often Jimmy's mother prompted him to begin listening to a tape as soon as he got in the car, thereby avoiding disruptive behavior altogether. These antecedent interventions reduced the aggression in the car to negligible levels.

It is important to note that the programs developed in both Jimmy's and Juanita's cases were created in partnership with their families. Their opinions, values, and strengths were considered. The interventions were developed to fit into existing and ongoing routines. The families were not required to set aside additional times to implement the interventions. Data were collected, and the children's progress was assessed on a continuing basis. Throughout all phases of support planning and implementation, the parents and other team members worked in partnership.

SUMMARY

Research supports the notion that parent education and home-based support are important components of PBS, and that teaching episodes can be incorporated into family routines and daily life. In this way, parents and other family members will not be required to rely solely on professionals for their child to receive ongoing intervention, and they will be equipped with the tools to empower them when handling problem behaviors, capitalizing on "teachable moments," and otherwise interacting with their child throughout the day. Furthermore, a lower rate of institutionalization occurs when parents participate in parent education programs (Mesibov & Schopler, 1983). In short, parents can provide effective individualized programs; however, there are a number of important considerations when team members are developing and implementing such programs. Assuring that assessment and interventions consider the ecocultural variables, and that parents and professionals develop a PBS plan as a team, will result in an increased likelihood that programs will be implemented and that gains will be maintained over time.

REFERENCES

Albin, R. W., Lucyshyn, J. M., Horner, R. H., & Flannery, K. B. (1996). Contextual fit for behavioral support plans: A model for "goodness of fit." In L. K. Koegel, R. L. Koegel, & G. Dunlap (Eds.), *Positive behavioral support: Including people with difficult behavior in the community* (pp. 81–98). Baltimore: Paul H. Brookes.

Allen, R. I., & Petr, C. G. (1996). Toward developing standards and measurements for family-centered practice in family support programs. In G. Singer & L. Powers (Eds.), *Redefining family support: Innovations in public–private partnerships* (pp. 57–86). Baltimore: Paul H. Brookes.

Bristol, M., Gallagher, J., & Holt, K. (1993). Maternal depressive symptoms in autism: Response to psychoeducational intervention. *Rehabilitation Psychology, 38,* 3–10.

Campbell, S., Cannon, B., Ellis, J. T., Lifter, K., Luiselli, J. K., Navalta, C. P., et al. (1998). The May Center for Early Childhood Education: Description of a continuum of services model for children with autism. *International Journal of Disability, Development and Education, 45,* 173–187.

Carr, E. G., Dunlap, G., Horner, R. H., Koegel, R. L., Turnbull, A. P., Sailor, W., et al. (2002). Positive Behavioral support: Evolution of an applied science. *Journal of Positive Behavior Interventions, 1,* 4–16.

Carr, E. G., Levin, L., McConnachie, G., Carlson, J. I., Kemp, D. C., Smith, C. E., et al. (1999). Comprehensive multisituational intervention for problem behavior in the community: Long-term maintenance and social validation. *Journal of Positive Behavior Interventions, 1,* 5–25.

Dunlap, G., Kern-Dunlap, L., Clarke, S., & Robbins, F. R. (1991). Functional assessment, curricular revision, and severe behavior problems. *Journal of Applied Behavior Analysis, 24,* 387–397.

Dunlap, G., Koegel, R., & Koegel, L. (1984). *Toilet training for children with severe handicaps: A field manual for coordinating training procedures across multiple community settings.* Santa Barbara: University of California, Santa Barbara.

Dunlap, G., & Robbins, F. R. (1991). Current perspectives in service delivery for young children with autism. *Comprehensive Mental Health Care, 1,* 177–194.

Dunst, C. J., & Paget, K. (1991). Parent–professional partnerships and family empowerment. In M. J. Fine (Ed.), *Collaboration with parents of exceptional children* (pp. 25–44). Brandon, VT: Clinical Psychology.

Dunst, C. J., & Trivette, C. M. (1994). Aims and principles of family support programs. In C. J. Dunst, C. M. Trivette, & A. D. Deal (Eds.), *Supporting and strengthening families: Vol. 1. Methods, strategies and practices* (pp. 30–48). Cambridge, MA: Brookline Books.

Dunst, C. J., Trivette, C. M., & Deal, A. G. (1994). Enabling and empowering families. In C. J. Dunst, C. M. Trivette, & A. G. Deal (Eds.), *Supporting and strengthening families, Vol. 1: Methods, strategies and practices* (pp. 2–11). Cambridge, MA: Brookline Books, Inc.

Forehand, R., & Kotchick, B. A. (1996). Cultural diversity: A wake-up call for parent training. *Behavior Therapy, 27,* 187–206.

Fox, L., Dunlap, G., & Philbrick, L. A. (1997). Providing individualized supports to young children with autism and their families. *Journal of Early Intervention, 21,* 1–14.

Frea, W. D., Koegel, L. K., & Koegel, R. L. (1994). *Understanding why problem behaviors occur: A guide for assisting parents in assessing causes of behavior and designing treatment plans.* Santa Barbara: University of California, Santa Barbara.

Gallimore, R., Weisner, T. S., Kaufman, S. Z., & Bernheimer, L. P. (1989). The social construction of ecocultural niches: Family accommodation of developmentally delayed children. *American Journal on Mental Retardation, 94,* 216–230.

Groden, G., Groden, J., & Stevenson, S. (1997). Facilitating comprehensive behavioral assessments. *Focus on Autism and Other Developmental Disabilities, 12,* 49–52.

Horner, R. H. (2000). Positive behavior supports. *Focus on Autism & Other Developmental Disabilities, 15,* 97–105.

Horner, R. H., & Carr, E. G. (1997). Behavioral support for students with severe disabilities: Functional assessment and comprehensive intervention. *Journal of Special Education, 31,* 84–109.

Koegel, L. K., Koegel, R. L., & Dunlap, G. (Eds.), (1996). *Positive behavioral support: Including people with difficult behavior in the community.* Baltimore: Paul H. Brookes.

Koegel, L. K., Koegel, R. L., Harrower, J. K., & Carter, C. M. (1999). Pivotal response intervention: I. Overview of approach. *Journal of The Association for Persons with Severe Handicaps, 24,* 174–185.

Koegel, L. K., Koegel, R. L., Openden, D., McNerney, E., Symon, J. B., & Sze, K.

(2003). *A model for increasing in-home services to children with autism.* Santa Barbara: University of California, Santa Barbara.

Koegel, L. K., Koegel, R. L., & Smith, A. (1997). Variables related to differences in standardized test outcomes for children with autism. *Journal of Autism and Developmental Disorders, 27,* 233–244.

Koegel, L. K., Stiebel, D., & Koegel, R. L. (1998). Reducing aggression in children with autism toward infant or toddler siblings. *Journal of The Association for Persons with Severe Handicaps, 23,* 111–118.

Koegel, R. L., Bimbela, A., & Schreibman, L. (1996). Collateral effects of 2 parent training programs on family interactions. *Journal of Autism and Developmental Disorders, 26,* 347–359.

Koegel, R. L., & Koegel, L. K. (Eds.), (1995). *Teaching children with autism: Strategies for initiating positive interactions and improving learning opportunities.* Baltimore: Paul H. Brookes.

Koegel, R. L., Koegel, L. K., & Schreibman, L. (1991). Assessing and training parents in teaching pivotal behaviors. *Advances in Behavioral Assessment of Children and Families, 5,* 65–82.

Koren, P., DeChillo, N., & Friesen, B. (1992). Measuring empowerment in families whose children have emotional disabilities: A brief questionnaire. *Rehabilitation Psychology, 37,* 305–321.

Lucyshyn, J. M., & Albin, R. W. (1993). Comprehensive support to families of children with disabilities and behavior problems: Keeping it "friendly." In G. H. S. Singer & L. E. Powers (Eds.), *Families, disability, and empowerment: Active coping skills and strategies for family interventions* (pp. 365–407). Baltimore: Paul H. Brookes.

Lucyshyn, J. M., Albin, R. W., & Nixon, C. D. (1997). Embedding comprehensive behavioral support in family ecology: An experimental, single case analysis. *Journal of Consulting and Clinical Psychology, 65,* 241–251.

Lucyshyn, J. M., Olson, D., & Horner, R. H. (1995). Building an ecology of support: A case study of one young woman with severe problem behaviors living in the community. *Journal of The Association for Persons with Severe Handicaps, 20,* 16–30.

Lucyshyn, J. M., Horner, R. H., Dunlap, G., Albin, R. W., & Ben, K. (2002). Positive behavior support with families. In J. M. Lucyshyn, G. Dunlap, & R. W. Abidin (Eds.), *Families and positive behavior support* (pp. 3–44). Baltimore: Paul H. Brookes.

Mahoney, G., Kaiser, A., Girolametto, L., MacDonald, J., Robinson, C., Safford, P., et al. (1999). Parent education in early intervention: A call for a renewed focus. *Topics in Early Childhood Special Education, 19,* 131–140.

Mesibov, G. B., & Schopler, E. (1983). The development of community-based programs for autistic adolescents. *Children's Health Care, 12,* 20–24.

Moes, D. (1995). Parent education and parenting stress. In R. L. Koegel & L. K. Koegel (Eds.), *Teaching children with autism: Strategies for initiating positive interactions and improving learning opportunities* (pp. 79–93). Baltimore: Paul H. Brookes.

Moes, D. R., & Frea, W. (2000). Using an assessment of family context to inform intervention planning for the treatment of a child with autism. *Journal of Positive Behavior Interventions, 2,* 40–46.

Moes, D. R., Koegel, R. L., Schreibman, L., & Loos, L. M. (1992). Stress profiles for mothers and fathers of children with autism. *Psychological Reports, 71,* 1272–1274.

Pfeiffer, S. I., & Nelson, D. D. (1992). The cutting edge in services for people with autism. *Journal of Autism and Developmental Disorders, 22,* 95–105.

Prizant, B. M., & Wetherby, A. M. (1989). Providing services to children with autism (ages 0 to 2 years) and their families. *Focus on Autistic Behavior, 4,* 16.

Risley, T. (1996). Get a life!: Positive behavioral intervention for challenging behavior through life arrangement and life coaching. In L. K. Koegel, R. L. Koegel, & G. Dunlap (Eds.), *Positive behavioral support: Including people with difficult behavior in the community* (pp. 425–437). Baltimore: Paul H. Brookes.

Robbins, F. R., Dunlap, G., & Plienis, A. J. (1991). Family characteristics, family training, and the progress of young children with autism. *Journal of Early Intervention, 15,* 173–184.

Ruef, M. B., Turnbull, A. P., Turnbull, H. R., & Poston, D. (1999). Perspectives of five stakeholder groups: Challenging behavior of individuals with mental retardation and/or autism. *Journal of Positive Behavior Interventions, 1,* 43–58.

Santarelli, G., Koegel, R. L., Casas, J. M., & Koegel, L. K. (2001). Culturally diverse families participating in behavior therapy parent education programs for children with developmental disabilities. *Journal of Positive Behavior Interventions, 3,* 120–123.

Schopler, E. (1989). Principles for directing both educational treatment and research. In C. Gillberg (Ed.), *Diagnosis and treatment of autism* (pp. 167–183). New York: Plenum Press.

Singer, G. H. S., & Irvin, L. K. (1991). Supporting families of persons with severe disabilities: Emerging findings, practices, and questions. In L. H. Meyer, C. A. Peck, & L. Brown (Eds.), *Critical issues in the lives of people with severe disabilities* (pp. 271–312). Baltimore: Paul H. Brookes.

Strain, P. S., & Hoyson, M. (2000). The need for longitudinal, intensive social skill intervention: LEAP follow-up outcomes for children with autism. *Topics in Early Childhood Special Education, 20,* 116–122.

Stiebel, D. (1999). Using to promoting augmentative communication during daily routines: A parent problem-solving intervention. *Journal of Positive Behavior Interventions, 1,* 159–170.

Turnbull, A. P., Blue-Banning, M., Turbiville, V., & Park, J. (1999). From parent education to partnership education: A call for a transformed focus. *Topics in Early Childhood Special Education, 19,* 164–172.

Turnbull, A. P., & Ruef, M. (1997). Family perspectives on inclusion lifestyle issues for people with problem behavior. *Exceptional Children, 63,* 211–227.

Turnbull, A. P., & Turnbull, H. R. (2000). *Families, professionals, and exceptionality: Collaborating for empowerment* (4th ed.). Columbus, OH: Merrill.

Vaughn, B. J., Clarke, S., & Dunlap, G. (1997). Assessment-based intervention for severe behavior problems in a natural family context. *Journal of Applied Behavior Analysis, 30,* 713–716.

Weiner, T. S., Coots, J. J., Bernheimer, L. P., & Arzubiaga, A. (1997). *The Ecocultural Family Interview.* Los Angeles: Ecocultural Scale Project.

Wetherby, A. M., & Prizant, B. M. (1992). Facilitating language and communication development in autism: Assessment and intervention guidelines. In D. E. Berkell (Ed.), *Autism: Identification, education, and treatment* (pp. 107–134). Hillsdale, NJ: Erlbaum.

CHAPTER 13

◆ ◆ ◆

Schoolwide Positive Behavior Support

◆

ROBERT H. HORNER
GEORGE SUGAI
ANNE W. TODD
TERI LEWIS-PALMER

On the whole, schools are good places. They are the most familiar and among the most influential of our public institutions. On any given school day, nearly 25% of the U.S. population is attending, teaching, or administering schools (Tyack, 2001). The history of schools, however, is marked by shifting expectations and ever-changing practices. Today parents and school boards expect schools to (1) deliver improved academic performance, (2) build social competence, and (3) ensure safety. They are being asked to do more with less and to do it quickly. Schools also are expected to be successful with a wider range of children. Children in schools today

Development of this chapter was supported by a grant from the Office of Special Education Programs, with additional funding from the Safe and Drug Free Schools Program, U.S. Department of Education (No. H326S980003). Opinions expressed herein are our own and do not necessarily reflect the position of the U.S. Department of Education, and such endorsements should not be inferred. For additional information regarding the contents of this chapter, contact Robert H. Horner (*robh@oregon.edu*).

come with a wide range of skills and from an increasing array of cultural, financial, and social contexts (Fuchs & Fuchs, 1994). Children with disabilities and children with problem behaviors are part of this diversity.

This chapter addresses the challenges posed by students with problem behaviors, and the emerging approach to school discipline represented by *schoolwide* positive behavior support (PBS). The thesis of this chapter is that traditional, "get-tough" approaches to discipline do not address the needs of modern schools (Skiba, 2002). As the expectations for schools have evolved, the need has developed for a broader, more proactive approach to addressing the wide array of behavioral challenges now present in our schools. Schoolwide PBS represents a practical response to this need. It emphasizes prevention of problem behavior, active instruction of adaptive skills, a continuum of consequences for problem behavior, assessment-based interventions for children with the most intractable problem behaviors, the implementation of organizational systems to support effective behavioral practices, and the use of information to guide decision making. We describe in this chapter (1) the need for a new approach to discipline, (2) the research foundation for schoolwide PBS, (3) an overview of schoolwide PBS procedures, (4) the empirical support for this approach, and (5) implications for future research and school reform.

THE NEED FOR A NEW APPROACH
TO DISCIPLINE IN SCHOOLS

Aggression, bullying, insubordination, disruption, vandalism, noncompliance, withdrawal and truancy continue to be major concerns in schools (Dwyer, Osher, & Warger, 1998; Shinn, Stoner, & Walker, 2002). In fact, problem behavior has been among the top concerns of educators for over 20 years (Horner, Diemer, & Brazeau, 1992; Rose & Gallup, 1998). Skiba and Peterson (2000) report that not only is antisocial behavior increasing, but it is directly hindering academic achievement. These findings are consistent with the U.S. Surgeon General's recent report documenting that although major crime by youth is in decline, the rate of disruptive and defiant behavior has risen (U.S. Department of Health and Human Services, 2001).

The traditional responses to problem behavior in schools have been punishment and exclusion (Gottfredson, Gottfredson, & Hybl, 1993; Tolan & Guerra, 1994). Children engaging in problem behaviors receive reprimands, loss of privileges, office discipline referrals, detentions, suspensions, Saturday school, and expulsions. This approach emphasizes reducing our "tolerance" for antisocial behavior, and removing children who fail to respond to reprimands, detentions, and office discipline referrals. The assumption is that reactive, get-tough responses will deter future occurrences of problem behavior; teach and encourage students to engage in prosocial, adaptive behavior; or simply remove disruptive students so that others can benefit. Students who maintain patterns of problem behavior are referred to alternative education programs, placed in special education, or simply expelled. However, the focus on "zero-tolerance" policies has been ineffective (Skiba, 2002). Although short-lived reductions in problem behavior have been noted (McCord, 1995; Patterson, Reid, & Dishion, 1992), Mayer and his colleagues (Mayer, 1995; Mayer & Butterworth, 1979; Mayer, Butterworth, Nafpaktitis, & Sulzer-Azaroff, 1983) describe the overall effects of toughened school discipline as *increases* in vandalism, truancy, tardiness, and aggression. In effect, when schools are made more aversive, the result is more disruptive behavior. This evidence does not argue against the use of clear, consistent consequences for problem behavior, but it indicates that reactive consequences alone will not result in safe and orderly schools, especially for students who present the most severe problem behavior challenges. An alternative approach is needed.

THE FOUNDATION FOR SCHOOLWIDE PBS

PBS is the integration of valued outcomes, behavioral and biomedical science, empirically validated procedures, and systems change to enhance quality of life and minimize/prevent problem behaviors (Carr et al., 2002; Sugai, Horner, et al., 2000). The foundation for *schoolwide* PBS lies in the application of these features to the whole school context in an effort to *prevent*, as well as change, patterns of problem behavior.

Historically, behavior support in schools has been reserved for those students who demonstrate problem behaviors (Sugai & Horner, 2002). But if schools are to meet current challenges, an expanded focus on preventive, as well as reactive, behavior support will be needed. Walker and his colleagues (Walker et al., 1996; Walker & Shinn, 2002) offer a prevention model of behavior support adapted from public health efforts that integrates intensive behavior support for individual students with prevention efforts for all students (Larson, 1994; National Research Council & Institute of Medicine, 1999; Shonkoff & Phillips, 2000). The overall design of this model, as depicted in Figure 13.1, involves a three-tiered approach. The initial tier focuses on *primary prevention*, targets all children, involves all adults, applies to all settings, and covers all times. The aim is to actively teach appropriate behavior, and through this preventive instruction to build a coherent social culture that is predictable and reinforcing, yet quickly responsive to problem behavior. The primary prevention effort assumes that all children need behavior support (Evertson & Emmer, 1982;

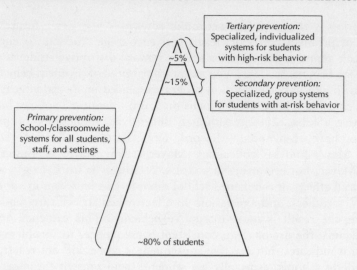

FIGURE 13.1. The three-tiered model of prevention for school discipline.

Sprick, Sprick, & Garrison, 1992; Weissberg, Caplan, & Sivo, 1989). Every child entering school should receive clear instruction on what is acceptable and unacceptable, and ongoing recognition when he or she engages in appropriate behavior.

The _secondary prevention_ tier in the prevention model focuses on children who are at risk for problem behavior, but for whom intensive, individualized intervention is not necessary. The emphasis in secondary prevention is on increasing the intensity of behavior support for students who need more than primary prevention. These students have histories of problem behavior associated with academic failure, limited family and community supports, disabilities, membership in deviant peer groups, health-related complications, poverty, and so forth. These students also have limited access to the protective supports that are needed to buffer them against these risk factors—for example, special education, health and medical care, welfare support, preschool and child care, and stable family support (Gresham, Sugai, Horner, Quinn, & McInerney, 1998; Walker, Colvin, & Ramsey, 1995; Walker & Shinn, 2002). Children with high risk factors are less likely to respond to primary prevention efforts and remain at risk for developing durable patterns of problem behavior unless they receive additional assistance. A growing number of secondary-level interventions are demonstrating change in student behavior, both socially and academically (Crone, Horner, & Hawken, 2004; Davies & McLaughlin, 1989; Dougherty & Dougherty, 1977; Hawken & Horner, 2003; Leach & Byrne,

1986; Lewis, Colvin, & Sugai, 2000; March & Horner, 2002; Nelson, Martella, & Galand, 1998).

The *tertiary prevention* tier of the prevention model is reserved for children with the most intense behavior support needs. These students typically receive individualized, comprehensive supports, as described in this book. The design of intensive, individual behavior supports has been the most durable focus of research efforts (Eber & Nelson, 1997; Scott & Eber, 2003). Results are encouraging; they suggest that when individualized planning is blended with functional assessment, comprehensive support plan design, adequate personnel and resources, and active use of data for decision making, impressive changes can be observed in the behavior of children (Carr et al., 1999; Didden, Duker, & Korzilius, 1997; Ingram, 2002; O'Neill et al., 1997; Todd, Horner, Sugai, & Sprague, 1999).

To date, the three-tiered prevention model has been a heuristic offered by Walker and his colleagues to guide the design of behavior support in schools and to emphasize the need for multiple behavior intervention efforts (i.e., primary prevention with the whole school; secondary prevention with smaller groups of at-risk children; and intensive, individualized intervention with selected students). As indicated in Figure 13.1, it is estimated that approximately 80% of students in a school will respond to primary prevention efforts, and their behavior will remain within social norms; an additional 15% will respond to secondary prevention efforts; and a final 5% will require the intensive, individualized interventions associated with the tertiary level of prevention (Sugai & Horner, 1994).

Office discipline referrals have been identified as a useful form of information to describe the disciplinary status of a school within the three-tiered model, because the data are generally available in schools and reflect the overall status of problem behavior (Irvin, Tobin, Sprague, Sugai, & Vincent, 2004; Sugai, Sprague, Horner, & Walker, 2000; Tobin, Sugai, & Colvin, 2000). Office discipline referral data are especially useful if they are contextualized—that is, if (1) how they are used in a schoolwide system is clearly and operationally defined; (2) definitions of problem behavior are mutually exclusive and comprehensive; (3) agreements exist about what constitutes an office discipline referral; (4) formal and efficient systems are in place for collecting, storing, summarizing, and reporting the data; and (5) overt processes are in place for regular and systematic evaluation and action planning. Recently, Sugai (2002) reported descriptive office discipline referral data supporting the validity of the three-tiered model. These data are provided in Figure 13.2 and display the average proportion of students with different rates of office discipline referrals for the 2002–2003 school year for 321 elementary schools from 13 states, as reported through the School-Wide Information System (SWIS; May et al., 2000). Schools

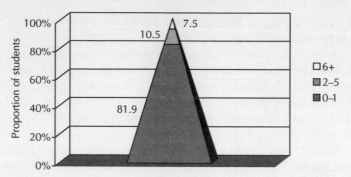

FIGURE 13.2. The mean proportion of students with varying rates of office discipline referrals across 321 elementary schools for the 2002–2003 academic year. Data from Sugai (2002).

included in this database had at least 1 year of data, received training on the features of useful and informative systems for managing and using office discipline referral data, and had at least some schoolwide PBS practices in place.

A total of over 143,400 office discipline referrals were recorded. Each school reported the percentage of enrolled students with 0–1 office discipline referrals, the percentage of students with 2–5 referrals, and the percentage with 6 or more referrals. The means across the 321 schools indicated that on average, 87% (SD = 10) of students had 0–1 office discipline referrals, 9% (SD = 6) had 2–5 referrals, and 4% (SD = 5) had 6+ referrals. These patterns suggest that the three-tiered model may have applications to understanding what prevention-based approaches might look like in schools. The contributions of the three-tiered prevention model for school discipline design have been (1) recognition that behavior support needs to include a *schoolwide* component; and (2) appreciation that investment in primary prevention efforts will both decrease the proportion of students who need more intense support, and increase the likelihood of successful intervention with those students receiving tertiary prevention support (Colvin, Kame'enui, & Sugai, 1993; Epstein et al., 1993; Nelson, Colvin, & Smith, 1996; Taylor-Greene et al., 1997).

Taken together, a growing body of research offers guidance for responding to violence and disruption in schools. The foremost message is that punishment and exclusion are ineffective if they are not paired with prevention efforts (Gottfredson, Karweit, & Gottfredson, 1989; Mayer, 1995; Tolan & Guerra, 1994). The companion message is that a combination of primary, secondary and tertiary prevention of problem behavior through schoolwide PBS can make a substantive difference (Chapman &

Hofweber, 2000; Colvin & Fernandez, 2000; Lohrman-O'Rourke et al., 2000; Nakasato, 2000; Nelson, Martella, & Marchand-Martella, 2002; Nersesian, Todd, Lehmann, & Watson, 2000; Sadler, 2000; Taylor-Greene et al., 1997; Taylor-Greene & Kartub, 2000).

FEATURES OF SCHOOLWIDE PBS

Schoolwide PBS blends four key elements: *outcomes, practices, systems,* and *data use* (see Figure 13.3) (Sugai & Horner, 2002). The first feature (and the foundation) of schoolwide PBS is a focus on *student outcomes.* Schools are expected to be safe environments where students learn the academic and social skills needed for life in our society. The basic goals of any system of schoolwide PBS must be to provide the behavioral assistance needed to achieve these outcomes. Schools should be able to define measurable standards for student achievement, social behavior, and safety. The academic standards that now drive school reform will not be achieved without also attending to the behavioral climate of schools.

The second feature of schoolwide PBS is the use of *research-validated practices.* These include the curriculum, classroom management, instructional procedures, rewards, and contingencies that are used on a daily basis to build and sustain student competence. In other words practices are what teachers use to build and influence student behavior, and are the grist of classroom and behavior management efforts (Alberto & Troutman, 2003; Heward, Heron, Hill, & Trap-Porter, 1984; Jensen, Sloane, & Young,

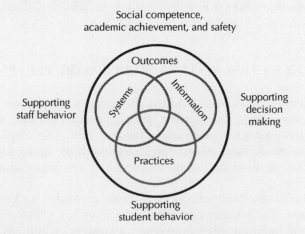

FIGURE 13.3. Four defining elements of schoolwide PBS.

1988; Kame'enui & Darch, 1995; Kazdin, 1982; Kerr & Nelson, 1983, 2002; Vargas, 1977; Wolery, Bailey, & Sugai, 1988). Schoolwide PBS is based on practices that have evidence supporting their impact on student behavior. Schools often are criticized for adopting a practice without careful consideration or empirical documentation that the practice is (1) related to change in valued student outcomes, (2) efficient and feasible, (3) cost-effective, or (4) based on sound educational/behavioral theory (Carnine, 1997; Peters & Heron, 1993). Schoolwide PBS is defined in part by the adoption of research-validated practices that are tied to those outcomes most important for students.

The third feature of schoolwide PBS is an emphasis on the _systems_ needed to sustain effective practices. These are the _policies, staffing patterns, budgets, team structures, administrative leadership, operating routines, staff training, and action plans_ that affect the behavior of adults in schools. We believe that systems are essential for the sustained use of effective practices. All too often, educational innovations are implemented in schools only to be replaced by something "new" the next year (Latham, 1988). Schoolwide PBS includes attention to the systems that we hypothesize are needed to implement and sustain research-validated practices.

The fourth defining feature of schoolwide PBS is the active _collection and use of data for decision making_. Gilbert (1978) argues that no strategy is more efficient for producing change in an organization than the active collection and reporting of information about valued outcomes. Within schools, data should be collected about the academic performance, social competence, and safety of children. The data should be collected continuously and reported to the faculty, administration, teams, families, and students on a regular basis. Of greatest importance, the information should be used to make decisions on how to improve the school (Gilbert & Gilbert, 1992).

PRACTICES AND SYSTEMS FOR PRIMARY PREVENTION

Other chapters in this book address the detailed procedures (functional behavioral assessment, intervention design, implementation, and adaptation) that are used to provide individualized PBS. The emphasis in this chapter is on the primary prevention elements (those applicable to all students, all staff, all times, and all locations) within the larger schoolwide PBS approach.

Schoolwide discipline efforts have been advocated and studied since schools began. The primary prevention efforts within schoolwide PBS borrow from and build on this strong store of knowledge and advice (Colvin,

Sugai, & Kame'enui, 1994; Comer, 1985; Gottfredson, 1987; Gottfredson, Gottfredson, & Skroban, 1996; Knoff, 2002; Mayer et al., 1983; Sprick & Nolet, 1991; Sulzer-Azaroff & Mayer, 1994; Weissberg et al., 1989). From this literature, five practices and six systems variables emerge as important for effective and sustained implementation of schoolwide PBS efforts (see Table 13.1).

Practices

In schools that are behaviorally successful, the environment is predictable, positive, and consistent. Children know the behavioral expectations of the school, receive instruction on how to be behaviorally successful, and are acknowledged and supported in their efforts to apply that instruction. Problem behaviors are strongly discouraged. Consistent consequences for misbehavior are delivered. But active instruction and behavior support, not the delivery of negative consequences, are viewed as the primary strategies for changing student behavior. The specific practices used to achieve primary prevention within schoolwide PBS follow.

Define Schoolwide Behavioral Expectations

The first practice is to identify five or fewer, brief, positively stated behavioral expectations that are presented in a memorable format and posted throughout the school. These expectations should capture the major social values of the school and reflect the language of the local community. The behavioral expectations are the big concepts that guide the behavioral curriculum and social standards of the school. Behavioral expectations adopted in schools from Maryland to Hawaii include examples such as: "Be respectful," "Be responsible," "Be kind," "Do your best," "Follow directions."

TABLE 13.1. Practices and Systems of Primary Prevention within Schoolwide PBS

Practices	Systems
• Define expectations	• Team-based implementation
• Teach expectations	• Administrative leadership
• Monitor and encourage expected behaviors	• Documented commitment
• Prevent and discourage problem behaviors	• Adequate personnel and time
• Collect and use data for decision making	• Budgeted support
	• Information system

Behavioral expectations are always defined in positive terms. A common error is to define behavioral expectations in terms of what *not* to do (e.g., no hats in class, no running in the hall, no bullying). The number of problem behaviors we would like children to avoid is large and unwieldy. When the core positive behavioral expectations are defined, all problem behaviors become examples of not following the positive expectations. For instance, bullying behavior is an example of not being respectful; dropping trash in the hall is an example of not being responsible. Defining the desired behavioral expectations makes the development of appropriate behavior, rather than the suppression of an infinite array of undesirable behaviors, the focus of discipline efforts.

Defining schoolwide behavioral expectations, however, is more than building a list that goes in the school discipline handbook. Students are expected to know and practice the schoolwide behavioral expectations. The expectations should be posted in at least 80% of the public spaces in the school and regularly reviewed as themes relevant throughout the school day. In one elementary school, the three behavioral expectations were "Be respectful," "Be responsible," and "Be safe." To help children remember the expectations, the staff presented the expectations as the "Three B's" and used a bumblebee motif in displays and presentations. In a middle school, the staff identified five behavioral expectations and presented them to the students as the "High Five" (Taylor-Greene et al., 1999). The goal is to arrange displays of schoolwide positive expectations, so that any individual can identify the behavioral expectations within 5 minutes of entering the school.

Teach the Behavioral Expectations

As is true of all educational concepts, the schoolwide three to five behavioral expectations will become relevant only if they are tied to very concrete behaviors and actively taught in practical contexts. Learning the expectation to "be respectful," for example, will not change student behavior until that concept is tied to specific behaviors. The teaching of behavioral expectations occurs differently at different age levels and in different parts of the country. Some middle schools, for example, teach behavioral expectations during the first 1–2 days of school. Students rotate through stations in the school to learn how the behavioral expectations apply for the classroom, cafeteria, gym, hallway, or bus area. In elementary schools, the training of behavioral expectations may occur through an initial assembly and then in classroom cohorts through multiple 15- to 20-minute sessions spread over the first 4–6 weeks of schools. In addition, behavioral expectations may be revisited periodically throughout the school year.

Effective curricula for teaching behavioral expectations have the following main features: (1) opportunities and schedules for teaching across multiple locations in the school, (2) presentations of appropriate behavior contrasted with inappropriate behavior examples, and (3) the opportunity for all students to perform or practice appropriate behavior and be acknowledged for correct performance.

Designing the curriculum for teaching behavioral expectations is typically a task organized by the faculty team responsible for schoolwide discipline, and completed by the whole faculty. Elsewhere, we (Horner, Sugai, Lewis-Palmer, & Todd, 2001) have described one effective process in which the team builds a matrix with behavioral expectations on one side and school locations on the other (see Figure 13.4). In each cell of the matrix, the faculty identifies the one or two specific appropriate behaviors that would be representative and important to the context or culture of the school, and that best illustrate the expectation in a specific setting. For example, one faculty selected "raising your hand before speaking" as the best example of being respectful in class. Another identified "wearing appropriate shoes" as the best example of being responsible in the gym. A third faculty identified "waiting behind the red line" as the best example of being safe in the bus area. The list of "best examples" for a specific location (e.g., cafeteria) becomes the curriculum for teaching the behavioral expec-

	Classroom	Gym	Hallway	Playground	Bus area
Be safe	Follow directions	Follow directions	Walk Open doors slowly	Go up ladders and down slides	Wait behind the red line
Be respectful	Raise your hand to talk Hands and feet to self	Follow rules of the game Return equipment at bell	Hands and feet to self	One-minute rule for sharing equipment Wait for your turn	Hands and feet to self
Be responsible	Bring books and pencil to class Do homework	Participate Wear appropriate shoes	Keep books, belongings, and litter off floor	Stay within the recess area	Keep your books and belongings with you

FIGURE 13.4. A curriculum matrix for teaching schoolwide behavioral expectations.

tations in that location. The teaching is done by taking the children to that location; reviewing the big behavioral expectations (the main concepts); and then teaching the concepts by (1) showing the best example(s) of doing it the "right way," and then (2) contrasting that with an example of how *not* to behave. The contrasting, or "negative," examples allow teachers to define what is not being respectful or responsible. Negative examples are always presented as a contrast to doing things the correct way (see Becker, Engelmann, & Thomas, 1975, or Engelmann & Carnine, 1982, for a review of using negative teaching examples). Instructional sessions always end by students having an opportunity to perform appropriately, and receiving feedback and recognition for correct performance. An example of the teaching plan format is provided in Figure 13.5.

Instruction on behavioral expectations has been successful when a person can stop random students in the hall, ask them whether they know the expectations, and find that at least 80% of the students can name both the expectation and what it means for a specific location.

Monitor and Encourage Performance of Expected Behaviors

The old adage that one should never teach something that is not reviewed and rewarded on a regular basis is just as true for behavioral expectations as it is for identifying the subject of a sentence or applying the Pythagorean theorem. In schools that are behaviorally successful, every adult carries an ongoing obligation to acknowledge appropriate student behavior. This acknowledgment should be provided in multiple forms; in classrooms, as well as in hallways and playgrounds; and by secretaries, custodians, educational assistants, and administrators, as well as teachers. Acknowledging appropriate behavior may take the form of tangible rewards or simple verbal statements. Regardless of the medium by which it is carried, the students should receive the message that their behavior is valued and appreciated. The message is of importance; the method of extending this message should be appropriate to the developmental level of the students and the culture of the school.

The development of organized strategies for acknowledging appropriate student behavior is at the heart of creating a positive school environment, but it is a controversial topic. Some teachers and administrators express concern that formal systems of reward will tarnish behavioral expectations and leave students only willing to behave appropriately if they are promised rewards. Published texts, workshops, and credible research have emphasized the possibility that unnecessary rewards may have a damaging effect on building the self-guided motivation we all seek. However, Cameron and her colleagues (Cameron, 2002; Cameron, Banko, & Pierce, 2001; Cameron & Pierce,

Teaching Schoolwide Behavioral Expectations

Given: A location and three to five schoolwide expectations.

1. Review schoolwide expectations (labels and definitions).

2. Review rationale for expectations.

3. What do those expectations "mean" in this location?
   a. Positive examples (correct ways to behave—from matrix)
      -
      -
      -
      -

   b. Negative examples (to provide precision to the rules)
      -
      -
      -

4. Provide an activity that allows practice of appropriate behaviors.

5. Reward appropriate behavior.

FIGURE 13.5. Teaching plan format.

1994, 2002) provide a compelling review of the research foundation for these concerns, which presents a different picture. They find that although concern over the use of rewards provides great substance for media events, it is a poor foundation for policy and action. In fact, their meta-analysis documents that (1) rewarding students for appropriate behavior is likely to facilitate, not hinder, their performance of desirable behaviors in later contexts; and (2) the far greater danger is the creation of school environments with low rates of positive feedback from adults. In essence, children in our schools are at greater risk of being underrewarded than overrewarded. Designing classroom and school settings to ensure that there are frequent and compelling rewards for appropriate academic and social behavior is a critical feature of successful schools.

The design of strategies for acknowledging appropriate student behavior should fit the age level of the students and provide predictable as well as unexpected rewards, tangible as well as social rewards, small as well as substantive rewards, and frequent as well as infrequent rewards. The goal is to create a positive environment where children have a high rate of positive contacts with adults, where adults are consistently reminding students that appropriate behavior is valued, and where students view the setting as behaviorally predictable and positive. In other words, the goal is to provide students with (1) a clear and predictable road map for social success, (2) the training and support to follow that map, and (3) immediate and clear feedback when they deviate from the successful path.

A school can claim to have an effective system for acknowledging behavioral expectations if at any time at least 80% of students interviewed indicate that they have received some form of recognition for behaving appropriately within the previous 10 school days.

Prevent and Discourage Problem Behaviors

A clear, fair, consistently applied continuum of consequences for problem behaviors is appropriate and important (Darch & Kame'enui, 2004). This continuum should include distinct and operational definitions of "minor" and "major" problem behaviors, as well as appropriate consequences that vary in intensity and are linked to the severity of the minor and major problem behaviors. Most schools have a list of the problem behaviors that result in negative consequences from adults. Those schools that are most effective clarify which problem behaviors should be managed in class and which should result in an office discipline referral. They also have clear problem behavior definitions that are operational, mutually exclusive and exhaustive, so staff and faculty are able to be consistent. Finally, they use information about patterns of problem behavior to guide decisions about school discipline.

The major messages are these: (1) Build a continuum of consequences that are clear, fair, and easy to administer; (2) instruct the students early in the school year about appropriate behavior, as well as the consequences for inappropriate behavior; (3) implement the consequences with consistency; (4) do not ignore escalating problem behavior; and (5) above all else, do not expect negative consequences to result in substantive change in behavior patterns. The purposes of consequences for problem behavior are to (1) maintain safety, (2) prevent inappropriate behavior from escalating, (3) prevent inappropriate behavior from being rewarded, (4) provide a clear message to the student (and observers) that his or her behavior is unacceptable, and (5) allow instruction and normal activity in the school to move forward.

For 80% of students in most schools, instruction on behavioral expectations, and use of low-intensity consequences for misbehavior, will be sufficient to maintain appropriate behavior. For the 5–15% of students who are at greater risk for problem behavior, negative consequences will often be ineffective. In some cases, consequences that are intended to be negative (e.g., being sent to the office) will function as rewards for the student; in other cases, the complex contingencies that maintain problem behavior (including those from home and peers) will be unaffected by the school consequences. For these students, formal intervention, active instruction, and a more comprehensive response to their behavioral needs will be required to produce a functional effect (Walker et al., 1995). In many ways, the system of negative consequences for problem behavior is designed to "keep the lid on" and allow the school day to move forward. Real behavior change is unlikely to result from a simple system of negative consequences.

Collect and Use Data for Decision Making

The fifth practice for schoolwide primary prevention is the efficient gathering and use of data for decision making (Horner, Sugai, & Todd, 2001). Collecting information that will allow evaluation and ongoing self-improvement is among the most professional of educational activities. Schools are ever-changing environments. If change is to be guided by a commitment to student outcomes, efficiency, and sound documentation, then a reliable system for gathering and using data is essential (Carnine, 1992, 1995, 1997).

Effective primary prevention requires that the school faculty, the school team, individual teachers, administrators, and related service personnel have information about student behavior. The most common unit for summary of behavioral data is that of the individual student. If Jason is identified as having problems, then a record is developed to assess his attendance, grades, office referrals, suspensions, and so forth. Within a primary prevention approach, the faculty and schoolwide team will also regularly review the behavior patterns for the whole school. At least every 2 weeks, the schoolwide team should review the frequency of office discipline referrals organized (1) per day and per month, (2) per type of problem behavior, (3) per location in the school, (4) per time of day, and (5) per child. The information reviewed by the team should be as recent as 48 hours old, accurate, and displayed in graphic form rather than via a table of numbers. An emerging set of evaluation reports suggests that with accurate and timely data, schoolwide teams perceive improved effectiveness in identifying problem patterns early, as well as in developing practical and effective strategies for supporting appropriate student behavior and decreasing problem behavior (Ingram, Horner, & Todd, 2002). Efficient systems for gathering, summarizing, and reporting office discipline referral information are available in web-based information systems (May et al., 2000; *www.swis.org*), as well as through a growing array of district-based management systems.

The central messages are these: (1) Effective, schoolwide behavior support involves gathering and using data about the whole school; (2) the data need not be rigorous research data, but can be summaries of the data typically collected in schools; (3) the data should be reviewed regularly (weekly, monthly) by the team, administration, and staff; and (4) most importantly, the data should be used for active decision making. Decisions about adoption of new behavior support programs, continued use of existing programs, and allocation of staff time to change behavior support efforts should be guided by local information. The challenge of designing a positive social culture is an ever-evolving process. Efficient gathering and use of information for decision making is a key tool for navigating this process successfully.

Systems to Support and Sustain Effective Practices

Schoolwide PBS emphasizes the organizational systems needed to support implementation and sustained use of effective practices. Too often, effective practices are introduced without the systems-level support needed to carry them forward. Schools that have been successful in implementing the three tiers of schoolwide PBS have incorporated the following system features.

Team-Based Implementation

A schoolwide effort requires the active involvement and design of a local school team. The schoolwide team is typically composed of five to nine individuals who represent the administration, the teaching faculty, and related service personnel. Where appropriate, including parent, student, and neighborhood representatives can be helpful in establishing a community voice and securing commitments. The team will then benefit from the multiple perspectives and creative problem solving of these groups. The key features of team-based implementation are that the schoolwide team (1) operates with effective procedures (e.g., agenda, scheduled meeting dates, action planning, meeting minutes); (2) invests in building the common vision, terminology, and experience that allow the individuals to function as a team; and (3) gathers, reports, and uses outcome data for continuous development and improvement of the behavior support efforts in the school.

Administrative Leadership

Schoolwide PBS efforts require the clear and consistent support of the school administration. This must involve not just statements of support, but active participation on the behavior support or school climate team. The role of senior administrators in school buildings is not well appreciated. The principal and vice-principal can shape the level of opportunity for innovation and development (Colvin & Sprick, 1996). Participation by administrators gives the team authority in making decisions related to personnel and budget, as well as scheduling, integrating, and prioritizing multiple initiatives.

Documented Commitment

Commitment to use schoolwide PBS begins with commitment to the education of all children, including those with problem behavior. As such, the first level of documented commitment is agreement about a common purpose or mission statement for the school. This statement should express a belief about the importance of academic excellence, effective teaching practices, developing character and social competence, and contribution to building a caring and productive community. In addition, improving the behavioral climate of the school should be (1) ranked as one of the top three goals for the school, (2) supported by at least 80% of the faculty, and (3) given at least 3 years to be fully implemented.

Efforts at school reform often ignore the value of establishing broad commitment to the goals of, vision of, and need for a reform before moving to define specific activities. No action-planning process should be initiated without a thorough assessment of what is in place and what needs to be improved. Similarly, clear and measurable outcomes should be identified that reflect the conclusions from the assessment and serve as the basis for evaluating implementation progress.

Adequate Personnel and Time

A major trend in schools across the United States over the past 10 years has been a reduction in the number of adults per pupil. This reduction can affect allocation and quality of instructional time; number of opportunities to respond; quantity and quality of interactions among teachers, students, and parents; and other factors that have an impact on the school and classroom climate and on academic outcomes. Teacher, staff, and administrator minutes are precious. The natural response to the growing expectations and dwindling hours of adult time is to cut the time allocated to all activities.

To implement schoolwide PBS successfully, a team needs to meet at least every other week to review data and make programmatic decisions. The meeting needs to last at least 45 minutes and be a regular, valued part of school operations. Although the amount of time needed to implement and sustain schoolwide PBS efforts will differ from school to school, a clear systems feature of successful schools has been the investment in precious adult time to organize and manage the schoolwide effort. Kame'enui and Carnine (2002) indicate that schools must learn to "work smarter, not more." This translates into the following recommendations: (1) Prioritize, (2) invest in a few (two or three) initiatives at a time, (3) adopt practices and strategies that have a proven record of achieving desired outcomes, and (4) monitor implementation continuously and directly to enable timely improvements and enhancements.

Budgeted Support

Schoolwide PBS is an investment in the improved educational experience of children and the efficient use of teacher/staff time. This investment, however, will require funding for at least the following: (1) development of the team, (2) time for the faculty to build the schoolwide training curriculum, (3) support for preparing staff for implementation (staff development), and (4) materials and rewards for acknowledging appropriate student behavior.

Information System

Just as a key practice for schoolwide PBS is the use of information for decision making, a key systems variable is the development of an efficient information system to deliver those data. One of the responsibilities of the team and administration within a school is to devise an inexpensive strategy for gathering, summarizing, and using behavioral information. An array of computer applications is becoming available to enter and organize data. In general, the system needs to allow easy data entry; to permit access to graphic displays of schoolwide (as well as individual student) data; and to provide teams, faculty, and administrators with accurate and recent data (i.e., no more than 48 hours old).

THE EFFECTS OF SCHOOLWIDE PBS

We have presented the rationale and foundation of schoolwide PBS. We also have reviewed the major practices and systems for primary prevention within the schoolwide PBS approach. An important concern, however, is the extent to which these practices and systems are already being used by schools and are associated with changes in student problem behavior and student academic performance. Research efforts are in progress to provide rigorous experimental analysis of these questions. For the present, we are left with encouraging, descriptive, small-scale studies that help us respond to common questions.

How Can a Team Determine Whether a School Is Using Schoolwide PBS?

In an effort to help schoolwide teams examine the extent to which they are using schoolwide PBS practices, two instruments have been developed. The Effective Behavior Support Self-Assessment Survey (EBS Self-Assessment) is a four-part survey used by schoolwide teams and whole faculties to self-evaluate the extent to which PBS practices are used at the schoolwide, classroom, and individual-student levels (Todd et al., 1999). The School-wide Evaluation Tool (SET) is a more rigorous, 28-item research tool administered on site by an external reviewer to document use of schoolwide primary prevention practices and systems. For example, to assess whether behavioral expectations have been defined, the observer reviews written documents and then looks to see whether the expectations are posted in public locations throughout the school. To assess whether students have been taught the behavioral expectations, the observer reviews teaching curriculum materials and asks a sample of students to identify the expectations. To assess whether a viable information system is being used, the observer reviews current data reports and the minutes of meetings in which data were used for active decision making. The SET produces a total score and seven subscale scores for elements such as "behavioral expectations taught," "appropriate behavior rewarded," and "information used for decision making." A school is considered to be using schoolwide PBS when the SET results indicate both a total score of 80% and a "behavioral expectations taught" subscale score of 80%. The reliability and validity of the SET have been examined and found acceptable (Horner et al., 2004).

The SET has been used to assess the status of schoolwide PBS efforts in schools before and after technical support was provided. Of interest is the fact that across a total of 61 schools in Hawaii (n = 29) and Illinois (n = 32) that were self-selected to receive technical assistance in schoolwide PBS, none were found to meet the SET implementation criteria prior to receiving support (mean total SET score = 36). These data suggest (but do not prove) that schoolwide PBS practices may not be an active part of many schools, and that an appropriate focus of school improvement plans may be to self-evaluate the extent to which schoolwide PBS is being used.

Can Typical Schools Make the Changes Needed to Adopt Schoolwide PBS?

A related concern must be the extent to which schools are able to adopt schoolwide PBS. It is one thing to demonstrate that procedures are effective, and another to demonstrate that they can be adopted with fidelity in typical school contexts. This is a concern of special importance when schoolwide systems are advocated. Figure 13.6 provides descriptive results from 22 schools in an Oregon school district that has been using school-wide PBS for over 5 years. Elementary and middle schools in the district were self-selected to receive technical assistance to adopt schoolwide PBS procedures. As part of the process, each school received a SET evaluation prior to receiving technical assistance and was reassessed at least a year after technical assistance was provided. The data indicate that the 22

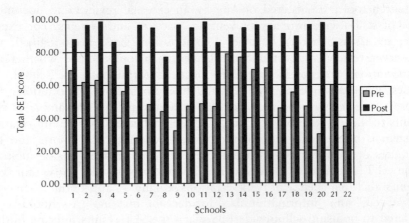

FIGURE 13.6. Percentages of schoolwide PBS implementation as measured by the School-wide Evaluation Tool (SET) across 22 elementary and middle schools.

schools scored an average of 53.9 (total) on the SET prior to receiving support and an average of 91.5 a year after receiving support. These results were not collected within the context of an experimental design, and no attribution can be made about the link between technical support and change in SET scores. The data do, however, document that at least some typical schools are capable of implementing the schoolwide PBS practices.

Does Implementation of Schoolwide PBS Practices and Systems Affect Student Problem Behavior?

Schools adopting schoolwide PBS typically use conventional, educational outcome measures to assess student impact. Changes in rates of office discipline referrals, attendance, suspensions, and expulsions are often used as indices of improvement. It is important to note, however, that each of these measures is affected not only by student behavior, but by adult decision making and the overall management systems within a school. With these caveats, there remains agreement that reduction in the student behaviors leading to office discipline referrals, suspensions, and expulsions is generally desirable. A strong argument can be made that office discipline referrals are important and useful indicators of the social health of a school (Irvin et al., 2004).

Schools providing pre–post information about adoption of schoolwide PBS are reporting 20–60% reductions in office discipline referrals and suspensions following full implementation (Lohrman-O'Rourke et al., 2000; Luiselli, Putnam & Sunderland, 2002; Sadler, 2000; Taylor-Greene & Kartub, 2000; Taylor-Greene et al., 1997). Figure 13.7 provides pre–post office discipline referral results from four elementary schools and three middle schools in Oregon that met schoolwide PBS implementation criteria between the academic years 1999–2000 and 2001–2002. Each school demonstrated reductions in its rate of office discipline referrals per 100 students following implementation of schoolwide behavioral expectations. On average, the seven schools reported a 45% reduction in office discipline referrals from the year prior to implementation to the year immediately following implementation. The three schools reporting a second year of implementation demonstrated sustained improvement.

The documentation of sustained effects is of special importance. The history of educational reform is characterized by brief innovations that fade after 1–2 years (Latham, 1988). The emphasis on schoolwide *systems* is intended to promote durable change, and initial results suggest that durable change is possible. In Elmira, Oregon, Fern Ridge Middle School (grades 6, 7, 8), under the leadership of Susan Taylor-Greene, has been using schoolwide PBS since the 1995–1996 school year. The rate of office disci-

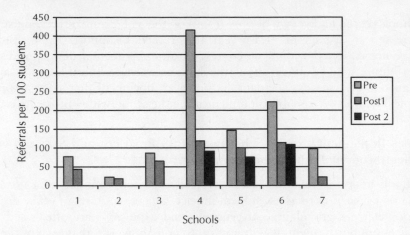

FIGURE 13.7. The rates of office discipline referrals per 100 students before and after implementation of schoolwide PBS (pre and post) for seven schools.

pline referrals per 100 students per year for the period 1994–2002 is provided in Figure 13.8. These data document a >40% reduction in office discipline referrals during the initial year of schoolwide PBS adoption, and sustained effects (65% reduction in office discipline referrals) over 7 years of continued implementation.

A more detailed analysis of the effects of schoolwide PBS on the behavior of students has been compiled by research reports provided by Cushing (2000), Smith (2000), and Todd (2002). Lisa Cushing developed

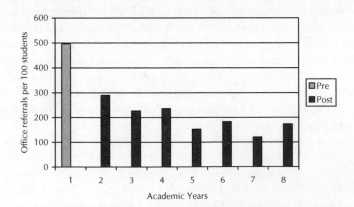

FIGURE 13.8. Rates of office discipline referrals per 100 students at Fern Ridge Middle School prior to and after adoption of schoolwide PBS (pre and post).

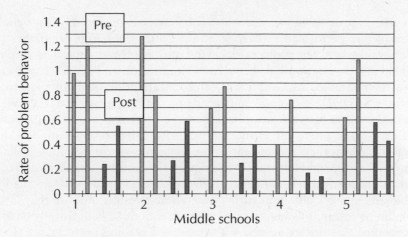

FIGURE 13.9. Direct observation rates of problem behavior before and after implementation of schoolwide PBS.

a direct observation measure of student social behavior to assess the rate of problem behavior and the conditional probability of different social consequences for problem behavior in schools (Cushing, Horner, & Barrier, 2003). Smith used this measure to collect ongoing social behavior data at the same time that the SET was used to assess the extent to which schools were implementing schoolwide PBS procedures. A result from these efforts allows comparison of direct observation rates of problem behavior collected in cafeterias and hallways for five middle schools. Data were collected twice in the spring prior to training in schoolwide PBS (pre), and again in the Fall and Spring of the following year when schoolwide PBS procedures were being used (post). Figure 13.9 provides the results from this comparison, demonstrating reduction in the rate of observed problem behavior as schools adopted schoolwide PBS. These results suggest that changes in office discipline referral rates reported by each of these schools were associated with real changes in the rates of problem behaviors observed in various settings of the schools (e.g., hallways, cafeteria).

Are Schoolwide PBS Practices Related to Change in Student Academic Performance?

The primary mission of schools is to help children acquire academic skills. Although considerable debate remains about the most appropriate way to assess academic performance, a concern relevant to the present chapter is whether improvement in student social behavior is related to improvement in academic performance (Barriga et al., 2002). Research examining the relationship between problem behavior and academic gains has demonstrated inverse relationships between (1) aggression and academic achievement (Williams & McGee, 1994), and (2) attention-deficit/hyperactivity disorder (ADHD) symptoms and academic gains (Faraone et al., 1993). The association between schoolwide social culture and academic gains has been of special interest in elementary schools, where intense emphasis has been placed on the development of literacy skills in early grades. Kellam, Mayer, Rebok, and Hawkins (1998) report results from a randomized control group analysis examining the effects of schoolwide PBS on reading achievement for children in early grades. Their results indicate that introduction of research-validated reading interventions in behaviorally chaotic classrooms was *not* associated with improved reading performance. Only when the same reading interventions were linked with schoolwide PBS were significant academic gains obtained. The basic message is that academic and behavioral supports must be intertwined. Children will not learn to read by being taught social skills, but they also will not learn to read if a good curriculum is delivered in a classroom that is disruptive and disorganized. Effective education involves a solid behavioral foundation, an empirically validated curriculum, and sound instruction.

Recent descriptive data support the value of combining academic and behavior support practices (Watson, 2003). One school district in Oregon that uses schoolwide PBS has 19 elementary schools, all of which were implementing an approved, phonics-based reading program. Between the 1997–1998 and 2001–2002 academic years, 13 of these schools chose to adopt and use schoolwide PBS. The schools were not randomly assigned, and no experimental design was employed. Watson compared the percentage of third graders who met the state reading standards in each school for 1997–1998 with those meeting the same standards in 2001–2002. The changes in percentages of students meeting the state reading standards over this time period for the 13 schools adopting schoolwide PBS are provided in the top panel of Figure 13.10. The similar change scores for the 6 schools that did not adopt schoolwide PBS are provided in the lower panel of Figure 13.10.

It is important to recognize that the data provided by Watson are purely descriptive and could be associated with a range of variables. They do, however, provide documentation of changes consistent with those patterns reported by Kellam et al. (1998). Combining behavior support and effective instruction may be an important theme for school reform in the United States. Further, controlled analysis of the combined value of academic and behavioral supports is needed.

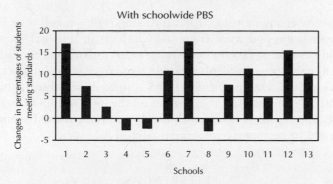

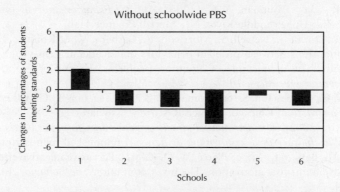

FIGURE 13.10. Changes in the percentages of students meeting state reading criteria for third grade in elementary schools from academic year 1997–1998 to academic year 2001–2002. Thirteen schools (top panel) adopted and used schoolwide PBS during this period, and 6 schools (bottom panel) did not.

SUMMARY

Schoolwide PBS is an approach to school discipline that incorporates specific practices and systems designed to produce socially important and sustained improvement in the behavioral culture of a school. The approach is based on a three-tiered model of prevention that incorporates different levels of support, depending on the need a student exhibits. The application of PBS at the whole-school level is now occurring throughout the United States. Preliminary, descriptive information suggests that schools are able to implement the approach when they receive appropriate technical assistance; that once the practices and systems are implemented, they endure; and that these practices and systems are associated with socially important improvements in children's behavioral and academic gains.

PBS is the emerging rubric for addressing problem behavior in school, home, community, and work contexts. Chapters in this text focus appropriately on the role of PBS for improving behavior support for individuals. The present chapter extends this message to a larger scale. Support for individuals is essential, but insufficient if PBS is to have broad social impact for all students. We suggest here that extending the logic of PBS to larger social systems (e.g., schools) is both feasible and necessary if the benefits of this approach are to become an integrated part of our society.

REFERENCES

Alberto, P. A., & Troutman, A. C. (2003). *Applied behavior analysis for teachers* (6th ed.). Upper Saddle River, NJ: Merrill/Prentice Hall.

Barriga, A., Doran, J., Newell, S., Morrison, E., Barbetti, V., & Robbins, B. (2002). Relationships between problem behaviors and academic achievement in adolescents: The unique role of attention problems. *Journal of Emotional and Behavioral Disorders, 10,* 233–240.

Becker, W. C., Engelmann, S., & Thomas, D. (1975). *Teaching 2: Cognitive learning and instruction.* Chicago: Science Research Associates.

Cameron, J. (2002). *The detrimental effects of reward hypothesis: Persistence of a view in the face of disconfirming evidence.* Unpublished manuscript.

Cameron, J., Banko, K. M., & Pierce, W. D. (2001). Pervasive negative effects of rewards on intrinsic motivation: The myth continues. *The Behavior Analyst, 24,* 1–44.

Cameron, J., & Pierce, W. D. (1994). Reinforcement, reward, and intrinsic motivation: A meta-analysis. *Review of Educational Research, 64,* 363–423.

Cameron, J., & Pierce, W. D. (2002). *Rewards and intrinsic motivation: Resolving the controversy.* Westport, CT: Bergin & Garvey.

Carnine, D. (1992). Expanding the notion of teachers' rights: Access to tools that work. *Journal of Applied Behavior Analysis, 25*(1), 13–19.

Carnine, D. (1995). Using research to bolster student learning. *School Administrator 52*(6), 10–14, 16.

Carnine, D. (1997). Bridging the research-to-practice gap. *Exceptional Children, 63,* 513–521.

Carr, E. G., Dunlap, G., Horner, R. H., Koegel, R. L., Turnbull, A. P., Sailor, W., et al. (2002). Positive behavior support: Evolution of an applied science. *Journal of Positive Behavior Interventions, 4*(1), 4–16, 20.

Carr, E. G., Horner, R. H., Turnbull, A. P., Marquis, J. G., McLaughlin, D., McAtee, M. L., et al. (1999). *Positive behavior support for people with developmental disabilities: A research synthesis.* Washington, DC: American Association on Mental Retardation.

Chapman, D., & Hofweber, C. (2000). Effective behavior support in British Columbia. *Journal of Positive Behavior Interventions, 2*(4), 235–237.

Colvin, G., & Fernandez, E. (2000). Sustaining effective behavior support systems in an elementary school. *Journal of Positive Behavior Interventions, 2,* 251–253.

Colvin, G., Kame'enui, E., & Sugai, G. (1993). Reconceptualizing behavior management and school-wide discipline in general education. *Education and Treatment of Children, 16,* 361–381.

Colvin, G., & Sprick, R. (1996). *Administrative support and the implementation of school-wide discipline.* Unpublished manuscript, University of Oregon.

Colvin, G., Sugai, G., & Kame'enui, E. (1994). *Curriculum for establishing a proactive school-wide discipline plan: Project PREPARE.* Eugene: University of Oregon.

Comer, J. (1985). The Yale–New Haven Primary Prevention Project: A follow-up study. *Journal of the American Academy of Child Psychiatry, 24,* 154–160.

Crone, D., Horner, R. H., & Hawken, L. S. (2004). *Responding to problem behavior in schools: The behavior education program.* New York: Guilford Press.

Cushing, L. S. (2000). *Descriptive analysis in the school social culture of elementary and middle school students.* Unpublished doctoral dissertation, University of Oregon.

Cushing, L. S., Horner, R. H., & Barrier, H. (2003). Validation and congruent validity of a direct observation tool to assess student social climate at school. *Journal of Positive Behavior Interventions, 5*(4), 225–237.

Darch, C. B., & Kame'enui, E. J. (2004). *Instructional classroom management: A proactive approach to behavior management* (2nd ed.). Upper Saddle River, NJ: Merrill.

Davies, D. E., & McLaughlin, T. F. (1989). Effects of a daily report card on disruptive behaviour in primary students. *Journal of Special Education, 13*(2), 173–181.

Didden, R., Duker, P. C., & Korzilius, H. (1997). Meta-analytic study on treatment effectiveness for problem behaviors with individuals who have mental retardation. *American Journal on Mental Retardation, 101*(4), 387–399.

Dougherty, E. H., & Dougherty, A. (1977). The daily report card: A simplified and flexible package for classroom behavior management. *Psychology in the Schools, 14*(2), 191–195.

Dwyer, K., Osher, D., & Warger, C. (1998). *Early warning, timely response: A guide to safe schools.* Washington, DC: U.S. Department of Education.

Eber, L., & Nelson, C. M. (1997). School-based wraparound planning: Integrating services for students with emotional and behavioral needs. *American Journal of Orthopsychiatry, 67,* 385–395.

Engelmann, S., & Carnine, D. (1982). *Theory of instruction: Principles and applications.* New York: Irvington.

Epstein, M. H., Nelson, C. M., Polsgrove, L., Coutinho, M., Cumblad, C., & Quinn, K. P. (1993). A comprehensive community-based approach to serving students with emotional and behavioral disorders. *Journal of Emotional and Behavioral Disorders, 1,* 127–133.

Evertson, C. M., & Emmer, E. T. (1982). *Preventive classroom management.* Alexandria, VA: Association for Supervision and Curriculum Development.

Faraone, S., Biederman, J., Lehman, B., Spencer, T., Norman, D., Seidman, L., et al. (1993). Intellectual performance and school failure in children with attention deficit hyperactivity disorder and in their siblings. *Journal of Abnormal Psychology, 102,* 616–623.

Fuchs, D., & Fuchs, L. (1994). Inclusive schools movement and the radicalization of special education reform. *Exceptional Children, 60*(4), 294–309.

Gilbert, T. F. (1978). *Human competence: Engineering worthy performance.* New York: McGraw-Hill.

Gilbert, T. F., & Gilbert, M. B. (1992). Potential contributions of performance science to education. *Journal of Applied Behavior Analysis, 25,* 43–49.

Gottfredson, D. C. (1987). An evaluation of an organization development approach to reducing school disorder. *Evaluation Review, 11,* 739–763.

Gottfredson, D. C., Gottfredson, G. D., & Hybl, L. G. (1993). Managing adolescent behavior: A multiyear, multischool study. *American Educational Research Journal, 30,* 179–215.

Gottfredson, D. C., Gottfredson, G. D., & Skroban, S. (1996). A multimodel school based prevention demonstration. *Journal of Adolescent Research, 11,* 97–115.

Gottfredson, D. C., Karweit, N. L., & Gottfredson, G. D. (1989). *Reducing disorderly behavior in middle schools.* Baltimore: Center for Research on Elementary and Middle Schools.

Gresham, F. M., Sugai, G., Horner, R. H., Quinn, M. M., & McInerney, M. (1998). *School-wide values, discipline, and social skills.* Washington, DC: American Institutes of Research and Office of Special Education Programs.

Hawken, L. S., & Horner, R. H. (2003). Evaluation of a targeted group intervention within a school-wide system of behavior support. *Journal of Behavioral Education, 12*(3), 225–240.

Heward, W. L., Heron, T. E., Hill, D. S., & Trap-Porter, J. (1984). *Focus on behavior analysis in education.* Columbus, OH: Merrill.

Horner, R. H., Diemer, S. M., & Brazeau, K. C. (1992). Educational support for students with severe problem behaviors in Oregon: A descriptive analysis from the 1987–1988 school year. *Journal of The Association of Persons with Severe Handicaps, 17*(3), 154–169.

Horner, R. H., Sugai, G., Lewis-Palmer, T., & Todd, A. W. (2001). Teaching school-wide behavioral expectations. *Report on Emotional and Behavioral Disorders in Youth, 1*(4), 77–79, 93–96.

Horner, R. H., Sugai, G., & Todd, A. W. (2001). "Data" need not be a four-letter word: Using data to improve school-wide discipline. *Beyond Behavior, 11*(1), 20–22.

Horner, R. H., Todd, A. W., Lewis-Palmer, T., Irvin, L. K., Sugai, G., & Boland, J. B. (2004). The School-wide Evaluation Tool (SET): A research instrument for assessing school-wide positive behavior support. *Journal of Positive Behavior Interventions, 6*(1), 3–12.

Ingram, K. (2002). *Comparing effectiveness of intervention strategies that are based on functional behavioral assessment information and those that are contraindicated by the assessment.* Unpublished doctoral dissertation, University of Oregon.

Ingram, K., Horner, R. H., & Todd, A. W. (2002). *Program evaluation of the School-Wide Information System (SWIS).* Unpublished manuscript.

Irvin, L. K., Tobin, T. J., Sprague, J. R., Sugai, G., & Vincent, C. G. (2004). Validity of office discipline referral measures as indices of school-wide behavioral status and effects of school-wide behavioral interventions. *Journal of Positive Behavior Interventions, 6*(3), 131–147.

Jensen, W. R., Sloane, H. N., & Young, K. R. (1988). *Applied behavior analysis in education: A structured teaching approach.* Englewood Cliffs, NJ: Prentice-Hall.

Kame'enui, E. J., & Carnine, D. W. (2002). *Effective teaching strategies that accommodate diverse learners* (2nd ed.). Upper Saddle River, NJ: Merrill.

Kame'enui, E. J., & Darch, C. B. (1995). *Instructional classroom management: A proactive approach to behavior management.* White Plains, NY: Longman.

Kazdin, A. E. (1982). Applying behavioral principles in the schools. In C. R. Reynolds & T. B. Gutkin (Eds.), *The handbook of school psychology* (pp. 501–529). New York: Wiley.

Kellam, S. G., Mayer, L. S., Rebok, G. W., & Hawkins, W. E. (1998). The effects of improving achievement on aggressive behavior and of improving aggressive behavior on achievement through two prevention interventions: An investigation of causal paths. In B. Dohrenwend (Ed.), *Adversity, stress, and psychopathology* (pp. 486–505). Oxford: Oxford University Press.

Kerr, M. M., & Nelson, C. M. (1983). *Strategies for managing behavior problems in the classroom.* Columbus, OH: Merrill.

Kerr, M. M., & Nelson, C. M. (2002). *Strategies for addressing behavior problems* (4th ed.). Upper Saddle River, NJ: Merrill.

Knoff, H. M. (2002). Best practices in facilitating school-based organizational change and strategic planning. In A. Thomas & J. Grimes (Eds.), *Best practices in school psychology—IV* (pp. 235–252). Silver Spring, MD: National Association of School Psychologists.

Larson, J. (1994). Violence prevention in schools: A review of selected programs and procedures. *School Psychology Review, 23,* 151–164.

Latham, G. (1988). The birth and death cycles of educational innovations. *Principal, 68*(1), 41–43.

Leach, D., & Byrne, M. (1986). Some "spill-over" effects of a home-based reinforcement programme in a secondary school. *Educational Psychology, 6*(3), 265–276.

Lewis, T. J., Colvin, G., & Sugai, G. (2000). The effects of precorrection and active supervision on the recess behavior of elementary school students. *Education and Treatment of Children, 23,* 109–121.

Lohrman-O'Rourke, S., Knoster, T., Sabatine, K., Smith, D., Horvath, B., & Llewellyn, G. (2000). School-wide application of PBS in the Bangor Area School District. *Journal of Positive Behavior Interventions, 2*(4), 238–240.

Luiselli, J. K., Putnam, R. F., & Sunderland, M. (2002). Longitudinal evaluation of behavior support intervention in a public middle school. *Journal of Positive Behavior Interventions, 4*(3), 182–188.

March, R. E., & Horner, R. H. (2002). Feasibility and contributions of functional behavioral assessment in schools. *Journal for Emotional and Behavioral Disorders, 10*(3), 158–170.

May, S., Ard, W., III, Todd, A. W., Horner, R. H., Glasgow, A., Sugai, G., et al. (2000). *School-Wide Information System.* Eugene: Educational and Community Supports, University of Oregon.

Mayer, G. R. (1995). Preventing antisocial behavior in the schools. *Journal of Applied Behavior Analysis, 28,* 467–478.

Mayer, G. R., & Butterworth, T. (1979). A preventive approach to school violence and vandalism: An experimental study. *Personnel and Guidance Journal, 57,* 436–441.

Mayer, G. R., Butterworth, T., Nafpaktitis, M., & Sulzer-Azaroff, B. (1983). Preventing school vandalism and improving discipline: A three year study. *Journal of Applied Behavior Analysis, 16,* 355–369.

McCord, J. (Ed.). (1995). *Coercion and punishment in long-term perspective.* New York: Cambridge University Press.

Nakasato, J. (2000). Data-based decision making in Hawaii's behavior support effort. *Journal of Positive Behavior Interventions, 2*(4), 247–251.

National Research Council & Institute of Medicine. (1999). *Risk and opportunities: Synthesis of studies on adolescence.* Washington, DC: National Academy Press.

Nelson, J. R., Colvin, G., & Smith, D. J. (1996, Summer–Fall). The effects of setting clear standards on students' social behavior in common areas of the school. *Journal of At-Risk Issues,* pp. 10–17.

Nelson, J. R., Martella, R., & Galand, B. (1998). The effects of teaching school expectations and establishing a consistent consequence on formal office disciplinary actions. *Journal of Emotional and Behavioral Disorders, 6,* 153–161.

Nelson, J. R., Martella, R., & Marchand-Martella, N. (2002). Maximizing student learning: The effects of a comprehensive school-based program for preventing problem behaviors. *Journal of Emotional and Behavioral Disorders, 10*(3), 136–148.

Nersesian, M., Todd, A., Lehmann, J., & Watson, J. (2000). School-wide behavior support through district-level system change. *Journal of Positive Behavior Interventions, 2*(4), 244–247.

O'Neill, R. E., Horner, R. H., Albin, R. W., Sprague, J. R., Storey, K., & Newton, J. S. (1997). *Functional analysis of problem behavior: A practical assessment guide* (2nd ed.). Pacific Grove, CA: Brooks/Cole.

Patterson, G. R., Reid, J. B., & Dishion, T. J. (1992). *Antisocial boys.* Eugene, OR: Castalia.

Peters, M. T., & Heron, T. E. (1993). When the best is not good enough: An examination of best practice. *Journal of Special Education, 26,* 371–385.

Rose, L. C., & Gallup, A. M. (1998). The 30th annual Phi Delta Kappan/Gallup poll of the public's attitude toward the public schools. *Kappan, 79,* 41–56.

Sadler, C. (2000). Effective behavior support implementation at the district level: Tigard–Tualatin School District. *Journal of Positive Behavior Interventions, 2*(4), 241–243.

Scott, T. M., & Eber, L. (2003). Functional assessment and wraparound as systemic school processes: Primary, secondary, and tertiary systems examples. *Journal of Positive Behavior Interventions, 5*(3), 131–143.

Shinn, M., Stoner, G., & Walker, H. M. (Eds.). (2002). *Interventions for academic and behavior problems: Preventive and remedial approaches.* Silver Spring, MD: National Association of School Psychologists.

Shonkoff, J. P., & Phillips, D. A. (Eds.). (2000). *Report: Board on children, youth and families, commission on behavioral and social sciences and education.* Washington, DC: National Academy Press.

Skiba, R. J. (2002). Special education and school discipline: A precarious balance. *Behavioral Disorders, 27*(2), 81–97.

Skiba, R. J., & Peterson, R. L. (2000). School discipline at a crossroads: From zero tolerance to early response. *Exceptional Children, 66*(3), 335–356.

Smith, B. (2000). *Problem behavior within the context of peer delivered consequences.* Unpublished doctoral dissertation, University of Oregon.

Sprick, R. S., & Nolet, V. (1991). Prevention and management of secondary-level behavior problems. In G. Stoner, M. R. Shinn, & H. M. Walker (Eds.), *Interventions for achievement and behavior problems* (pp. 519–538). Silver Spring, MD: National Association of School Psychologists.

Sprick, R., Sprick, M., & Garrison, M. (1992). *Foundations: Developing positive school-wide discipline policies.* Longmont, CO: Sopris West.

Sugai, G. (2002, October). *School-wide positive behavior support.* Paper presented at the National Forum on schoolwide PBS, Naperville, IL.

Sugai, G., & Horner, R. H. (1994). Including students with severe behavior problems in general education settings: Assumptions, challenges, and solutions. In J. Marr, G. Sugai, & G. Tindal (Eds.), *The Oregon Conference monograph* (pp. 102–120). Eugene: University of Oregon.

Sugai, G., & Horner, R. H. (2002). The evolution of discipline practices: School-wide positive behavior supports. *Child and Family Behavior Therapy, 24*(1–2), 23–50.

Sugai, G., Horner, R. H., Dunlap, G., Hieneman, M., Lewis, T. J., Nelson, C. M., et al. (2000). Applying positive behavior support and functional behavioral assessment in schools. *Journal of Positive Behavior Interventions, 2*(3), 131–143.

Sugai, G., Sprague, J. R., Horner, R. H., & Walker, H. M. (2000). Preventing school violence: The use of office discipline referrals to assess and monitor schoolwide discipline interventions. *Journal of Emotional and Behavioral Disorders, 8*, 94–101.

Sulzer-Azaroff, B., & Mayer, G. R. (1994). *Achieving educational excellence: Behavior analysis for achieving classroom and schoolwide behavior change.* San Marcos, CA: Western Image.

Taylor-Greene, S., Brown, D., Nelson, L., Longton, J., Gassman, T., Cohen, J., et al. (1997). School-wide behavioral support: Starting the year off right. *Journal of Behavioral Education, 7*, 99–112.

Taylor-Greene, S., Brown, D., Nelson, L., Longton, J., Gassman, T., Cohen, J., et al. (1999). *The High Five Program: A positive approach to school discipline.* Elmira, OR: Fern Ridge Middle School.

Taylor-Greene, S. J., & Kartub, D. T. (2000). Durable implementation of school-wide behavior support: The High Five Program. *Journal of Positive Behavior Interventions, 2*(4), 233–235.

Tobin, T., Sugai, G., & Colvin, G. (2000, May). A guide to the creation and use of discipline referral graphs. *NASSP Bulletin, 84*(616), 106–117.

Todd, A. (2002, May). *School-wide behavior support outcomes.* Paper presented at the annual meeting of the Association on Behavior Analysis, Toronto.

Todd, A. W., Horner, R. H., Sugai, G., & Sprague, J. R. (1999). Effective behavior support: Strengthening school-wide systems through a team-based approach. *Effective School Practices, 17*(4), 23–37.

Tolan, P., & Guerra, N. (1994). *What works in reducing adolescent violence: An empirical review of the field.* Boulder: Center for the Study and Prevention of Violence, University of Colorado.

Tyack, D. (2001). Introduction. In S. Mondale & S. Patton (Eds.), *School: The story of American public education* (pp. 1–10). Boston: Beacon Press.

U.S. Department of Health and Human Services. (2001). *Youth violence: A report of the Surgeon General.* Washington, DC: U.S. Government Printing Office.

Vargas, J. S. (1977). *Behavioral psychology for teachers.* New York: Harper & Row.

Walker, H. M., Colvin, G., & Ramsey, E. (1995). *Antisocial behavior in public school: Strategies and best practices.* Pacific Grove, CA: Brooks/Cole.

Walker, H. M., Horner, R. H., Sugai, G., Bullis, M., Sprague, J., Bricker, D., & Kaufman M. J. (1996). Integrated approaches to preventing antisocial behavior patterns among school-age children and youth. *Journal of Emotional and Behavioral Disorders, 4,* 194–209.

Walker, H. M., & Shinn, M. R. (2002). Structuring school-based interventions to achieve integrated primary, secondary, and tertiary prevention goals for safe and effective schools. In M. R. Shinn, G. Stoner, & H. M. Walker (Eds.), *Interventions for academic and behavior problems: Preventive and remedial approaches* (pp. 1–26). Silver Spring, MD: National Association of School Psychologists.

Watson, J. (2003, May 14). *Report to the 4J School Board.* Eugene, OR: 4J School District.

Weissberg, R. P., Caplan, M. Z., & Sivo, P. J. (1989). A new conceptual framework for establishing school-based social competence promotion programs. In L. A. Bond & B. E. Compas (Eds.), *Primary prevention and promotion in the schools* (pp. 255–296). Newbury Park, CA: Sage.

Williams, S., & McGee, R. (1994). Reading attainment and juvenile delinquency. *Journal of Child Psychology and Psychiatry, 35,* 442–459.

Wolery, M. R., Bailey, D. B., Jr., & Sugai, G. M. (1988). *Effective teaching: Principles and procedures of applied behavior analysis with exceptional students.* Boston: Allyn & Bacon.

Index

♦

ABC analysis. *See* Antecedent–behavior–consequence analysis
Academic performance
  functional assessment, 132, 134–135
  problem behavior inverse relationship, 382
  schoolwide positive behavior support effect, 381–383
Accountability for problem behavior, 297–298
Accountability in teams
  problem-solving approach, 99
  sharing of, 77
Acting-out behaviors
  communicative function, 29
  examples of, 295–297
  response interventions timing, 293–297
Action plan, 93–94
  development in teams, 93
  key elements, 93–94
Adaptive skills. *See* General adaptive skills instruction
Advocacy, in self-determination movement, 8
Age appropriateness, response interventions, 282
Aggression
  aversive procedures side effect, 279, 282
  communicative function, 32
  communicative skill deficits link, 32

Alternative skills instruction, 60–62, 237–274. *See also* Replacement skills
  in behavior support plan, 58–62, 271, 273
  case examples, 270–274
  conceptual framework, 238–239
  in coping and tolerance, 255–261
  general adaptive skills, 261–268
  in home and community settings, 347
  limitations, 240
  long-term effectiveness, 61
  meaningful outcomes, 319
  outcome patterns, 320
  purpose of, 60–62, 240
  replacement skills, 238–255
Analogue functional analysis, 190–193
  advantages and limitations, 191–193
  in hypothesis testing, 190–193
  procedure, 190–191
Anecdotal notes
  example of, 146
  in information gathering, 145–146
Anger control training
  case example, 266–267
  description of, 260
Antecedent–behavior–consequence (ABC) analysis
  and antecedent identification, 170–174
  case examples, 161–162, 170–174
  information collection format, 145–147
  observation form example, 147